THE BRAVEST

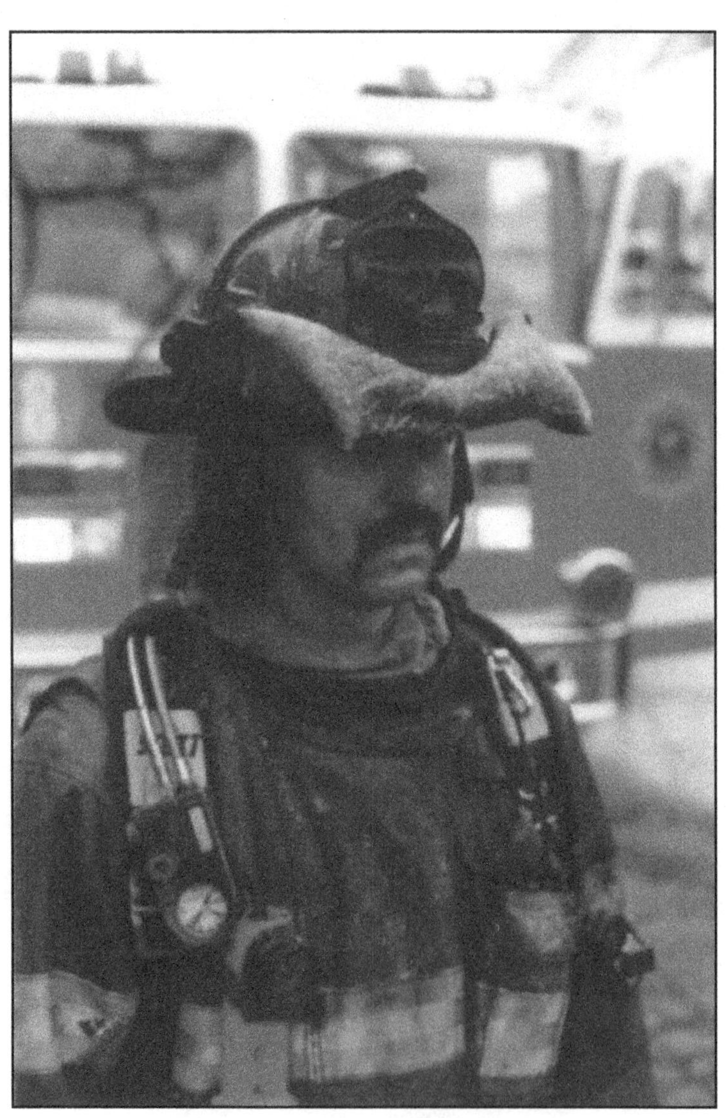

For those brave souls who relentlessly sacrifice for others; serving daily and courageously maneuvering amongst the flames to tame the beast. To the first-in, the glory hounds, the under-appreciated and unrecognized heroes of the fire service. The ones who rush in to save complete strangers because it's the right thing to do, even at the cost of their own peril. This book is for you.

Contents

Disclaimer

The stories in this book represent the author's views and personal experiences. Other people involved in the actual events or incidents may or may not recall them the same way. The perspectives and descriptions relayed herein may contain sensitive and offensive information to some readers. Certain well-respected institutions, public offices, and agencies are discussed in this book. At no point does the author intend to defame or maliciously destroy the general public's trust in these great institutions.

When necessary, the names and identifying characteristics of the people involved have been changed to protect their privacy. In these cases, any resemblance to actual persons is purely coincidental. The conversations contained in this book are from the author's recollections and are not intended to represent verbatim transcripts. Rather, they are retold in a way that reflects the author's perceived essence of the dialogue. The events portrayed in this book are a recollection of the author's life and experiences.

This book is not intended to be a firefighting instructional manual. Professional firefighters should use their best judgment in the fireground scenarios they are faced with. In the social situations presented, the reader should likely do the exact opposite of the author's actions—to proceed through life in a favorable light as viewed by peers and family members. Ultimately, the author wishes to convey his own personal experiences as a Firefighter/EMT and raise public awareness of the life choices and emergency situations first responders around the world are confronted with every day.

The story follows a mostly chronological path through the author's career, with chapters loosely based on significant events, or on certain subject matter to add levity and break up the monotony of the nearly constant emergency runs filled with chaos and trauma. This book was written for the firefighting professional stuck in the grind, without a voice, to let everyone know what's really going on out there. It's as if the author were sitting down with them, enjoying a cup of coffee and a cigarette between calls at the firehouse, having a typical, foul-mouthed discourse on the intricacies of the fire service. For the civilian reader, if at any time during the perusal of this material they feel woozy, lightheaded, or nauseated, the author wishes to remind them to take a deep breath. In and out. Always remember to breathe. It's the first thing we did when we got here, and it's the last thing we'll do before we leave.

INTRODUCTION

A Chat with the Smoke Eater

Forbidden secrets of a legendary profession were revealed that night at the Hangar 13 airport tavern. A flash of lightning and a crackling thunderclap disrupted the conversations of delayed passengers, all killing time, bellied up to the bar. In an instant, the mood changed from casual discourse about family and career to shocking revelations of mind-blowing consequence.

It began with a seemingly innocent question…

"Fireman, eh…so what's the worst thing you've ever seen?" the stranger asks.

With a flip of my wrist, the whiskey vanishes from my glass and burns down my throat. The buzzing airport terminal seems to pause and hold its breath, waiting for a response.

"You don't really wanna know," I reply, hoping to deflect the sadistic query. He's just making rhetoric. He doesn't know. If he did, he wouldn't have asked.

The question tends to come up when people find out I'm a firefighter. I'm somewhat used to it now, after twenty years. Tonight, the stranger insists on an answer, citing the tavern's abundant collection of spirits and our impending three-hour weather delay.

"Sure. Why the hell not?" I say. Giving in to his persistence, I counter with, "What do you want to know?"

"It's your story," he says. "You pick."

Where to begin? First, a signal to the barkeep for refills and chasers. We're going to need them. Here we go.

The real estate at the top of a firefighter's worst-things-ever list is often crowded, and it can be difficult to choose one event. I've found—most of the time—leading with human carnage in these scenarios tends to either shut the conversation down immediately or blossom it into a more profound understanding of the insane things we've been through.

For instance, there's the car accident with the eighteen-year-old boy, where his skull was cut clean through horizontally, his body slumped over in his driver's seat. His bits of minced brain matter sitting in the cereal bowl of what's left of the lower part of his cranium. His drunk friends sitting on my ambulance bench seat, flicking what looks like wax worms off their clothing. Not having the slightest idea they're pieces of their dead friend's brain stuck to them. My partner, explaining to them bluntly: "That's your buddy's brains."

Stuff like that? The barkeep arrives with more refreshments. *Keep them coming please.*

In the heart-wrenching irony genre, there's the entire family that died when their pick-up drifted off the highway on the way home from a high school volleyball game. Their teenage daughter was ejected from the vehicle as it barrel rolled repeatedly down an embankment and finally came to rest, crushing her body under the weight of the truck's roof. Her naked, lifeless legs sticking out in the snow while Swedish House Mafia blasted from the upside-down truck's stereo, on repeat: "Don't you worry, child, Heaven's got a plan for you."

In the morbidly grotesque category, we have mothers lighting their children on fire. That's always a crowd pleaser. I actually have *two* of those stories. Or there's severed limbs. I've got all kinds of these. My personal favorite was the human tongue lying alone in the middle of the highway. Or maybe it was walking down the train tracks at midnight, in the pouring rain, carrying a woman's entire leg—which was surprisingly heavier than it looked.

There's the drunk homeless man I was trying to help, who told me he was going to rape and murder my family. Or the baby floating in the toilet, still connected to the mother's umbilical cord, that I had to fish out from urine and feces, cut the cord, and do CPR on, while the 300-plus-pound mom sat there smoking a cigarette explaining she had no idea she was even pregnant. The kid didn't end up making it. Though certainly not for a lack of resuscitative efforts on our part.

I've seen a woman jump twelve stories to her death, landing on the concrete directly in front of me. I learned firsthand that human bodies splatter quite a bit farther than they do in the movies. Imagine a pumpkin or a watermelon dropped from a similar height, and a juicy one at that. Now you've got the picture. They're exceedingly messy, those calls.

I've buried nine of my active-duty coworkers, all from job-related injuries in varying degrees. I've witnessed twenty-six of my fellow colleagues become physically disabled to the point of being unable to continue in the profession. I've literally touched *thousands* of dead and dying human beings and tried my very best to save them on what always tended to rank as the worst day of their lives. With failure rates that beg the question: Why even try at all?

Is it body fluids? Or maybe corpses? Or maybe corpses leaking body fluids? Perhaps it's none of the above. I've seen criminal politics and betrayal in government that rivals all the human tragedy and carnage, in terms of deplorable actions and spiraling consequences. Maybe it's folks backstabbing their best friends, backdoor deals, or the ignorant traditions of "isms" like racism, sexism, or nepotism. I've seen plenty of those, too.

I've got thousands of stories that come to mind when someone asks that question. So please do us all a favor—don't ever ask a soldier, or a firefighter, or a cop, or a nurse about the worst thing they've ever seen. Have some respect for the sea of human tragedy they swim through every time they wake up and go to work. Understand that, for them, certain smells, like the raw sweetness of blood mixed with alcohol, can bring about horrific memories.

Just driving down random streets or the mere passing mention of a name can uncover intense moments of heroism and heartache. The *last* thing they need is someone asking them to recount what they've desperately tried to bury down deep just so they can sleep at night. Best to say something patronizing, like, "Thank you for your service," or something honest and heartfelt, such as, "Holy shit, why *the fuck* would you want to do that with your life?"

"Fascinating," the stranger says as he orders the next round. "Tell me more."

"What was your name again?" I ask, my suspicion growing.

"Trent," he says after a sip of whiskey. "Trentin Quarantino. I'm a filmmaker. I love a good story, and it sounds like you have one. Please, continue."

For me personally, the *why* was the pension and the benefits. That's the mantra that kept me going. When I was twenty-two hours into a twenty-four-hour shift and hadn't eaten or slept since arriving at work, that's what I kept telling myself. *The pension and the bennies*. They can do anything to me for twenty-four hours, but then it's my time.

Of course, sometimes our relief person would be late, and we'd catch another alarm right at shift change before they arrived. Then it would be twenty-five or twenty-six hours, but hey, at least it wasn't a *normal* job. We were freakin' heroes. We had to tell ourselves things like that to keep pushing forward and hopefully make it through to the retirement finish line.

We never really stopped to think about the sheer number of intensely visual and emotional traumas happening to us over the course of a twenty-four-hour period. Not while wading through them, knee deep in a bloody pile of guts, and with the adrenaline of the call still surging through our veins. By the time I checked in with my family in the evening, I'd have already forgotten half the calls we'd made earlier in the day. It was mind-numbing and surreal.

We'd hop from hospital to call, and back again, sometimes without even being able to finish a written run report. Simply dumping our patient in a bed, giving the ER nurse an abbreviated verbal report, and then dashing off to the next emergency scene. Only to do it again three or four more times before lunch. By dinner time, I was numb from all the trauma I'd seen and cruising on autopilot. By nightfall I'd have a full-blown case of sleep deprivation, complete with that heavy metallic taste in my mouth and the thousand-yard stare.

I'd try hard to stay focused as we screamed through the city streets, going lights and sirens at 70 miles per hour, trying to get the kid who was dying in the back of our sled to definitive medical care. Drugs, alcohol, sex—nothing felt real anymore. It was like a dream I just couldn't wake up from. A nightmare honestly, but none of us really understood how fucked up it was until we stepped away and looked back on it all. Twenty-four hours of trauma at a time, back-to-back, over and over, in a seemingly endless cycle of chaos and human tragedy.

"I wanna hear everything," Trent said.

"Everything." I throw back a shot of whiskey.

"Beginning to end. I wanna hear it."

"You're a sick fuck, you know."

"So I'm told." He raises his glass into the air. "To great stories!"

"As you wish." We tap our glasses and begin the journey.

In 1998, I hired into the fire department of a capital city in a Midwestern state. Our department ran around 30,000 calls a year, with fire-based EMS. When I hired on, the pension and the benefits were the best around. Our retirement wage, or FAC (final average compensation), was 80 percent of our highest two years' average salary, with health care, dental, and vision insurances for our immediate family for life. After twenty-five years of service, we'd be eligible to retire. It seemed like the fastest route to being able to do what I wanted to do, when I wanted to do it. Man, was I stupid.

All that's gone now, whittled away by politicians, corrupt union officials, and the ballooning legacy costs of the rust belt cities and their shrinking economies. For those outside of the Northeast and Midwest, the rust belt is a region that once flourished with manufacturing businesses. Where, after WWII, virtually anyone could get a decent-paying job. Now, it's characterized by declining industry, vacant factories, and population numbers stuck in a freefall.

The only thing I could see at the time was a chance to be somebody, retire early and somewhat comfortably, and have an exciting profession that was new every day. The true cost of becoming a firefighter is rarely talked about. It's exacted in heavy tolls on our families, our own mental and physical health, and frequent hospital visits and funerals for our coworkers.

So, let's get right into it, then. This is a tell-all about my experiences as a U.S. firefighter in the late 1990s and early 2000s. *All* of it. The good, the bad, and the ridiculously ugly. Don't get me wrong. I *love* the fire service. The only time I've felt really, truly alive in this life was when I was on the fireground. There's an adrenaline rush like I've never felt before or since, running into a situation to help while everyone else is running away. Certain people operate heroically well in moments of chaos. Those same people often falter terribly in basic, everyday social situations. The things that work well in the firehouse and on the fireground—much like on the battlefield—don't translate very well into home life, and vice versa.

To be clear, I'm not spilling my guts about everything I've seen in my twenty-plus years as a Firefighter/EMT to upset the civilian populace or because I'm angry at the profession. Hell,

I'd still like to be a firefighter after this comes out. Looking back on the things I've witnessed and the oceans of craziness I swam through, this has to happen. There's simply no other way for me to deal with the enormous pile of shit in my head, than to throw open the closet door and let it all spill out onto the floor.

While compiling the list of events worthy of inclusion, the sheer number of noteworthy traumatic experiences had me shaking my head, wondering how I wasn't a drooling vegetable rocking back and forth in the corner of a psych ward somewhere. So, for the sake of healing, posterity, and the general public's greater understanding, I present my skeletons.

I'd like the professionals to enjoy this for what it is: a straight look at the experiences many of us have lived. Spending countless nights, holidays, and birthdays away from our loved ones. Being a part-time parent, problem-solver, hero, teacher, student, chef, janitor, launderer, accountant, inventory manager, mechanic, chauffeur, street doctor, therapist, tour guide, surgeon, landscaper, hydraulic engineer, pharmacist, disciplinarian, business manager, babysitter, et cetera, et cetera, makes for a peculiar view of the world, and only a select few individuals have successfully navigated the perilous waters of a U.S. fire service career.

The fire department lifers may not like what I'm doing, but at least they'll know I'm being honest. I want folks to get a glimpse of the true joys of what it really feels like to be a firefighter in a big city. I'd like the civilians to understand that people are not always heroes; they're human beings. They fuck up and struggle with things. They aren't always honorable. They're just like everyone else. I'd like to convey, as best I can, the strange delights of the language, patois, and macabre sense of humor found on the front lines.

I'm *not* the guy with all the letters behind his name. I didn't take administrative classes while my peers were grinding it out in the trenches. This is about street-level emergency management. Where we do what needs to be done to accomplish the task at hand. After twenty-plus years in the business, I've been from the heights of heroism down to the depths of despair and back again. So I know a few things, and I'd like to bring the world on a ride-along.

Of course, there's always the chance this could end my career in the fire service. There will be horror stories: on-duty drinking, drugs, screwing in the fire stations, unsavory revelations about industry practices, but I simply won't deceive *anyone* about the life as I've lived it. For me, firefighting has been a long love affair, with moments both heavenly and horrendous. Whether rescuing a family from an inferno, being seduced by my officer, getting a rare CPR save, or smoke boxing the ladder truck with marijuana while cruising through the city, the fire service has always been a wild adventure for me. And I hope it is for you, too.

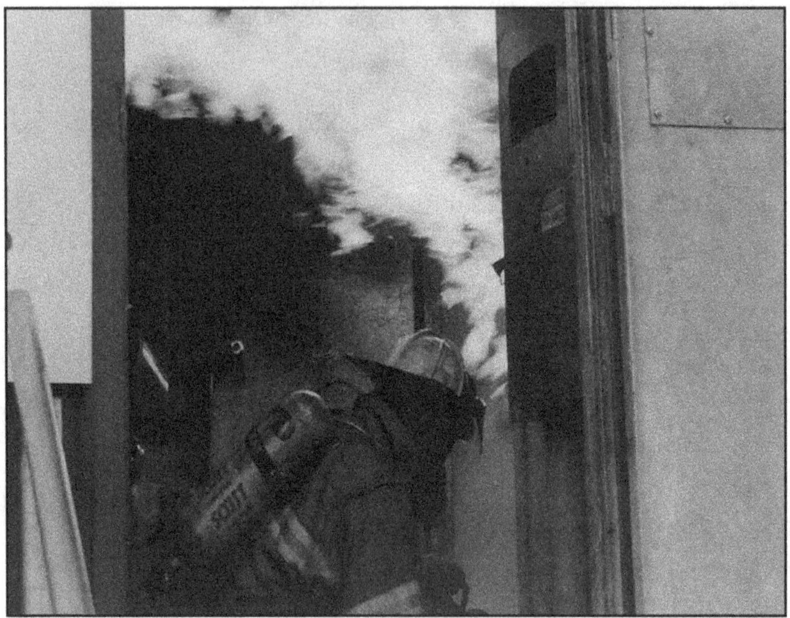

Flashover training

Chapter 1

In the Beginning (The Background Check)

Born and raised in the city I worked in, I thought I knew pretty much everything there was to know about the place. It seemed like a quiet, friendly spot to live. After hiring into the fire department, I realized just how many godawful things happened that the general public never even knew about. Somehow most of it simply disappeared. Failing to pass through the filters of the media censors or the powerful local political figures, whose personal agendas didn't fit well with the full disclosure and release of the information I'd been privy to.

My father, Richard—we'll call him Dick—was both a preacher and a politician, which made for a unique and twisted upbringing. With me as a young child in tow to his evening committee meetings, we'd mingle with local celebrities, like governors, mayors, legislators, senators, county commissioners, city council members, and departmental heads of staff. I had a somewhat privileged—albeit religiously sheltered—childhood. My folks split up over my father's burgeoning political ambitions (and his inability to keep his dick in his pants) when I was eleven years old. That divorce was the single most terrible and influential incident that clinched my apprehension towards hypocrisy and its many practitioners.

My mother and I spent the next two years living in her friends' and family members' basements. While out one evening, she met a man at a bar—once again named Richard. We'll call him Dick #2. This sleazeball of a man seduced her, and within ninety days they were married, and we moved in with the guy. He was arrested a month later for distribution of child pornography, domestic assault, fraud, and a parole violation because it turned out he was a previously convicted sex offender. Background checks, people. Run those background checks.

When the police came to our home to investigate, they informed my mother that Dick #2 was a notorious con man who'd meet single mothers, marry them, drain their bank accounts, and violate their children. My mother had fallen victim to his scheme, along with a dozen or so other women who'd had their entire life savings stolen. Fortunately, I still had my virginity intact by the time they'd caught the sick motherfucker in a pedophile sting operation.

The marriage was annulled, and Mom moved us into our thirteenth home in as many years. She soon met another man at a bar, and—wait for it—you guessed it: his name was Richard. Dick #3 was a tall hillbilly character with long hair and a handlebar mustache who taught me how to hunt and fish, the joys and pains of blues and classic rock music, and was more of a father to me than my own absentee padre had ever even attempted to be. That's three Dicks in three years for those who are counting.

Not surprisingly, I rebelled often through my mostly fatherless pubescent years and somehow managed to graduate from high school with a 3.75 GPA and a preferred walk-on football invitation to the local university. Pursuing a degree during the day and partying my ass off at campus keggers all night proved to be a difficult proposition. So when my ex-girlfriend and former high school sweetheart—we'll call her Sonya—advised me she was pregnant and the baby was mine, I decided to drop out of college and get a job to support my new family. It seemed like the responsible thing to do at the time.

I found work as a union construction laborer on commercial projects around the capital city. During a lunch break one day, I asked my aging superintendent what his thirty-plus years in the industry had taught him, and if he had any advice for a young laborer just starting out.

He told me, "Son, you're never going to become wealthy working for someone else," and encouraged me to start my own business, confessing that was his greatest regret.

A few months later, Sonya miscarried with our child. Now I was stuck with a job and a relationship and didn't really want either of them. My overly religious upbringing was ringing in the back of my head that I needed to be there and stick around for the poor girl. That I should just stay the course and keep working hard on both my career path and the relationship, just like my grandparents had done.

It was an outdated mode of thinking that held romantic notions of nostalgia for me, and while ethically and morally right according to how I'd been raised, I should've recognized it as my only chance to run and pursue my dreams. Hindsight being clearer than foresight, I stuck around and tried to make the best of an awful situation.

Sonya's father was an independent flooring installer and offered to teach me his trade. That was the path of least resistance to business ownership, as my construction super had suggested. After a year-long apprenticeship, I became a flooring installer. I subcontracted from the local home improvement stores and was making more money than ever. Sonya and I married, and we purchased a house in a decent neighborhood. Life was good.

That summer I helped a high school buddy of mine, RP, install his uncle's new hot tub. Uncle Rudy was an engineer at the capital city's fire department, and he suggested we submit our applications to become firefighters. He explained he only worked around ten days a month and could retire after twenty-five years of service with a pension and benefits. It sounded like a good plan, and I could continue my self-employed contracting business on my days off. So I gave it a shot and did as Uncle Rudy advised.

The process to becoming a firefighter consisted of written and psychological tests, a physical ability test, and an oral interview. I scored well on the written and psych tests—without any formal training—and advanced to the physical ability portion. We were assigned into groups of four candidates and began our progression through the fire department's obstacle course.

It was actually quite fun, like an *American Gladiator* or *Ninja Warrior* challenge, and I found the many obstacles to be intriguing tests of skill and strength. I did well on the physical agility course and progressed onward to the interview process. Ultimately, I was passed over because of a lack of Fire and EMS (emergency medical services) certifications. The rejection was disappointing. However, I was determined to make it happen on the next hiring cycle.

I worked my flooring contractor job during the day and enrolled at the local community college for EMT (emergency medical technician) school at night. There was a motley mix of flunkies and weirdos in the classes. A middle-aged body builder named Paul, a slutty blonde named Sarah (who always sat next to me and whispered in my ear during tests about her adventures with phallus-shaped fruits and vegetables), a kid named Clevenger who uncannily resembled Sloth from *The Goonies*, and a guy named Steve who spoke like John Wayne were some of the more notable characters there.

The classes were taught by local firefighter and paramedic instructors who all worked at the various local fire departments, making it perfect for obtaining professional references. Willy P and Wardo both held firefighter positions at the same fire department I sought employment with. After proving myself worthy in their classes, they both agreed to be listed on my résumé.

Nearing the end of the semester, we were required to complete ride-alongs with actual ambulance service providers. Since the community college was right across the street from the largest fire-based EMS service in the area, we rode with our instructors' employers. There, it was an incestuous relationship at best, full of nepotism and a good ol' boy, you scratch my back and I'll scratch yours, mentality. Fathers, sons, brothers, and cousins—there were scores of relatives that worked together at the fire department. It appeared to me straight away, that if one greased the right palms, one could do anything they wanted there.

As I sat in the ambulance, parked out in front of Fire Station 1 on one particular ride-along day, Firefighter/EMT John Lohan and I completed the daily inventory. John was explaining to me how things *really* worked in the back of the ambulance.

"Hell, sometimes, when the poor motherfucker's been dead for a while, but we gotta work the ol' bastard to keep the family appeased, we'll just stop CPR (cardiopulmonary resuscitation) while the sled rolls to the hospital. Then we'll pick it back up on arrival, when the doors open, and transfer the poor stiff to the ER," he revealed.

"Geez, are you kidding me?" I asked.

"Naw, man, crazy shit goes down here. You're about to find out," he forecasted, like a firefighting, psychic Miss Cleo.

Personally, I never saw this happen at any point during my watch over the next twenty-plus years. At the time, my head spun with images of potential negligence and lazy EMS providers scamming the unsuspecting public. It was unfathomable to me then and still is today. It turns out that individuals in the fire service are just a microcosm of our society as a whole. There are good people and bad people, and a sea of variants in between.

With our ride-alongs completed, we practiced relentlessly for the upcoming state licensing exams.

"Universal precautions. Overview the scene," we began. (We had to verbalize all our actions. If not, they'd say we hadn't done it and dock us points.)

"Safe scene," the instructor replied. "Johnny here has a hole in his head from a GSW (gunshot wound). He's unconscious."

"I'd take C-spine control and check his vital signs. Open his airway with the modified jaw-thrust technique. Look, listen, and feel for breathing," I explained.

"He's breathing five times a minute; agonal respirations," the instructor advised.

"Checking for further injuries," my partner said, as he patted down the torso, arms, and legs of the pretend victim.

"Remember the genital sweep," I said.

"He's got a boner," the instructor nonchalantly replied.

This is medically known as a priapism and can be an indicator of a spinal cord injury.

I finished the scenario with, "We'd C-collar and backboard our patient using the log-roll technique, maintaining C-spine control, then administer high-flow O_2 via non-rebreather mask. Load and go, and continue to monitor his vitals en route to the nearest trauma center."

Later in my career, I'd joke how, in my opinion, the genital sweep was the most underutilized field technique in EMS. Literally, after EMT school, nobody did it. Probably because it was highly inappropriate to touch our patient's privates, even with the back of our hand, as it was taught. That tiny little maneuver was an auto-fail at the state licensing test if we didn't verbalize it in *every* simulated scenario. It was just one of those late-career observations that was glaringly true, yet nobody seemed to find funny, or even care. Just to clarify: it was obvious if a patient had a tent pole in their pants. Touching it was *not* necessary.

I reapplied to the fire department at the next hiring cycle, bugged the shit out of the fire chiefs on a weekly basis to the point they stopped answering my calls, and sought out influential professional references. I passed the state licensing exams and received my EMT license a month before the next municipal hiring cycle. With a passing score on the city's written test and a green light on the psychological exam, I progressed onward to the physical ability test. I knew that something needed to set me apart from the masses of applicants this time around.

The fire department offered practice times for the physical ability test for two weeks prior to the actual testing date. I showed up every day and ran the obstacles over and over. I asked the proctors and training staff for helpful hints and techniques to shave seconds off my time and began making friends with fire department employees. I ran two miles a day and cut my cigarette smoking down to a half a pack a day.

I asked the fire department training staff for professional references and got them. Buzz was beginning to trickle up the chain of command, and on the day of the test all the Fire Administration chiefs showed up to watch my performance. I'd shattered all the existing course records in my practice runs, and now it was time to make it official.

The physical agility course was a veritable gauntlet of demanding obstacles, simulating things we were likely to encounter on the fireground. I donned full turnout gear, bunker coat, bunker pants, clunky firefighting boots, and SCBA (self-contained breathing apparatus). It all started with a charged 2 ½″ hose line drag for a hundred feet.

I ain't gonna lie, those bad boys are heavy. Water weighs eight pounds per gallon, and I had a hundred feet of damn near 3″ hose filled with it. I learned to keep my momentum going—don't slow down—and if the hose coupling hooked a crack in the pavement, I needed to have enough speed to rip a chunk of concrete out of the sidewalk or it would stop me cold. Like shoveling snow on a sidewalk when the blade hits a crack and jams the handle into your guts.

After the hose drag across the parking lot and into the tower, I lifted a sixteen-foot roof ladder off a five-foot-high wall rack, and carried it on my shoulder, across the tower. It was designed to be like removing a ladder from the side of the fire truck. Many candidates struggled with this one. Some were too short to reach it; others didn't have enough upper body strength to lift it off the wall rack. Some would try for a minute, then just give up and walk off the course.

Like the pros did, I shouted, "Ladder coming through!" so people around me knew to be careful. At the other side of the building, I wedged the foot of the ladder against the wall where it met the floor and yelled "Checking for overhead obstructions!" I raised it up, hand over hand, then adjusted the bottom of the ladder out to the proper 75-degree climbing angle by having my toes touching the bottom of the ladder, then extending my arms and fingertips to touch the rails in front of me. The proctor gave me the thumbs up, and I took the ladder down in reverse order. Hollering again, "Ladder coming through!" as I carried it back across the room and hefted it onto the rack where I'd found it.

Next, I picked up an accordion-folded, fifty-foot length of 2 ½″ hose, threw it over my shoulder, and walked on top of two-by-fours stood up on their ends, and spaced sixteen inches apart, for about twenty feet, simulating walking across exposed floor joists. Then I turned around at the end of it and came back. After that, I dropped the hose bundle and crawled under a three-foot-high chute for twenty feet, grabbed a 150-pound dummy, and then crawled back under the chute, dragging the dummy behind me, to the start.

Back on my feet again, I had to pull down on a pole with a forty-five-pound weight attached to a pulley, twenty-five times, from full arm extension above my head, to hands just below the waist, to simulate pulling ceilings down during overhaul operations. After that, I climbed four stories up a stairwell, and then walked twenty feet through a room, and out to the fire escape.

There, I had to pull a rope that was tied to a 2 ½″ nozzle on the ground below, hooked to one hundred feet of dry hose, hand over hand, all the way up the four stories and over the fire escape railing.

Then it was back down the stairs and across the training tower floor, where I had to carry a roll of 2 ½″ hose for fifteen feet, up and over a two-step platform, walk another fifteen feet around a cone, then back across the platform to where I'd first picked up the hose roll. I set it down and grabbed the second of three items.

Next was a smoke ejector carry, up and over the platform, around the cone and back. Then, finally, a fire extinguisher carry, over the platform, around the cone and back, and I was done with the obstacle course. Everyone had to take two mandatory thirty-second breaks. One before ascending the stairs, and the second after we came back down.

The average time for a participant on the course was around eleven minutes. Thirteen minutes was the maximum time for passing the test. After training hard and practicing the obstacles daily for the previous two weeks, I smoked the ability course record, set by then Lieutenant Matthew Hawk at 7:43, by 22 seconds at 7:21. The record still stands today, decades later. All the recruit candidates congratulated me, so did the chiefs, while the firefighters in attendance looked on in amazement at the history they'd just witnessed.

Oddly enough, there were two firefighters named Bill Jacobson on the fire department when I hired on. One was nicknamed Tiny Paws because of his abnormally small hands and large, portly stature. The other was known as Stinky Bill, after his unique ability to take a shower and then smell like liver and onions fifteen minutes later.

Firehouse nicknames most often either poked fun at the physical characteristics of a person or were simply a shortened version of the person's name. As in B Lil for Brad Lilly, or Hawk for Matthew Hawk. If we were a probationary member, we were either newbie, new kid, probie (short for probationary firefighter), or FNG—the fucking new guy.

Tiny Paws, a captain at the time, came straight up to me after I ran the course and asked if I was related to Jack Lilly. Still out of breath, I acknowledged he was my grandfather—a local Police Commissioner when he'd passed away from a heart attack in 1980. Tiny Paws said he'd made that emergency call and performed CPR on my grandpa, but that he was already dead. I thought that was a heck of a first thing to say to a guy when you've just met them. But that's how some firefighters are. Not very big on the social skills.

There was still more to be done at the candidate testing grounds that day. The next item on the checklist of physical capabilities was a one-hundred-foot ladder climb on one of the aerial trucks. The department needed to rule out any fear of heights in their new crop of firefighter candidates. With its ladder fully extended and positioned at the proper and ideal 75-degree climbing angle, I waited for my turn. After putting on the ladder belt—a thick hunk of leather with a giant steel clip called a carabiner—I climbed up to the turntable of an old Seagrave ladder truck. The engineer gave me the signal, and up the ladder I went.

As I scaled the rungs higher and higher, the ladder began to bounce up and down. Pro tip: The key to climbing an aerial ladder is to have a slow and steady rhythmic step. If the ladder starts to bounce, one has to change the pace of their steps and lighten the impact of their weight. Things finally smoothed out and I reached the tip of the ladder at just under a hundred feet in the air.

That's almost ten stories up, and the ladder at the tip was just slightly bigger than a common, household extension ladder at that point. I could see the next towns over in all directions. The wind was blowing steady, and it felt cool against the sweat on my face, as it swayed the top of the ladder in a circular motion. I swear I could see the curvature of the Earth out at the horizon, but maybe I was just imagining things.

I clipped my ladder belt carabiner onto the rung in front of me and pushed the call button on the intercom. "All set," I said.

"OK, come on down," the voice from the speaker replied.

Going back down hand over hand, I noticed there was quite an offset between the ladder flys, and if one wasn't prepared for it, they could easily go to step down on a rung, and it would be a good four or five inches farther in than the previous one. If I wasn't hanging on tight when I transitioned to the next ladder fly, I could lose my footing and fall. So with intense focus and determination, I soon reached the bottom and disembarked from the turntable. It felt good to be back on solid ground again.

The final test was a search of a smoke-filled room about twenty feet long by twenty feet wide, or four hundred square feet, with random furniture strewn around haphazardly. The proctor had hidden a baby doll somewhere inside and it was my job to enter, search, and rescue the baby. In addition to a fog machine pumping simulated smoke into the room, the Scott mask we had to wear was covered with a hood to eliminate all sense of sight. Behind me, some of the candidates compared their completion times for the evolution. Thirty seconds to a minute seemed to be the average times for the group. As I stood by blindly at the door, the instructor explained the drill and asked if I was ready to begin. I confirmed with a gloved thumbs up and he opened the door.

I hit my knees as the door slammed shut and began to swing my arms across the floor in front of me. Through the thick firefighting gloves my mind attempted to create a mental picture of what I was touching. A couch, a wall, a bed, a baby doll… a baby doll! My hand closed around a plastic leg, and I dove backward to where the door had been.

Flopping out onto the asphalt, the instructor stopped the clock at seven seconds. "That's bullshit!" he yelled.

Wardo was one of hairiest guys I've ever met. Like a walking Wookie. This guy could go trick-or-treating with his family in street clothes and win best gorilla or grizzly bear costume. He drank a twelve pack of Mountain Dew every day and it showed through in his hyperactive speech. He was a certified fire instructor, my EMT course instructor, and an engineer on the fire department.

"You saw me put that doll there," he yelled.

"Honest, I can't see shit, sir," I offered.

"Do it again, and this time, turn around and face the other way. I'm gonna hide it good."

He disappeared into the search room and when he emerged, sounded confident I'd have a tougher go of it this time. We readied at the door, and I began again, this time searching left, instead of right, along the wall. I felt a table and a baby doll under it. Flying out the door with the child in hand, it was like déjà vu.

"That's bullshit!" Wardo screamed, louder than the first time. "Five fucking seconds! What the fuck? You *lucky* son of a bitch!"

I advanced to the final interview process, and was hired on October 5, 1998, in a class of nineteen recruits. Those lucky nineteen, out of an initial 1,347 applicants, received letters requesting confirmation calls accepting the position of Firefighter Trainee, and I immediately obliged. Our group met at city hall in the council chambers for the official welcoming committee of department heads from the Personnel, Finance, and Fire Departments.

We selected our insurances: health, dental, and vision policies for the whole family. We listed our beneficiaries in case we were killed in the line of duty. We chose our 457 deferred compensation plan and confirmed our level of contributions per paycheck. It was for real now, I was in. I was twenty-one years old, staring down a twenty-five-year commitment of work, to retire around age forty-six. I had no idea what I'd gotten myself into.

Chapter 2

The Fire Academy

When I arrived at my first day of the training academy, my personal vehicle was a white seventeen-foot-long Ford Econoline XL van, the preferred mode of transportation for any respectable flooring installer. The other trainees took to calling it the "Shaggin' Wagon." But the only shaggin' going on in it was the 1970s shag carpet being removed and hauled away from my clients' homes, I assured them. The rear windows were decorated with dozens of square bumper stickers from the local Christian radio station, arranged in the shapes of two giant crucifixes.

When I went out to the club, it was to a Christian nightclub called Visions. Church was Saturday night at Visions, and then again Sunday morning at Faith Wesleyan, a church my grandparents were founding members of. Bible study was every Wednesday night. My wife and I said prayers at meals and bedtime, and any other time we needed to talk to the man upstairs. The books I read were the Bible and devotional studies that linked to passages in the Bible. On flooring jobs, our crew listened to Christian music and never cursed. We sang in the church choir and tithed 10 percent of our weekly earnings. I was a good young man. Naïve, innocent, and good.

As probationary firefighters, we spent the next two weeks being immunized from all manner of human diseases, put through the rigors of simulated fireground activities, and tested on our EMS skills in ACLS (advanced care life support) class, so we could be officially certified to operate an ambulance in the Tri-County Medical Control Authority. Some of the recruits in our class were seasoned ambulance pros who had years of experience under their belt. Others, like me, had never made a real emergency run outside of ride-alongs in school.

The ACLS instructors were brutal. I recall one of them—we'll call him BJ—destroying my confidence when I described the process of measuring an oropharyngeal airway as the distance from the tip of the nose to the angle of the jaw.

"Bullshit! What the fuck, probie?" he yelled, as everyone in the classroom turned to look. "Hey, everybody, this new kid just mis-measured an oral airway on my grandmother and ripped her fucking trachea apart."

The previously buzzing room fell silent, and I felt the urge to shit my own pants from the intense shame and embarrassment.

"You just killed my grandma, you *fucking* idiot probie. Nice job, asshole," BJ said, leaning in so he could look me square in the eyes, his biceps bulging and about to rip through his powder blue uniformed shirt sleeves.

I glanced at the blond girl next to him and noticed she was smiling dreamily at BJ while he explained to me how "it's either the center of the mouth to the angle of the jaw, or the corner of the mouth to the tip of the earlobe." He made sure to finish with a "dumbass" for emphasis.

What a douche, I thought. It's not *that* big of a difference in length. It was tolerable.

At the end of the day, we received our American Heart Association CPR certifications. I remember the instructor explaining how the rhythm of chest compressions for effective adult CPR could easily be timed correctly by singing in our heads the Bee Gees song "Staying Alive." "Ah, ah, ah, ah, stayin' alive, stayin' alive"—that was the compression pace we wanted. Then when the chorus kicked in with "stayin' aliiiiiii-hiiiiiiii-ayaiiiiiiii-iiiiiiive," we administered two breaths of high-flow O_2 via bag valve mask, resuming chest compressions with the following verse. So, there you go. Just in case you ever find yourself pumping away on someone's chest.

For the next three months I reported on weekdays to the fire department's Training Tower, an imposing complex of buildings and training simulators in the middle of town. My instructors were Chief of Training Mike Buzynski—aka Two-Shoes, because he showed up to work one day, still drunk, wearing two different shoes; Captain Victor Johnson—aka Big Vic, because of his sense of self-worth and large physical stature; and Captain Theresa Avery—aka Donkey Gums, because she had short teeth and abnormally long gums.

We were strictly forbidden to have cell phones or pagers on us during academy training hours. However, I'd received an exemption from Donkey Gums, who'd been made aware my wife could go into labor for our first child at any moment. Big Vic was giving a presentation on the different types of smoke ejectors, and when and how to use them effectively, when my cell phone rang in my pocket.

It was just like the jelly doughnut scene from *Full Metal Jacket*, with Big Vic as R. Lee Ermy, the drill sergeant. Big Vic stopped his presentation and slowly turned around. "What the *fuck* was that?" he asked slowly and with better enunciation than any of us had ever heard from him before.

"That was my phone, sir. My wife's gone into labor, and I need to leave," I replied.

"You've gotta be *shittin'* me, probie!" Big Vic yelled. "Where the *fuck* do you get off bringing a phone into my classroom? I'll have your ass for this!"

"Captain Avery gave me permission, sir," I explained, as Big Vic's eyes bulged and the throbbing veins in his forehead gave me a visually accurate pulse rate of 140 beats per minute.

"Get out of my classroom, new kid!" Big Vic screamed as he pointed at the door. "Get out and don't come back until you have proof. I want a goddamn chunk of her placenta when she delivers it! You hear me, probie? Get the *fuck* out of my classroom!"

I scrambled to collect my belongings and rushed off, arriving home just in time to help Sonya into the car. Then her water broke on the way to the hospital. And that, my friends, is why I highly recommend leather seats in your personal vehicle. For their ease of cleaning. Amniotic fluid has a way of soaking into those cloth seats and just ruining that new car smell. My first daughter was welcomed into the world later that evening. I returned to the fire academy the following day—sans placenta—and resumed my place in the class.

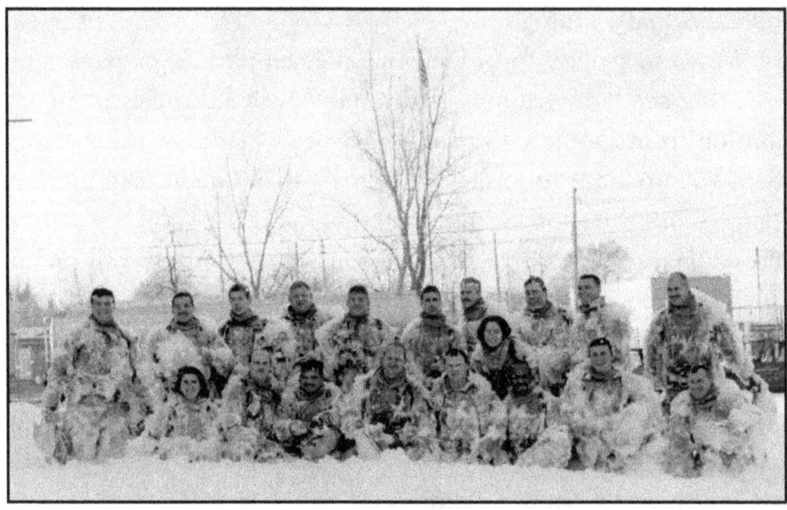

The author is front row, second from right

We were learning to use AFFF (aqueous form filling foam) that day, and there's a great photo of the whole class covered in the stuff. We all crowded into the burn room and the instructors opened the roof hatch, douching all the probies in bubbles. When the room was filled to capacity, we opened the door and gathered in close for the training academy's photo tradition.

There was a Halloween party a few weeks later at the Polish Hall. The Squid Band was playing, and this was my first official fire department function. The Squid Band was a group of local firefighters who'd formed a cover band. They were actually pretty good, and their parties were always epic. As trainees still, we were mere ghosts to the hundreds of active-duty firefighters that filled the building to capacity that night. We watched and learned.

It was pure craziness: the band was playing, people were dancing, firefighters were kissing and screwing nurses and cops everywhere we looked, beer and liquor were flowing, and everybody was having a blast. It was pure debauchery, and I drank it all in with my fellow recruit trainees by my side. We partied all night long, and as the sun crept over the horizon, we were left infatuated with what we'd gotten ourselves into. This was the life!

The day soon arrived when we were to draw for seniority in rank. I sat next to "Rotten" Ron (rotten because he was incorrigible with his constant sexual innuendoes) and told him I had a feeling I was going to draw number one. The union official reached into a fire helmet filled with folded paper and drew my name first! I smacked Ron on the arm and hurried to the front of the class as instructed. Next, the union rep brought out a second helmet and told me to draw a number. Surprised, I reached in and handed him one of the folded pieces of paper.

"Number sixteen," he announced, as my name was written on the blackboard near the bottom of the group. Ron laughed out loud, and I sulked back to my seat. The union guys told us the double-blind draw was the fairest way to select positions for seniority in rank, but it sure didn't seem so fair to the ones who got stuck at the back of the seniority line.

Later, it would mean the difference of seven additional years in the ambulance rotation between recruits one and nineteen, and two-thirds of our class being unable to make the rank of battalion chief by retirement age, negatively impacting their FAC, or retirement income. Such a small thing it seemed at the time, yet it had such far-reaching consequences. Seniority in rank determined nearly everything in the career fire department.

Five of us had been hired without Fire I and II State Certifications and were required to stay in the fire academy for another three months, then test out. We received a training wage of $17,841 per year, which worked out to around $423 bi-weekly after taxes and insurance. Not much to live on or raise a family with, considering I'd been making five times that as a flooring installer. But it was all about the pension and the benefits for my family, and we were determined to make ends meet for a while.

The other fourteen recruits were immediately released into the stations for deployment where they were needed most: being tossed to the wolves on the meat wagons, or ambulances. An infusion of fresh blood meant an extra couple of days off the sleds for the other veteran firefighters already in the ambulance rotation. A collective sigh of relief went through the entire department as the added personnel made the workload easier on all ranks.

Two-Shoes and Big Vic were rarely seen or heard from at this point of the fire academy. They were most likely at a bar or in a staff meeting and then the bar, so it was pretty much Donkey Gums and the Fab Five Trainees from 8 to 4 p.m. every weekday. We had classroom time for study and tests, book work, training videos, and the occasional guest speaker for specialty firefighting topics. We did practical training at the simulators outside on the tower grounds, where we'd learn and practice hands-on firefighting techniques. If there were any major incidents in the city, we'd all pile into the training academy minivans and respond to the scene to assist with the cleanup, better known as overhaul activities.

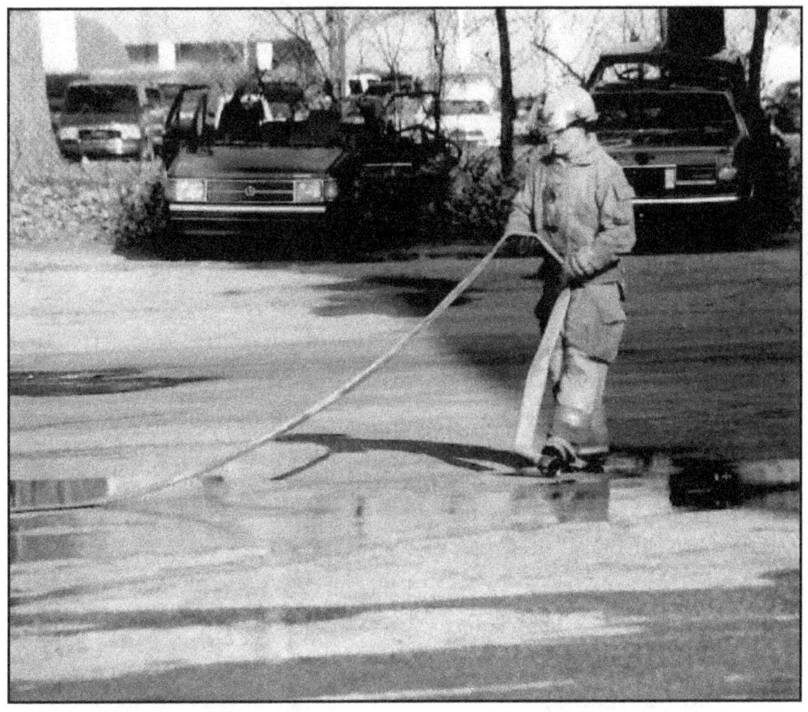

The author breaking down 2 ½" hose after a training evolution

For the most part, toward the end of the academy our afternoons were spent watching TV, playing basketball or football in the parking lot, and smoking cigarettes on the roof of the four-story tower. Donkey Gums could easily bum three to five smokes a day off me, after she'd blazed through her own pack-a-day habit. We learned she'd injured her back on duty from a slip and fall in an icy training tower parking lot and transferred to the training division right before we'd all hired on. She was only there until her line-of-duty disability was approved and kicked in. So life was easy when it was just us there, which was most of the time.

True story: At one of the fire department golf outings, ol' Two-Shoes was pulled over after leaving the course and arrested for DUI. He was excited to see an off-duty battalion chief arrive at the police station a short while later and approach his cell.

"Hey, thanks for coming to get me out of here!" he joyfully exclaimed.

"Move over," said the battalion chief, who'd just been arrested himself for the same thing and consequently joined his compadre in the drunk-tank lockup of the county jail until they'd both sobered up enough to drive home.

There was a garage fire at the end of my street one day. Just as I was arriving home from the academy, neighbors alerted me to the smoke coming from down the road. There was heavy smoke showing from behind the house, so I pulled my turnout gear from the trunk of my car, put it on, and walked over. Thinking I'd do whatever I could to help the incoming crews out.

The first due company, Engine 5, arrived with Captain Rob Thompson (later chief of the entire department and then a state senator) and Firefighter Brent Gillette.

"Who the fuck are you?" Gillette asked me as he stepped off the tailboard with a 2 ½" hose line on his shoulder.

"Brad Lilly, new recruit. I live right here. How can I help?" I said.

"Help me stretch the kinks out of this hose," he told me.

So, I did, and soon found myself in the yard, backing up the nozzle crew as they made entry into the fully involved garage fire. The officer somehow ended up with the nozzle, then turned to me and said, "Here." He handed me the fucking nozzle. I had no station assignment, no crew, no SCBA, but fuck it, I had the nozzle! I sprayed the 2 ½" hose stream at the raging beast and soon the fire was out.

As I tried to sneak through the smoke and out the garage door I'd come in, someone grabbed me by the back of the collar.

"Who the *fuck* are you?" the safety officer growled.

"New recruit Brad Lilly, sir. I live right down the street. Just trying to help, sir."

"Get the *fuck* off my fireground, *NOW*!" he yelled.

I hauled balls back to the road, where Gillette was getting a fresh air bottle.

"Who'd you say you were?" Gillette asked.

"Nobody. Gotta go!" I said and took off for home.

A few minutes later, the battalion chief was knocking at my door.

"Hey, Chief, come on in," I said, not knowing if I was completely fucked out of a career path or not.

"It's Brad, right?"

"Yes, sir," I answered, handing him a glass of cold water.

"Don't get me wrong," he said, taking a sip, "you did a hell of a job out there today, and I wish I had fifteen guys like you every time we rolled out to a fire. But let me explain why what you did today was stupid and could *fuck* every single one of us out of a job."

He went on to cite the lack of accountability and personal protective equipment for me, the dangers of freelancing and just doing whatever I wanted to on the fire scene, then finished with a dissertation on the difference between volunteer and career firefighters. How, by just deciding to show up there while not on duty, I made a solid case for paid on-call firefighters and that's not the way things work around here. We were union strong, he said, and the career guys who came before us had fought long and hard for the benefits we enjoyed today.

I listened and apologized for being naïve, thanking him for taking the time to teach me. Crisis averted. One can avoid a lot of problems in life if they just accept responsibility for their actions. Don't try to justify them. Just own up to it and apologize. People respect that shit and most of them understand everybody makes mistakes. It's not a loss if we learn from it.

Shortly before graduation, the department was slated to give the media a press release on the latest recruit class to graduate from the fire academy. The plan was to light one of the vehicle extrication training cars on fire and have a crew put it out with a hose line. The car was selected and positioned prominently in the middle of the training tower parking lot. Hoses were hooked to the hydrant and charged. Rotten Ron and I manned the hose line together. The plan was, he and I would advance the line to the car, Ron would smash the window with a Halligan tool, and I'd open the nozzle and put the fire out. It sounded easy enough.

Crews from two of the local TV stations arrived, and when they were set up, Donkey Gums lit a road flare, tossed it into the car's back seat, and shut the door. Pretty soon the car was rolling with flames, and we got the green light. The pretend director in my head yelled, "Action!" We moved the hose line into position and Ron brandished his Halligan tool—its silver adze spike gleaming in the mid-morning sunlight. He reached back and swung hard into the window. It wasn't quite hard enough, though, and the Halligan just bounced off the window glass.

I tried hard to hold back the laughter, being on film and all, and hit Ron with a barely audible, "Set your purse down, Sally."

Ron gave me the evil eye, then pulled back for another try. This time he shattered the glass. Hilariously, though, his gloves were wet from the leaky hose line, and the Halligan tool slipped right through them, disappearing through the broken car window and into the inferno.

He looked down at his empty hands for a moment, wishing longingly for a "Cut!" call from the pretend director. Realizing none was forthcoming, he stepped behind me to back up the hose line while I extinguished the raging vehicle fire. The news piece was a success, thanks to some wonderful editing, and there were celebratory cheers from all around our table of recruits at the local pub after it aired on the six o'clock news broadcast that evening.

We graduated from the academy on December 7, 1998, and I finished with one of the highest point totals and grade percentages in recent history, with a 98 percent on my written exams and a 99 percent on the practical tests. We were now officially certified in Fire I and II through the State Board. The training officers allowed us to stay home with our families for the next week while we awaited our station assignments and official release into the world of chaos and carnage.

December 18, 1998, was the swearing-in ceremony for our entire class of nineteen, with plenty of pomp and circumstance. Reporters and camera crews, the mayor and his department heads, the battalion chiefs, and our immediate family members enjoyed the ceremonies with *way* too much clapping and hand shaking.

We received our station and shift assignments, and officially became probationary firefighters. I was assigned to red 1 Kelly—the best shift, in my opinion—stationed at number three firehouse right in the downtown area. The union guys all said we could practically murder somebody and not get fired from this job. I found out later just how true that actually was.

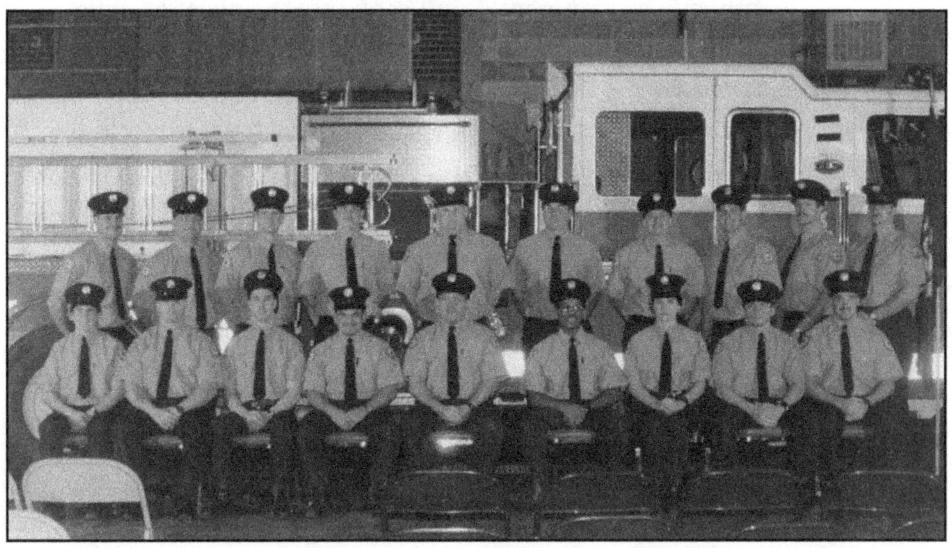

Graduation day. Author is front row, second from right.

Chapter 3

The School of Hard Knocks—Year One

No amount of classroom instruction or simulation can adequately prepare a human being for the traumas they will face as a first responder. I imagine it's that way with combat, too. I worked 127 twenty-four hour shifts in that first year as a firefighter. Innocence, faith, ethics, and morals—all sank into the abyss and disappeared in this short time. The foundation of my existence up to this point was eroded. The things I'd previously believed in could not survive my new realization of how the world truly worked. It was both devastating and liberating.

This sheds light on just some of the experiences I went through in that first year on the job. These events changed me. They changed everyone who went through them—and not for the better. It's going on today all over the world as men and women swear an oath and earn a badge. Everyone should have a better understanding of the effects of these things. They say first impressions are extremely powerful. These were mine.

December 23, 1998, was my first twenty-four-hour shift, at Station 3, a single company engine house in the downtown area. It was a quiet shift, mostly spent learning about the daily station routine. Being so close to Christmas, however, many of the duties were canceled due to the holiday.

"Mean" Dean was my officer and said a grand total of two words to me during the entire shift—"yes" and "no." JT was the engineer, and he took me under his wing. He taught me a few easy meals to cook that first day and offered helpful advice at every turn after that. We'd be good friends our entire careers.

JT was known affectionately throughout the department as the "Porn King." His dormitory locker was packed full of it. He'd spend hours every shift watching it—sometimes in the upstairs lounge, sometimes downstairs in the dining room. I never understood how one could just sit there for twenty-four hours in a house full of guys and get all worked up with no release. Maybe that's why Mel (his wife and former exotic dancer) would come and visit every day, always in her high heels, and they'd disappear upstairs for a while.

Mean Dean was a Vietnam War veteran. He drank at the VFW hall when he wasn't on duty, and most days was completely pickled with a terrible hangover when he worked. He warmed up when there was a female in the firehouse, and it was only then that he transformed into a regular human being. He had a tendency to throw a pack of chicken breasts into our grocery cart and say that's what we were cooking him for dinner, regardless of what anyone else may be eating. He never offered any extra money for it, either.

The dirty yardbird, as he called it, needed to be prepared by being marinated in Zesty Italian dressing, seasoned with garlic, salt, and pepper, then grilled until the juices ran clear when poked with a meat fork. He was a man of few words, but if we fucked up his chicken tits (in reference to the chicken *breasts*), he wouldn't speak to us for days. He enjoyed his naps in the brown chair during the afternoons, so JT would go upstairs and watch porn while I studied streets and tended to the phones and kitchen duties. There were a few uneventful fire alarms and a handful of ambulance assists—nothing spectacular to write home about that first day.

The next shift, on Christmas Day, I met Engineer Grant Kostrzewski (better known as Koz) and Captain Chuck Sanders. Both amazing men. These two were total ass kickers on the fireground, and they taught me an immense body of knowledge about doing battle with the beast, how to get the best fireground jobs, and how to truly enjoy a career in the fire service. That evening we responded to a fatal fire—fourth engine in. In the Windmill Village trailer park, a victim had been discovered after the fire was extinguished. Merry *fucking* Christmas.

Trailer fires tend to go up quick and burn through fast. There's usually only one way in or out. The victim was in a back bedroom, the farthest room from the exit, and was found on the floor, beneath a mattress, attempting to shield herself from the heat and smoke. This tactic proved fatal for her. While we waited for the Fire Marshal to arrive, I stared curiously at her hard-boiled corpse; she was wearing only her underwear, and her skin was mottled, yellow, and bloated. It was my first Christmas in the station, and my first fatal fire. The first of many.

Roberta "Bobby" Franklin was a lesbian who, when I met her, was an angry at the world, fuck-you-motherfucker engineer at Station 4. She was the driver on my very first, first-in structure fire. It was after midnight, and we were all asleep in the common dorm when a full alarm came in. Two long tones on our alarm system meant a fire, followed by three short tones for an ambulance standby.

The dispatcher came on next and gave the address: an apartment complex in our *first due* (meaning we were the first unit to arrive). I sat up in bed and slid my feet into my fire boots, pulled my bunker pants up, and threw the thick suspenders over my shoulders as I rose from the bed. I made my way across the dorm and slid the pole, reviewing in my mind all the training of the past three months. I whipped my turnout coat on and climbed aboard the pumper, pounding the engine cowling twice with my fist so the engineer knew I was ready. The loud diesel motor roared to life, and we screamed off into the night.

My officer was Bud Adams. Everyone called him Bud the Fire Stud because he'd made so many fires—a *fucking* fire magnet, they said. I loved that dude. Damn near every time we rode together, we were battling the flames. His old lieutenant's helmet hangs on the wall today in my man cave. He was a former U.S. Marine and a helluva guy.

Tonight, he was popping my fire cherry, and like all first timers, I'd always cherish this moment. This was what I'd been waiting for since hiring on. What I'd trained so hard for—the opportunity to be a hero. As we turned onto Liberty Road, I looked through the windshield at the scene ahead of us. I could see the smoke rising and knew it was a real working fire. A thin, silver stream of smoke wafted up past the full moon in a cloudless night sky. It was beautiful. Bob Ross or Norman *fucking* Rockwell couldn't have painted a better picture of the smoke, backlit by the full moon, rising high into the air. It was absolutely perfect.

I howled with excitement as we pulled up to flames showing from the front door and Bobby hit me with a "*Jesus*, new kid, don't trip over your dick!"

Bud laughed and told me to pull the 1 ¾" pre-connect and meet him at the door to the involved apartment. Then he calmly gave his radio report, "Dispatch, Engine 4 on scene, three-story apartment building, smoke and flames showing from the ground floor apartment, Engine 4 stretching pre-connect, have the next engine in grab a hydrant, Engine 4 has command."

Rounding the truck to the engineer's side, I stepped up onto the running board and ran my forearm through the dangling loops of the folded two-hundred-foot crosslay, grabbing the Select-O-Matic nozzle in my other hand. I pulled hard and the pile of hose slid from its bed. I stretched it down the sidewalk, one building to the right, sizing up the burning structure we were about to enter—three stories, twelve apartment units.

The first hose loop pulled tight, so I dropped it and began heading back past the fire with the second loop, weaving around the building's occupants amassing on the front lawn. Bobby had the rig in pump and as I passed the truck, Bud advised everyone was out of the building. I flaked out the kinks from the hose and advanced the dry line up to the garden apartment door.

Kneeling down on the hose line behind the nozzle in case it was charged, I began putting my Scott mask on. We were right outside the door and the apartment had been left open by the fleeing tenants. Flames licked across the living room ceiling and out the front door over our heads. Bobby charged the line, and it became rigid and stiff beneath my knee. I donned my helmet, pulled on my thick firefighting gloves, and picked up the hose. After cracking open the bale and allowing the pressurized air to escape, water flowed from the nozzle.

Bud told me to close it and to watch the fire for a moment. It was beautiful and alive as it rolled over itself and moved in waves across the ceiling in hues of reds, yellows, and oranges. Bud, with his hand on my shoulder, calmly said to always watch where it's going, to see what it wants to do. Then he slapped me on the shoulder and said "Give 'er hell, new kid!"

As I pulled back the bale of the nozzle and directed the stream at the flames overhead, the fire immediately darkened down. We pushed forward into the apartment and extinguished the living and dining rooms. In the kitchen we found the seat of the fire and with a well-directed, straight stream shot at its base, the flames disappeared, and the battle was over.

Bud opened the sliding glass window to let the steam, heat, and smoke escape, then we headed down the hallway and checked the bedrooms for any victims. They were empty and clear of fire, and we opened the bedroom windows to ventilate the smoke. I set the nozzle down in the living room and we exited the apartment for a fresh tank of air.

We were passed by the second-in engine crew heading inside to pull walls and ceiling, checking for fire extension. After ensuring the fire was completely out, the other rigs cleared from the scene and returned to their firehouses. We stayed until the Fire Marshal showed up, to preserve the chain of custody for evidence regarding the point of origin or cause of the fire. Then we packed up our hoses and returned to the fire station. It was 03:00 hours and I couldn't sleep. My adrenaline was through the roof. I'd fought the dragon and won—easily. This was the beginning of my love affair with the fire ground.

Station 3 was an extrication focus station, and they had the *Jaws of Life* or the vehicle extrication tools. Firefighters use these tools to free people from the mangled remains of their crashed vehicles. Station 2 on the extreme north end of town and Station 4 on the far south side of town also had a set of these tools. The idea was that Station 3 made all the north end extrication responses with Station 2, *and* all the south end calls, with Station 4. That way we had two sets of life-saving spreaders, cutters, and rams rolling on every "pin-in" call—the term for a person trapped inside their vehicle. We sent two sets of tools to every extrication call, just in case more than one vehicle at the same scene required them.

Some of the highways that carved through our urban sprawl were recessed deep into the earth, with on and off ramps that merged with parallel streets running above and alongside them. Station 3 was located on one of these streets, overlooking the highway that cut through the heart of the city's downtown. On a warm spring afternoon, Mean Dean, JT, and I responded on a motorist who'd crashed into a bridge abutment on the highway, just west of the fire station.

We sliced through the backed-up traffic and rumbled onto the median's shoulder, rolling to a stop at the scene. I grabbed the EMS blue bag from the cabinet and approached the car from behind. There was just one unconscious man in the car, the driver. His body was completely beneath the steering wheel. His face was lying in a pool of blood on his seat, and he was blowing red blood bubbles in it, like a dying fish out of water. We referred to these as agonal respirations because they were usually the last few breaths of a person in agony about to die.

The guardrail he'd just driven through had peeled back the roof of his car like a sardine can about halfway back. The front end was obliterated, the doors were stuck shut, and the dashboard had collapsed down on him. Mean Dean radioed the extrication call in and I hauled the Jaws over to the car. JT set up the hydraulic pump and the hoses, then we went to work on popping the doors open and rolling the dashboard up and away from the man. We'd practiced this evolution dozens of times and could do the whole operation in just a few minutes.

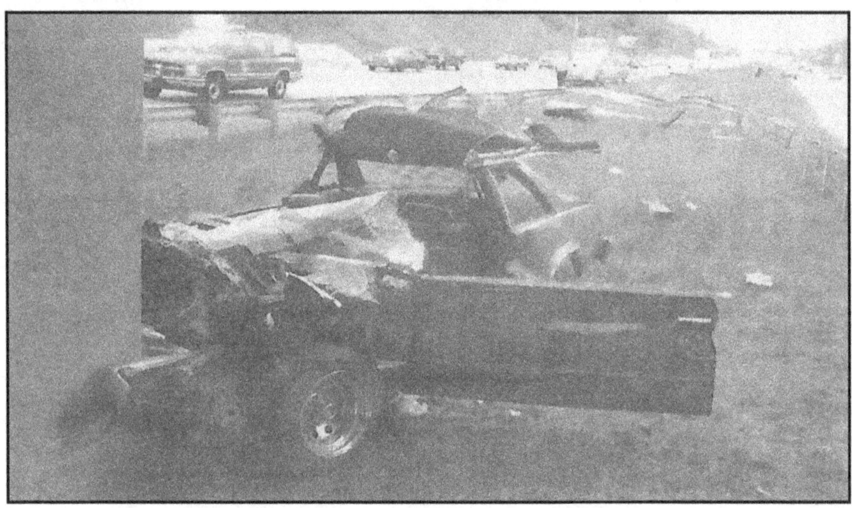

Everything went smooth on our end, and the medics had the man packaged for transport within the "Golden Ten Minutes" rule we have for our extrications. That's ten minutes from arrival on scene until transport to the hospital. The man still didn't make it. After twenty years in the business, we knew when we pulled up who was going to survive and who was already a K (short for KIA, or killed in action). I was new then, and had grandiose dreams that I could save everyone. If I could just do the right thing at the right time. I was wrong.

As spring yielded to the warmth of summer, Engine 3 was returning from a run, and we needed to stop by Station 1 to replace some EMS supplies after using them on a call. Sanders and Koz mingled with the downtown crews preparing lunch in the kitchen, while I secured the equipment. When it was time for us to leave, we began heading across the apparatus floor and out through the open garage doors. Koz stopped us just short from leaving the building and told Sanders he just couldn't let it happen.

"Ok… what do you want to do about it?" Chuck asked.

Koz turned to me and explained there were two firefighters and an engineer on the rooftop waiting to hit me with a bucket of water when I walked out. And how, if I had a set of nuts, I should go into the slop room, fill up a bucket of water, and climb to the roof to hit them with it instead. Sanders agreed with a sly smile.

I did as my crew advised. It was after all, practically a direct order *and* the size of my marbles were being judged. When I peered onto the roof from the hose tower door, Lenny Smith, Don Babcock, and Jughead, were all at the edge of the roof in front of me with their backs turned, watching for me to walk out below.

I snuck quietly across the roof to within a few feet of them and yelled, "Hey!"

Don Babcock was in the middle and when he turned around, I nailed him in the chest with the bucket full of water.

"Aw, heck no!" Lenny Smith cried, and all three of them drenched me with their buckets. They ran to the roof access door, closed, and locked it, trapping me on the rooftop. Jughead and

Babcock ran up and down the roof access stairs, shuttling buckets of water to Lenny, who then proceeded to open the door and fire them at me repeatedly.

Koz and Sanders were down on the street below honking the air horn on the fire engine and telling me to, "Hurry up, new kid," over the fire engine's PA system.

I leaned over the edge of the roof and yelled down, "They've got me trapped up here!"

It was around seventeen buckets later when they either got bored of it, or became tired from running the stairs, and left the roof door open. I snuck down the stairs and exited at the second-floor dormitory level hallway, where Don Babcock was waiting around the corner with one final bucket.

I held my arms straight out to the side and let him deliver it, unabated. Soaked to the bone, I shivered my way out to Engine 3 and rejoined my crew. I wondered if I wouldn't have just been better off walking out the garage doors to begin with. Either way, the precedent had been set. I wasn't afraid to tangle with the professional bullies when it came to firehouse pranks and had challenged them at their own game. I thanked Koz and Sanders for looking out for me and we headed back to Station 3 for a much-needed wardrobe change.

True story: Lenny Smith was a giant human being. A country boy who stood six feet five inches and weighed nearly 250 pounds of solid mass. Orval Jenkins was a petite man. At five feet six and 150 pounds, he relied on his brains rather than brawn to survive on the fire scenes. One night while brushing their teeth before going to bed at Station 1, Orval leaned over and spit his tooth paste right down Lenny's dark blue uniformed pant leg. Lenny looked down at his pants, then back at Orval. He calmly set his toothbrush on the sink, grabbed Orval by the back of the neck and belt, picked him up sideways, and wiped his pants off with Orval's squirming body. Then Lenny set the shocked Orval back on his feet without a word and finished brushing his teeth.

After twenty years in the business, I've touched more dead and dying bodies than I can remember. Some of them I knew personally. Some of them were my friends. My first was a good friend from high school. I was on Engine 8 one bright, sunny summer morning when an alarm came in for a young man hit by a falling tree.

We arrived first on scene to find my good friend, Corey Sanchez, lying on his back on the sidewalk with snoring respirations. As I rushed in to help, the distraught tree cutter beside him was explaining to me how, when he'd started his cut no one was there, and then as the tree trunk fell, he saw this guy just standing there, right in its path.

Corey's grandmother was crying and wailing hysterically in the front yard, cursing in Spanish at the tree cutter, whom she'd hired. Some of it I could understand, most of it I couldn't because of her sobs and gasping for air. Corey was unconscious and bleeding from an avulsion on the top of his head. I could see the white of his skull through his dark brown and bloody hair. He was posturing with his arms and legs folding in toward the midlines of his body. A large tree trunk about a foot in diameter and twenty feet or so long, lay beside him on the front lawn.

I recalled from EMT school how this was called decorticate posturing and was associated with a severe spinal cord injury. I took C-spine control and told my friend it was OK. That I had him, and we were here to help, to just relax. As I held his head between my hands and looked for other injuries, I could see he had a priapism (remember the genital sweep). I didn't know it at the time, but Corey was already gone. His body was just going through autonomic reflexes. His spirit had already left his vessel. We packaged him on the backboard and loaded him into the sled as it pulled up. He coded twice in the back of the ambulance while I drove the seven or eight blocks to the hospital. He was pronounced dead shortly after we arrived. I'd done everything right again, just like they'd taught me, and he still died. I prayed and sought revelation; however, peace and solace eluded me. The voice on the opposite end of the God hotline remained silent.

Occasionally we'd have to "rove" from our home station to another firehouse to fill in for an absent employee. This was my first rove to Station 5, a single company engine house with a medic unit. Jim Sparks was the boss and Spike Young was the driver. That evening, as I walked past the hose tower, I noticed Jim and Spike smoking a joint and drinking beer.

"Hey, new kid!" Sparks said as I walked by. "Get your ass in here. Pass him the joint, Young Dawg."

"Oh, no thanks," I said.

"Nah *fuck* that," Captain Sparks barked. "You hit that fucking shit right now, new kid, and drink this goddamn beer; that's a *fucking* order. You a fucking snitch? Are you a *fucking* snitch, new kid?" Sparks talked a mile a minute and cussed like a sailor.

"No sir," I said.

"Then hit that fucking shit now and show me. If you hit it, you can't snitch, cuz you'd be snitchin' on yourself, too."

Spike passed me the weed and I took a drag from the joint. Sparks cracked a can of beer and handed it to me.

"What happens if we catch a run?" I asked.

"You really think anyone *cares* if their rescuer is high?" Sparks replied. "They don't give a flying *fuck*. They just want to be saved."

We finished our beers, and I didn't snitch on them. I soaked up the machismo like a sponge and reveled in my newfound realization that one could do anything they wanted here. Know the right people, play the right cards, and anything was permitted. That was the first of many times I was directly ordered to smoke weed while on duty.

The ambulance was a nemesis where I worked. It was a meat grinder that chewed up new firefighters and spit them out. A zombie maker. It was known affectionately as "the sled," "bone box," "medic," "meat wagon," "bus," and "horizontal taxi." Sometimes, when we had a whiney patient, it was the wah-mbulance. Or, in impoverished neighborhoods, the bambalance. When I hired on, our department just purchased four large International rigs known as the Big Reds. The older, smaller ones that we had to switch into when our Big Reds broke down were called van-bulances.

As a probationary firefighter, I was in the ambulance rotation until I made the rank of engineer. That meant every three shifts or so, I staffed an ambulance. On the other shifts, I was assigned to either an engine company or a ladder company. I carried around a blue recruit notebook, for the officer to write a review of my performance in, at the end of each shift.

When new kids were just starting out on the ambulance, we rode with an FTI (field training instructor) who evaluated our skills and either cleared us for independent patient care or busted us back down to the academy for remedial training. They were sticklers for following protocol and with good reason. They explained how, on the ambulance, we represented our department and were tasked with saving the lives of our citizens in peril. This was in sharp contrast to the beer drinking and weed smoking I'd just experienced on Engine 5.

Out of Station 1, on a sultry summer evening, Jack "Agent" Mulder and I were on Medic 11. We called him Agent after the *X-Files* TV show character. An alarm came in around 21:00 hours and as we made our way to the sled, Dispatch accidentally toned out (the term for activating the fire station alarm system for a given unit) the other medic crew instead. Kevin Norwood and Sam Sullivan—the crew of the other ambulance—ran past us saying they'd take the call.

It was close to bedtime, and they didn't want to be "on deck" to take the next downtown EMS call. After 22:00 hours, Dispatch operated under the rule, "if you're out, you're up" for the downtown medic units. Meaning, if we were available for a call—still out of the station—and another alarm came in, it was an expected courtesy to let the other medic crew sleep for a while and for us to take two calls in a row. Agent told me not to let them beat us to what should have been *our* call, and the race was on. Kevin and I were both new kids riding with FTIs that day and were eager to impress our evaluators, so we followed orders without question.

We hopped into the cab of our sled, and I fired it up as Agent lit a cigarette. He always smoked on the way to calls. Pulling out of the station, we were neck and neck with the other medic. As we turned left, and then left again, I cut inside, into the oncoming traffic. Kevin swung wide around the corner. We were both flying down the street, side by side, lights and sirens, when the setting sun blinded us to the traffic light ahead that just turned red.

"Don't you let them beat us!" Agent hollered at me as I stood on the throttle.

Just then, the ambulance to our right slammed on its brakes and so did an elderly woman in a car traveling down the cross street to our right. Agent almost shit his pants and we both felt horrible knowing we'd just blown through an intersection and almost T-boned a little old lady—just so we could be the first ones to go to bed for the night.

There's a huge responsibility to bear as an equipment operator in the fire department. Civilians are depending on us to control our emotions and operate our apparatus with the general public's safety in mind. Lessons were learned that day. Those FTIs were responsible for teaching us the right way to do things. They shouldn't have been playing games with other people's lives. It was definitely a sobering moment.

There were five ALS (Advanced Life Support) ambulances at my department. Three in the south stationed at different firehouses, and two in the north, both housed at Station 1 downtown. It was expected we'd arrive at 06:15 hours to relieve the guy from the previous shift. Who was getting his nuts kicked in by emergency runs and had bags under his eyes so big they rivaled the giant duffel bag of turnout gear I'd just lugged to the rig and threw on the truck.

I'd take the other guy's gear off and either put it in his floor locker, or if he was a rover, leave it in a neat pile on the floor by the back of the truck. So when he stumbles out after the wake-up alarm at 06:30 and sees it, a sense of relief washes over his poor haggard soul. As he lays eyes on his personal gear, recently removed from the meat wagon, he knows his tour is over.

It was nothing to pull twenty or more calls in a twenty-four-hour shift. To not get a wink of sleep, and maybe have a nice dinner of hospital graham cracker packs, or saltines if one preferred. Thank God for the kind person who stocked the hospital's ambulance report writing room with water or hot coffee. They are hereby paid homage, bless their soul.

Hopefully, we could crank out that run report and turn it in to the emergency staff before Dispatch crackled across the radio, asking if we were available for another run. Hell, hopefully we weren't wheeling our patient in through the hospital doors when Dispatch called us.

Generally speaking, we were in the ambulance rotation until we made the rank of engineer. Folks on our department were making rank at around eight years when I hired on. I could do that, I told myself. My first ambulance shift I stayed up all night on purpose just to make sure I didn't miss a call. That was dumb. I'd lose the entire next day of my life if I fell asleep when I got home. And, even if I could manage to keep my eyes open, I was completely worthless to my family and any task that required a modicum of focus and coordination.

I learned quickly when we have down time in the firehouse, we take it. That shit is golden. If I made the rules, we'd have mandatory naps. We never knew when we were going to catch a cock knocker and be gone for hours. Then clear from that one and catch another, and another after that. Pretty soon the sun was rising over a pile of ashes that used to be someone's home. So screw anyone who thinks a firefighter sitting in a La-Z-Boy chair is a bad thing. That shit is earned.

Cock knockers were massive fires that usually entailed multiple alarms. The first alarm got the four closest engines, two ladder trucks, one battalion chief, one safety officer, and one medic. Every subsequent alarm brought an additional engine and ladder truck. So a three-alarm fire gave us six engines, four ladder trucks, a safety, a battalion, and a medic unit, at least in the city where I worked.

We found out what people are really made of at cock knockers. I suppose that's why they called them that. I've seen the firehouse loud mouths and braggarts turn pale, then run and hide at these ragers. I've both witnessed, and been a part of, a handful of guys who storm the castle, punch the beast in the mouth, execute perfection in their firefighting technique and make chaos become order. It's all in the initial actions. If the first-in crews do their jobs to the best of their ability, shit goes well. If not, well, then we're all going to be there for a while.

Cock knockers on the medic unit weren't all that bad. If we didn't have any victims to care for, we could get involved in the fireground activities. Changing SCBA bottles for the firefighters and setting up rehab stations with fresh water and dry towels were the usual activities on the sled. Maybe help a rookie flake the kinks out of a 1¾" pre-connect hose they were stretching to the door or throw a ground ladder to an upstairs window in case the interior crews had to bail out from the second or third story.

At least we weren't on some bullshit call like "Oh, I hurt my pinky toe three days ago and now it's really bothering me at 2:30 in the morning, and by the way, I can't walk so you'll have to carry me down three flights of stairs." The good firefighters on the medic understood the value of running a quality fireground rehab area and handled their air bottle changes with speed and accuracy, getting intel from the crews as they exited the structures. Making sure our compadres were ready to return to action quickly was key.

I'd pass the firefighters a cup of cold water and a towel as they came over for a bottle exchange. Then they'd turn around and lean forward slightly to expose the valve on the bottom of their Scott Pak. I'd close the valve and tell them to bleed the line. They'd hit the purge valve on their regulator and the air would rush out. I'd unscrew the supply hose coupling from the tank, release the harness clip, and slide the bottle out of the pack. I'd set the used bottle in the pile of empties, then grab a full one, opening the air valve to blast the dust cap off the threads, and with a *pop* the little blue cap would shoot off across the lawn or down the street.

Next, I'd slide the full tank into the harness, thread the hose coupling onto it, fold the harness clamp closed at the top, and ask if they wanted their tank open or closed. A slap on the shoulder to let them know I was done, and they were off. The whole time I'd be chatting them up with what's it like in there, how's it going—always encouraging them. It was like a *fucking* NASCAR pit stop and then they were off again. Thirty-second bottle changes. Yeah baby!

On the ambulance out of Station 1, Shana Proctor and I caught a cock knocker at one of the high-rise apartment buildings downtown. There was smoke showing from the ninth floor of the fourteen-story building as we turned the corner and pulled into the parking lot of the Ottawa Towers apartments. Residents were pouring out of the building, trying to escape the smoke that was filling their hallways and homes.

Ladder trucks backed up to the corners of the building and

started making rescue picks off the balconies. We instantly had multiple patients, so we transitioned into Medical Control and called for more ambulances to help transport, while we remained at the scene triaging the victims. The sun had set, and it was beginning to snow, so we set up our triage operation in the building's community room, just off the west stairwell on the ground floor. Since the fire was closer to the east stairwell, the west had been designated as the civilian evacuation stairs.

We had all kinds of elderly patients; some had fallen down the stairs, inhaled smoke and had DIB (difficulty in breathing), had sprained ankles, bruises, cuts, chest pains, burns, and all manner of boo boos and owwies. We were there for six hours treating patients. Damn near forty of them were transported. The worst was the fire victim in the apartment of origin. That was a tough one. Our crews had done their best, but she wasn't able to be saved that day. That was my first MCI (mass casualty incident), my first time as a Medical Control officer at one of these, and my first high-rise fire.

Shana was called Princess Fiona behind her back. By day, she was a semi-likable lesbian whose sarcasm and perverse sense of humor was mildly entertaining to be around. When the sun went down however, she went through a change—a metamorphosis—where she hated everything and everyone. She was like Fiona from Shrek, shape shifting into an ogre at night.

Marty Clevenger, the guy from my EMT school, whom everyone thought was legitimately mentally challenged and uncannily resembled Sloth from *The Goonies*, was nicknamed Shrek as well. So we had a Shrek and a Fiona in our department. Incidentally, Shrek would turn into an ogre, too, just like Fiona, if we referred to him as a window licker, a crayon muncher, or a paste eater, in reference to his kindergarten-like behavior and general intelligence level.

The five foot four inch Billy Engler was dubbed Lord Farquaad by his peers at the department because he drove a gigantic, lifted Ford F-350, and when he jumped out of it, he barely came up above the bumpers. In the movie, as Lord Farquaad dismounted his overtly large steed, Donkey and Shrek made offhand comments about him "compensating for something," and the comparison seemed similarly applicable to Billy. With the inclusion of Donkey Gums, the main character cast of the movie *Shrek* was effectively rounded out on our department with hilarious accuracy.

On the ambulance at Station 1, shortly after the New Year, Greg Mason and I were on Medic 11 together. It was late evening and twilight was upon us. We'd been steady, running almost constantly all day. The firehouse lights above kicked on, and the dispatcher called on us to respond on a young man having an asthma attack.

We arrived minutes later to find a twenty-one-year-old having difficulty in breathing. He said he'd used his rescue inhaler multiple times with no relief, that this was his first day out of prison, and he'd been celebrating by smoking weed and cigars with his friends and family. We applied high flow O_2 via non-rebreather mask and hurried him out to the ambulance.

Inside the sled, I set up an albuterol treatment as Greg listened for lung sounds. There were hardly any, and the young man was struggling more and moving less air with each shallow breath. He was sitting straight up and white knuckling the armrest rails on the cot. We called this posturing for breath. He was dying right in front of us.

I placed the albuterol mask over the man's face.

He struggled to stay conscious and fought against the mask, ripping it off his face trying to get more air into his lungs. Then his eyes rolled back in his head, and he fell over, unconscious. Greg called for an engine company to respond for a CPR in progress and I began chest compressions as Greg assembled the laryngoscope and attempted to drop an ET (endotracheal tube)—essentially a pipe between us and the patient's lungs.

Greg had trouble finding the patient's trachea because of his severely constricted airway, and he struggled to place the ET tube. After several minutes, and several failed attempts, we ended up just going with an oral airway. The engine crew arrived, and we headed to the hospital. Unfortunately, it was too late, and this young man passed away on his first day of freedom. That was my second time watching a human being die right in front of me, and not being able to save them. I felt like I should've been able to do more. It affected me terribly, deeply, and profoundly.

After that, I vowed to go to paramedic school and spent many hours on the intubation mannequin at Station 1, learning to start advanced airways. I learned little tricks like the Sellick maneuver or cricoid pressure, where one presses down lightly on the sides of the Adam's apple to help expose the vocal cords of the trachea, which are the landmarks for ET tube placement. I learned how to perform a cricothyrotomy in case an ET insertion ever failed again.

Back on Engine 3 one day, Peter McKinley had his first day acting captain, and Steve Bishop had his first day acting engineer. Occasionally, we'd act up one rank higher than our own if there were extra employees on duty at a lower rank and someone was needed at a higher rank. If we'd passed all the requirements for making the next rank and were just waiting on retirements for our promotion, we could act up, and seniority in rank determined the next actor.

So, to simplify, this was the very first day these two had acted at the next rank above their own. This would be one of the most legendary days of my career. It began with a late morning citizen assist at a state office building. The patient had ALS, or amyotrophic lateral sclerosis (better known as Lou Gehrig's disease), and just needed assistance from a toilet, back into his wheelchair. Or so Dispatch said.

We arrived on scene, and I grabbed the EMS blue bag. Together, we entered the building and made our way to the third-floor bathroom. The smell of fresh dookie slapped our nose holes hard as we approached the doors. This was a really nice bathroom. It had marble walls, a large foyer, three sinks, four stalls, and every goddamn surface had shit on it. It was like the proverbial shit had *literally* hit the fan. We could barely take a step without landing in human feces. I'd never imagined that amount of poop could come from one human being.

Expecting to find a gravitationally challenged heifer, I pushed open the last handicapped stall door to discover a tiny, frail man on the toilet. He said he just needed help wiping his ass and getting back into his wheelchair—which was also covered in shit.

I looked at Peter, who shrugged his shoulders and said, "It's good to be king," then simply walked out of the bathroom, leaving us to handle the patient and his massive ass-plosion.

Steve, who was also one of my ambulance FTIs, offered to hold the gentleman up while I cleaned his backside. Damn.

I thought about what it must be like to be in this guy's shoes, as I took the toilet paper and cleaned the ass-spackle from his crack. The smell was horrible. *Pension and the bennies, baby. Pension and the bennies*. Keep saying the mantra.

I finally smeared enough off to get his pants up and buckled them. Steve steadied him while I went to work cleaning his chair. The poor guy kept saying how sorry and embarrassed he was. I couldn't imagine. Once he was back in his powered wheelchair, the man didn't even try to navigate around the poop, he just rolled right through it, out of the restroom, and onto the carpet. We advised the security guard to call for a janitor on our way out. From that day on, Captain McKinley referred to me as "Shit Boy" every time he saw me.

That night was epic, though. One of the biggest cock knockers in the city's history was about to pop off, and I was on the second-due engine. Imagine an entire city block on fire; it was absolutely awesome! One of our off-duty dispatchers filmed it on a VHS camcorder. A three-story warehouse was fully involved, heavy timber, brick walls, close to ten acres of land just rolling with flames. The warehouse fire was started by vagrants lighting a pile of old tires to stay warm. It came in around 23:00 hours, and upon arrival it was more fire in one place than any of us had ever seen. Like a fucking volcanic eruption in the downtown area.

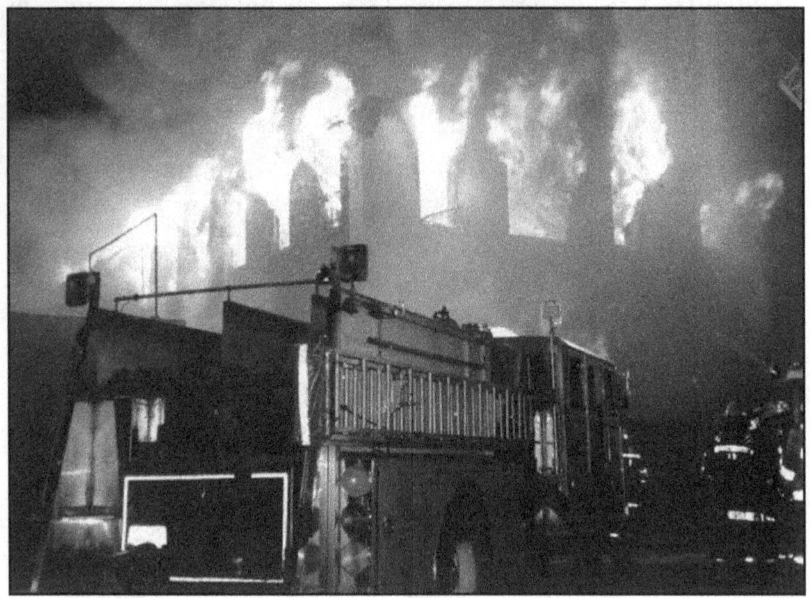

Warehouse fire

Our initial assignment was to supply Truck 8 on the west side of the building, along the railroad tracks. We hooked a hydrant for a water supply and ran a forward lay of 5" hose to where Truck 8 had set up, then we relay pumped into their supply intake. They raised their elevated master stream and began a *surround and drown* operation. That's just what it sounds like; put elevated ladders at the four corners of the structure, and flow 1,000 gallons per minute from the tip of each one, until the fire darkens down. We did this for several hours.

If we're going *hard from the yard*, or staying outside, we don't want to have anyone on the inside. It can make the interior conditions unpredictable and dangerous by flowing water through openings from the outside. Due to the amount of involvement by fire, and the potential for collapse, our chiefs determined a defensive strategy would be the best to start with.

With Truck 8 supplied with water from Engine 3, we pulled two 2" hoses from the bed and fitted them to the rear outlets over the tailboard. We looped them back on themselves, so the weight of the water-filled hose was greater than the back pressure created when the nozzle was opened, which was significant. Sometimes it could push us backward if the engineer had the pressure dialed up too high. Gating the nozzle bale down was also a good way to decrease the force if we ever needed to—if the hose was ever too difficult to handle.

The loop in the hose took the place of another firefighter backing us up—pushing into the nozzleman like doing a wall squat, back-to-back. Captain McKinley and I sat on the 2 ½" hose lines, directing water through the second story windows for hours. The fire was so hot it seemed to just laugh at us and continued devouring its heavy timber fuel load.

Around the north side of the building, Engine 8 hooked a hydrant to supply Truck 2. As it pulled away from the hydrant for the forward hose lay, one of the 5" supply line couplings caught the rear tire of a police cruiser that had parked just a little too close, attempting to block the road from civilian traffic. The police car spun violently in a wicked 360 that sent it flying back over to the curb where it belonged.

After hours of sitting on the hose lines, the battalion chiefs called the crews over to begin making plans for entry. The fire had darkened down considerably, and we gathered on the north side, near the main, three-story entrance with four other engine companies. We discussed the plan; to get to the seat of the fire with two 2 ½" hose lines, with two engine crews per line. As the ladder trucks ceased flowing water, we advanced our hoses through the burned-out interior of the warehouse. Rooms full of fire and stairways of cascading waterfalls met us as we made our way forward, into the red.

We came to a pair of closed double doors big enough to drive a car through. Kevin Norwood and I were each on a nozzle as the other crews forced the massive wooden doors open. On the other side the air was literally on fire. When they opened, four feet of water came rushing toward us, filling our boots, and washing some of the guys back down the hallway. We pressed on together and found the seat of the fire. With our two straight stream nozzles, directed at the base of the fire, the beast had no chance, and its appetite for destruction was finally quenched.

It was beautiful chaos. The one-way road on the north side of the building had to be shut down because we'd flowed so much water that the runoff had filled the three-lane roadway viaduct under the train trestle bridge with eight feet of water.

On the fourth alarm, Koz got Engine 7 stuck in the mud, created by the elevated master streams, just trying to arrive on scene. He buried that fucker up to the frame, dead in the water, right when he and his crew had just arrived. And it sat there, incapacitated in the mud, until the next morning when the sun rose over the fireground.

Trains kept on rolling by all night, passing mere inches away from Truck 8 and Engine 3 on the west side of the building. When we're that close to trains going full speed ahead, it's quite unnerving as the ground rumbles and shakes all around us.

The best cigarette I've ever had was on this fire, and I've been chasing it ever since. I climbed Truck 8 and stood for an hour, seventy feet in the air over a raging inferno, directing the elevated master stream into areas of heavy fire where the roof had collapsed. After having been there for a while and using only one hand on the toggle switch of the nozzle, moving it slowly back and forth, a cigarette to pass the time is simply perfect. The roaring flames, illuminating the blackness of night, perched over a volcano on a ladder. The best ciggy ever, period.

The old leather-lungers would rip their masks off as soon as the fire was extinguished and light up a cigarette. Their new-kid firefighters in tow, trying to emulate their masters, would often end up hacking and choking on the thick smoke still hanging in the air. Cigarette smoking, it seemed, made it infinitely easier to breath in the post-apocalyptic world of overhauling the fireground.

Later we'd learn about the dangerously elevated levels of hydrogen cyanide and carbon monoxide released during the incomplete burning of overhaul activities. Scott masks would be mandated until air monitoring by a safety officer could verify acceptable levels of carcinogens in the air. But for now, it was a "smoke 'em if ya got 'em" moment, so everybody lit up and pulled the plaster and lath walls and ceilings with our pike poles and ciggies hanging from our mouths. This was my first of many multiple-alarm fires, or cock knockers, if you prefer.

Sometimes, our firefighters referred to the stations in a possessive terminology. So instead of Station 1, it was simply Ones, or Station 3 was Threes. It became second nature to refer to them in this way and our spouses and family members were always questioning what the heck we were talking about; it made no sense to them. It was part of the fire service patois and if they weren't living it, they simply didn't get it.

The next morning, I'd traded a shift with a black shift firefighter at Threes and had to relieve myself. After being up all night at the fire, our engine returned to the firehouse to pick up the incoming crew. Then we rode back to fire scene, where I sat in a ladder truck bucket hosing down hot spots with Captain Larry Simmons, while an excavator demolished the building.

It wasn't all bad, though. Box 23, a group of civilian volunteers that responded to care for our firefighters on major scenes, had dropped off several dozen doughnuts and hot coffee for the responders that morning. Those folks were the best. If it was minus fifteen degrees, in the middle of the night, they'd be there at all the big ones, handing us a cup of warm cheer, a pair of dry gloves, or a slice of goodwill.

It wasn't until 15:00 hours when we finally left the scene and returned to the firehouse. Larry took pity on my poor soul and sent me to bed after we ate an Art's Bar pizza we'd picked up on the way home. That shit was the cheesiest. I couldn't tell you what happened for the next forty-eight hours. Pretty sure I slept through most of it.

When there's a new firefighter on the ambulance, and they're riding with an FTI, they take every patient, all day long. No alternating calls with their partner, or the paramedic takes all the advanced and the EMT takes all the basic patients. No, they take every goddamn one of them, all shift long. The FTI sits right there with them, watching their probationary ass the whole time, waiting for them to fuck something up so they can lambaste them in front of their peers.

The other firefighter on the three-person crew, they're the designated ambulance driver—aka third rider—for the whole twenty-four-hour shift. Later in my career, I learned that the third rider was the absolute best spot to be in if I had to ride the medic. It was like a reprieve from action with credit for time served. I didn't have to treat the patients, or write any run reports, all I had to do was climb aboard the sled and then drive it to the hospital. Easy peasy.

While I was in the hot seat being FTI'd, we caught a run to Main Street for a heroin overdose. It was mid-morning, and we were in the middle of a major weather event. It'd been snowing hard for the past twelve hours and there were ten inches of fresh powder on the ground. Engine companies were automatically dispatched on all EMS calls to help shovel a pathway for the ambulance crews to get their cots and equipment up to the doors.

Willy P and I arrived at the address just ahead of Engine 3. We trudged through the snow to the front door where a hysterical mother met us and led the way to the basement stairs. We all filed down the narrow, steep staircase and into a dimly lit room that opened up below. There was a mattress in the far corner of the basement floor with a three hundred pound, big-bearded man lying on his back, unconscious.

Willy P pulled open an eyelid and flashed his pen light back and forth while I checked for a pulse. His pupils were constricted and unresponsive to light, 15 beats per minute was the heart rate. He was breathing about four times a minute instead of the typical twelve to sixteen times. His mother advised he was a heroin addict, and judging by the needle still hanging from his arm, she was spot on with her assessment. Heroin, when overdosed, represses a person's respiratory drive and they become hypoxic, suffering from a lack of oxygen. If left untreated, they die.

We cracked our drug box and drew up the Narcan. Narcan counters the effects of the heroin and essentially cancels it out. It would wear off after a short while, though, so it was imperative to transport the patient to a hospital setting. We pushed it IM (intramuscular) into the guy's shoulder, and then tried to figure out how we were going to get him out to the ambulance. Willy P radioed the engine to shovel a path up the driveway and bring the cot around to the back door, as I dropped an oral airway (which he tolerated like a champ) and began to ventilate with a BVM (bag valve mask).

Rob "Dolph" Harrison was an enormous human being and was assigned to Engine 3 that day. He looked like Dolph Lundgren from *Rocky 4*. Remember Ivan Drago, the Russian guy (who was really a Swedish actor) that beat Sylvester Stallone to a pulp? Rob had the flat top hair and the guns to match. He suggested we use the blanket, taco the guy up in it, and four corner that bitch up the stairs, because there was no way we were getting a cot down there. We agreed and packaged the unconscious man for extraction. For all the pros out there, this was before the days of the Stair Chair—a device that supported the patient's weight when navigating stairways.

We hyperventilated the patient, knowing he'd be breathing on his own for a few minutes while we carried him, and with two guys at the head, and two guys at the feet, we hauled the man, wrapped in his own blanket, over to the base of the stairs. We paused to get a fresh grip on our corners and on the count of three, began our trek. It was tight. The steps were just wide enough for one average man to fit through. With two going up side by side, it was almost impossible to lift and climb.

About halfway up, Dolph went to lift, and his boot slipped off the step from all the snow and water we'd tracked in with us. His knee came crashing down on the corner edge of the stair. He howled in agony, and we had a man down. He was unable to continue the climb and required medical treatment himself. Willy P climbed over the patient and moved from the top spot to the bottom to replace Dolph. Now I had the entire top half of the blanket to myself.

I lifted so hard. One step at a time. Like this man's life depended on it. Because as far as I knew, it literally did. We got to the landing after an immense struggle and hoisted the patient onto the cot that was on the ground just outside the back door. We raised him up and rolled the loaded cot down the driveway to the ambulance, carefully staying in the path the engine company had cut through the snow. After hefting the man and the cot into the sled, I climbed in and began to reassess his vitals. I was soaked in my own sweat from the ordeal.

To my surprise, the Narcan had begun to take effect and cancel out the heroin. A sober man awoke, started gagging on the oral airway in his throat, wondering what had just happened, and where he was. I remember thinking that if we'd have just waited another five minutes in the basement, this dude could've walked himself out to the sled.

The paramedics always made it a point to explain to the overdosed patient just exactly *how* dead they were—right down to what degree of eternal damnation they'd just been saved from—hoping to guilt trip the patient into not shooting up heroin anymore. It never worked, but it was always fun to watch the various drug-shaming attempts anyway.

Dolph was being helped down the driveway, unable to walk on his own, as we pulled away in the ambulance. He'd fucked his knee all up. Torn a few ligaments, shredded some cartilage, and fractured his tibia. He was getting some paid time off for sure. This was my first heroin overdose, first major weather event on duty, and first line-of-duty injury I'd witnessed.

One of my earliest, first-in fires was out of Station 1. Lenny Smith was my officer and Don Babcock was the other firefighter on Engine 1. We'd discussed earlier in the shift that if we caught a fire, whoever's side of the truck it was on would pull the pre-connect hose. As we rolled up on the full alarm apartment fire, it was on Don's side, so he got to stretch line.

A two-story row of apartments ran along the left side of the parking lot for about two hundred feet. As Lenny gave his size up and Don pulled the dry hose line, I grabbed a set of irons (a flat-head axe and a Halligan bar), helped Don flake the kinks out, and together we advanced to the involved ground floor apartment. Fire was roaring out the open door and as we put our masks on and prepared for entry, the front picture window exploded, showering us in glass.

The hose line became rigid and Don opened the bale of the nozzle to let the air escape. When the water flowed, he sprayed the fire overhead and then made entry, swinging the fog nozzle in a circular pattern all over the living room. Lenny was in front of me, crouched low in the doorway with his hand on the back of Don's shoulder. Suddenly, Lenny stood straight up and fell backward into my arms, unconscious.

I caught him under his arms, and we fell over to our right. As I looked through his mask, his eyes were closed. I was yelling his name and shaking him, trying to wake him up. Then, just as fast as it happened, his eyes popped open, and he jumped back up and into position behind Don again. We pushed forward into the apartment and extinguished the fire.

Back outside, while getting a bottle change, I asked Lenny what the hell happened. He didn't even remember it. I noticed some silver metal slag on his shoulder and helmet, and we took a closer look. His ear was burned badly and blistered, and there was a puddle of cooled silver slag on his uniform shirt collar. Upon further inspection, his neck was burnt as well.

As best we could tell, when he was in the doorway leaning forward, the metal door frame had melted from the fire and dripped molten slag onto his ear and neck, causing him to pass out from the pain. To this day he doesn't remember fainting and tells me I'm just joshing him. Swear to God Lenny, if you're reading this, I will never forget your giant-ass falling on me.

Jughead and I were on Medic 11 and were called from the hospital to reports of a man who'd stabbed himself in the neck, jumped out of a moving vehicle, and was standing in the middle of a downtown intersection with a steak knife in his hand.

"Always an adventure," I said as we climbed into the sled and headed off.

En route we were advised by Spike Young, the captain on Engine 3, that one of us should hop in the back and get dressed in a Tyvek suit because there was, "a lot of blood."

Since Jughead was driving, I climbed in the back and began suiting up.

We pulled up at the scene, and I jumped out the back doors in my full-body exposure control suit to find Spike Young, who was rather short, talking to Demarius, who was a *fucking* GIANT, in the middle of the intersection. Demarius had a small steak knife in his right hand and was stabbing himself repeatedly in the chest saying he had demons in him, and they needed to get out.

He never even flinched as he sank the blade into his chest again, the handle bottoming out against his blood-soaked shirt, as he screamed "I need Jesus!"

"Hey, bro," I offered, "we all need Jesus." He looked down from the sky and fixed his gaze on me in my body condom.

"You!" he pointed at me, "Only you can help me. Nobody else!"

A collective sigh of relief ran through all the bystanders, cops, and firefighters as he pulled the steak knife from his chest and dropped it onto the ground. Jughead came around the ambulance with the cot and swung it into a chair. Demarius sat down and we laid him flat to load him into the meat wagon. It took three firefighters and two paramedics to lift this gigantic human being into position. I sat his head up and began to take his vitals while the other guys asked if I was all set.

Before I could answer, the doors slammed shut and I realized I was all alone with this man. He was so long his knees hung over the foot of the cot, and the middle of his torso was even with the top of the head of the cot. He was sitting on the floor and was taller than me sitting on the bench seat. As the ambulance pulled away, he looked at me again and explained how he needed Jesus because he had demons in him.

"And that's why you cut yourself?" I asked.

"Yes!" he replied. "I gotta get 'em out! They don't understand. I got demons in me!"

I could see three holes in his neck and at least four in his chest. One of the neck holes was whistling as he breathed and the skin around it moved like a balloon valve when one lets the air out. He'd cut his trachea with one of the knife wounds and was leaking air through his neck.

I asked if he'd let me put a bandage on the neck hole that was whistling at me.

He agreed. "Only you can take care of me, cuz you know we need Jesus!"

"You're goddamn right," I said, the irony of my words not lost on me as I placed a Vaseline gauze over the hole in his neck.

We were only a few blocks away from the ER now, so I explained I needed to call the hospital and let them know we were coming. He continued to yell about demons and Jesus, while I informed the triage nurse of our incoming very large, combative, psychotic patient.

As I ended the call and returned to patient care, I realized my new best friend had changed. He was more subdued (probably from shock) and the skin around his upper chest and neck had inflated, a lot. My man went from chiseled jock to a guy who now looked exactly like Eddie Murphy in *The Nutty Professor*. We called this subcutaneous emphysema, and basically, the pressurized air leaking from his lungs and trachea, couldn't exit through the open wounds anymore because of the seal created by the Vaseline-coated gauze, and was now traveling between his skin and tissues. We arrived and came to a stop in the hospital ambulance bay.

The look on Jughead's face was priceless when he opened the back doors to unload the patient, who no longer looked like the same patient he'd loaded up just a few minutes before.

"What? The man's got demons," I said as I pealed the gauze from the knife hole to release the air that was trapped between the layers of skin.

The folks at the hospital saved his ass; Demarius went on to star in college and was drafted into the NFL. He played at Miami, Minnesota, and Dallas for a time, until his demons finally caught up with him. This was my first of many times I treated an advanced patient as an EMT, acting above my level of EMS licensure.

On a rainy summer night, out of Station 1, Dolph and I responded to a diabetic emergency at one of the downtown high-rises. We loaded up the cot with our gear and walked toward the front door. To our left, about fifteen feet away, a TV smashed onto the pavement.

"Holy shit, it's raining TVs!" I yelled.

Dolph turned to me and said, "Five bucks says that's our guy."

As we stepped off the elevator on the eighth floor, we could hear more smashing and breaking of things and sure enough, Dolph was right. The man seemed surprised to see us as we entered his apartment and asked him how he was doing, if he was diabetic, and could we please check his blood sugar.

Half the items in his living room were either broken to pieces or had been thrown from his balcony window. He was covered in sweat, and Dolph calmed him down just enough to let us check his sugar. The glucometer read: 17. He wouldn't let us start an IV, so after some oral glucose and a few minutes of babysitting, he began to get his wits about him.

"Where's my TV?" he asked.

"In the parking lot," Dolph answered. "You threw it at us when we pulled up."

"I'm sorry," the old man offered.

"That's OK, I won five bucks because of it," Dolph said, winking at me.

The guy signed an AMA refusal for treatment after his blood sugar was at acceptable levels, and we witnessed him eat a PB&J sandwich I made for him in his kitchen while we waited. Then we hauled our equipment back down to the sled and drove off into the night.

On the way home, the streets were deserted. It was early morning and rain was cascading down in sheets. The radio was playing "Panama" by Van Halen. Dolph turned it up and started beating the steering wheel with his hands like a drum. Suddenly, Dolph stood on the brakes and cranked the wheel hard to the right. The ambulance rolled hard and hydroplaned sideways across the empty four-lane road. We slid in a complete 360, and as we spun back around to our original direction, Dolph slammed the throttle to the floor, and carried on down the road.

"You've gotta know what your rig can do, new kid!" he yelled over the music as I white knuckled the door handle and had my foot on the dash in a panic.

"Panama!" Dolph sang with the music, banging his head up and down.

Sometimes, our phone would ring on our day off with Operations calling. Operations was staffed by the officers at Station 1, and they did the scheduling for the whole department. If the phone call was between 06:30 and 07:30 hours, it was generally for a full shift of overtime. If it was outside of that time, it'd most likely be callback for a major incident, because someone went home sick, or for overtime the next day.

This time it was callback for a fire at one of the state office buildings downtown. It was a three-alarm cock knocker. I headed over to Station 8, hopped into a reserve engine, and headed to the scene. Upon arrival, we made our way over to staging. Our crew received an assignment to bring equipment, bottles, and tools up to the fourth floor of a six-story office building. Heavy gray smoke was rolling from the fifth-floor windows toward the west end of the building.

We loaded up as much as we could carry and entered the west stairwell. Hoses scaled the steps before us like intertwined snakes and it was precarious, weaving our way around obstacles and carrying heavy equipment. We arrived to find a flurry of activity on the fire floor. The fire had just been extinguished and crews were putting out hot spots and performing overhaul.

Matthew Hawk yelled, "Breaking glass!" Then he took his axe and smashed a ten-foot by ten-foot window to ventilate the smoke, raining glass five stories down below onto the courtyard.

He was probably the most prototypical bad-ass firefighter on our department. Handlebar mustache, fire academy instructor, and knew all the techniques to make a fire his little bitch.

Getting callback to fires means we're most likely going to be doing overhaul, putting out hot spots, or packing up hose. Which means we're probably cleaning up after the guys that just had all the fun. We stayed for hours, spreading tarps over furniture to protect it from water damage, emptying smoldering papers from filing cabinets and spraying them down, squeegeeing waves of water into the stairwells and out the door on the ground floor. It was a lovely waterfall of black, sooty water and tangled hose lines.

Willy P ended up slipping and falling down the stairs while trying to navigate descending the treacherous stairwell of spaghetti hose lines and cascading water. He ruptured multiple disks in his spine by landing on the base of his Scott Pak. This was the first of many callback fires for me, and the second line-of-duty injury I'd witnessed in just two months.

In the middle of the night, on Engine 3, we caught a run to Park Place for a woman who'd been hit by a train. The dispatch information was sketchy as the woman was near the tracks, midway between two city blocks. The road didn't really come close to the tracks in that area, so Park Place was our closest access point.

It was pouring rain and we were flagged down by a group of vagrants who'd found the woman. They explained she tried to kill herself by laying down across the tracks as a train approached. The train was long gone and most likely didn't even know about it. The woman was still conscious and missing her right leg just below the hip.

We applied a tourniquet and a trauma dressing as the medic crew from Station 1 arrived, backboarded the patient, and whisked her away to their sled. When the train rolled by, it cut her leg clean through the femur and sent her flying from the tracks. All the blood vessels shrank, closing off the bleeding and she survived. The medics tasked me with the job of locating the severed limb and packing it for transport, while they loaded the patient and started an IV.

Koz and I found her leg in the brush about thirty feet from where she'd been laying, and we wrapped it in a disposable blanket. There's something eerily sobering about walking down the train tracks at midnight, in the pouring rain, carrying a woman's severed leg in your arms. Adult human legs are much heavier than I thought they'd be. Just in case anyone ever has to.

I reunited the limb with its owner, then drove the ambulance the three blocks to the hospital while the medics were busy in the back. The surgeons were able to reattach her leg, but I'm pretty sure she walked away from the incident with a limp. Bad joke, I know. Sorry.

In October of my first year on the fire department, I was invited by Captain Chuck Sanders to the annual deer camp. This was a colossal camp attended by all the deer hunters on the department from both shifts. A few guys came that didn't even hunt, just to get away and enjoy the good times. It certainly wasn't for the trophy deer. The critters there were scrawny, more like dogs than deer. But at any rate, we all headed into the wilderness for a little guy time.

Camp was a conglomeration of large canvas military tents and campers. Some guys brought their own pup tents, but it was way too cold out for me. I slept on a cot in one of the canvas tents with a wood burning stove for warmth at night. The hunting was fine. I shot a doe my second day, and there were usually five or six out of the thirty or so guys there, who filled their tags each day.

In the evenings, tables were set up in the giant mess hall tent. Guys would bring their change jars from home and as the alcohol flowed, we began to play cards. The poker games alone were worth coming. Penny ante, all forms of poker. The dealer called the game and the rules. I learned an immense body of knowledge about playing poker from the old-timers there.

Lieutenant Carl Yankovic kept on saying great one-liners, like, "I'm in, I'd pay a quarter to see a monkey fuck," and other random stupid shit like that. All night and into the dawn, the men drank and played poker for spare change.

Around the campfire the second night there, I sank into an old, dirty couch we'd snagged from the roadside on the way into camp. Captain Dan Frank packed a hollowed-out deer antler pipe with weed and lit it up, passing it around the circle of men watching the flames. I declined and passed the antler when it came around to me and the proverbial turntable arm scratched the record, as everything around us suddenly ground to a halt. Dan was drunk as fuck and made a huge deal out of me not hitting the pipe.

"Hoooze yer captain new kid?" he slurred.

"Chuck Sanders," I replied.

He began yelling for Chuck, and when he found him, explained how I was such a vile, insolent, and ungrateful new kid, that I'd refused to hit the antler—the symbol of peace and fraternity that bound our clan of kinsmen together. Chuck smiled and winked at me, giving me the green light, and assuring me what happens on the island, stays there. For the sake of fraternity, harmony, and to restore the natural order of things, I took a pull.

I mentioned the young man with his skull cut clean through. Let's talk about that next. Sometimes, the engines roll along with the medics on what's known as an ambulance assist. Usually, it's for any situation where things could get crazy, and an extra set of hands could mean the difference between life or death. Or if a fire could occur, as in the case of a car accident.

When I roved out to old Station 6 for a shift, I had a crazy one of those calls that night. It was this poor kid's Happy 18th birthday/death day, and I was on Engine 61 with Lt. Spike Young and Engineer Stan Clemens. The thing I remember most about that one was pulling up to the scene in an open cab fire truck.

The old red bubble lights were illuminating the snowflakes that fell across the night sky backdrop. It was like fireworks going off all around me. Standing up and looking over the front of the cab roof as we sped through the darkness, I felt lucky to be one of the few in the world to experience this. The brisk winter air pierced my eyes and pulled me from my reflections as we rounded the bend on Seaway, a winding neighborhood street in the southwest corner of town.

Moments earlier, I'd been sound asleep in my bed when the alarm came in for a car versus tree. I sat up in bed, swung my feet into my bunker pants, slid the pole, and climbed onto the fire truck. The engine beside me roared to life as we sped away into the night.

We slowed to a crawl as we turned the corner on Seaway and the truck began to roll over large chunks of concrete that littered the entire width of the roadway. As we bounced farther along, I saw a tall light post made from concrete lying on the ground, partially blocking the road. We veered to miss the pole and came to a stop in the middle of a wide cul-de-sac.

The headlights of our rig were fixed on a white sedan, fitted squarely into a massive ten-foot diameter willow tree in the front yard of a house. I snagged my helmet from the engine cowling and stepped down from the truck. After grabbing the EMS bag, I joined Young Dawg at the front of the truck.

He told me to check the car for patients and he'd be looking for survivors in the yard since the passenger door was left open. I approached the car from the driver's side and switched on the Streamlight that was hooked to the chest pocket of my turnout coat.

Walking closer I could see a full, blood-red handprint against the white driver's side door. My hand gripped the Streamlight handle and directed its beam through the shadows and onto the driver. There was a body lying slumped down in the driver's seat, leaning slightly against the door. My light shone brightly across his head. It was cleanly sliced open by the section of concrete light post he'd driven through, and he'd taken a direct hit to the face—right about even with the eyes—cut straight back. The top of his skull was missing.

His brain was completely exposed, in what resembled to me, a bowl, made up of the bottom half of his skull. He didn't move and neither did I. The sweet smell of beer and blood seduced my senses for the first time ever and I was stunned. Caught in the immense gravitational pull of the moment, my mind struggled to recognize and comprehend exactly what was in front of me. I froze, locked in time. Who knows how long I was there? I don't.

Young Dawg reached over and shut my light off. "Don't look at that" he ordered, snapping me back to reality. "Did you see the handprint? We have another patient somewhere."

I reached over top of the young man and put the car in park. Then I removed the keys from the ignition and threw them onto the passenger seat.

We began to knock on the doors of the neighboring houses, asking if they'd seen anyone, when Clemmy yelled from a nearby porch, "Hey, over here!"

We discovered a teenage girl and boy in the house, and both appeared to be unhurt, though they admitted being drunk. I took their vitals as we waited for the ambulance to arrive. Young Dawg gave the incoming sled an update over the radio. Moments later, the medic unit rolled up out front and we walked the patients out.

Firefighter/Paramedic Bruce Owens (later assistant chief of the entire department) not so gingerly informed the intoxicated minors of the true nature of the sticky bits they were flicking onto his ambulance floor. They wailed as Bruce slapped them hard with his sober stick. It was their friend's 18th birthday, and they explained he'd been drunk and doing about 75 miles per hour through the neighborhood when he hit the curve, the pole, and then the tree.

The teens caught a ride to the hospital in the ambulance, the birthday boy got a ride in the coroner's van, and I rolled home in my open cab fire truck. The warmth of the engine cowling drifted through my turnout coat while the droning vibrations of the motor beside me numbed my mind as it wrestled with the tragedy I'd just witnessed.

Those are just a few of the highlights from my first year on the job. It was a crazy time filled with sublime moments of losing my innocence and learning how the firefighting game was played. I was a rookie and saw more shit in that first year than I could have possibly fathomed. There's simply no way to adequately prepare someone for what I'd experienced in that first year. I needed a completely different skill set to survive the onslaught of emergency chaos. The mold of the character type who always does the right thing in every circumstance was broken. I was naïve to the way the real world worked, and it was glaringly and painfully obvious to everyone. Monumental changes were inevitably forthcoming.

Chapter 4

Station Life

At one point I calculated it out. Over the course of a twenty-five-year career, at roughly ten days a month on duty, when all's said and done at retirement eligibility age, a career firefighter will have spent roughly eight continuous years of their life in a fire station. That was eight years away from my family, away from nights in bed with my wife, away from school events and tucking my kids into bed. It was like a mandatory eight-year prison sentence I'd voluntarily agreed to for the financial security of my family.

It didn't always feel like a jail sentence, though. There were times of pride and joy, of helping people and making a difference in their lives. But there's a lot of crazy shit that goes on that nobody on the outside those big garage doors really knows about or understands.

There's a delicate balance of social skills and administrative hierarchy that demands precise timing and intricate coordination of speech, intonation, and emotional engagement. If one is to survive and flourish in the firehouse environment, they must thicken their skin, remain vigilant, and always beware of both predator and prey alike. What follows is my best attempt at explaining the sanctum sanctorum of the fire service. That holy of holies one may have seen on a tour of the joint but could never experience its true nature until they've passed through the rites of initiation and been welcomed into the fold of the family.

If we were assigned to an engine or a ladder company at our department, typically only about 10 percent of our on-duty time was spent on fire scenes. The other 90 percent was spent either on EMS calls, at the station, the garage, the grocery store, PR gigs, or training evolutions. If we were an ambulance jockey or a pecker checker for the shift, we were gone with the wind all day. Lucky—if by the grace of the run gods—we made it back to the firehouse for meals, to watch the big game, or catch a few hours of sleep. If an engine or medic crew happened to have a light day, it was never mentioned or talked about until shift change the following morning for fear of jinxing the whole damn thing.

Shift change was a flurry of activity, with twice the normal amount of people milling around the station, sipping coffee, bitching about things, spreading rumors, and making wise cracks. It happened every day between 6:30 and 7:30 am. The hour-long shift change allowed for adjustments to be made, and in case someone called in sick or had to act up a rank at another station, it offered some leeway for drive times and re-racking of the running chart.

Upon arrival, I'd check the board near the station entrance to see my spot on the rig for the day. If I was roving to another station, my name was written at the bottom. Next, I removed the gear of the person from the previous shift who was in my assigned seat on the rig. Then I placed their gear neatly in their locker, or if they were a rover, on the floor in a neat pile behind the truck. Then it was time to check my equipment. Chance favors the prepared mind.

I turned on my SCBA and confirmed the tank's pressure was sufficiently full. Then I closed the valve and slowly bled the regulator to verify the low-pressure alarm engaged. When the line was empty, I made sure the motion sensor began to chirp and engaged after thirty seconds of inactivity on the SCBA. This would alert the RIT (Rapid Intervention Team) crew to my location if I was unconscious in a fire.

Once the Scott Pak was inspected, I clicked my mask into the regulator and placed the rest of my gear in its proper places. My helmet hung on the hook near my seat. Two Incident Command passport accountability tags with my name and number were placed on the officer's helmet with my rig identifier. My turnout coat hung on the grab bar outside my door with my Nomex hood either draped over the collar or over my bunker pants and boots at the floor, near my door.

Next, I attached the radio and Streamlight I'd removed from the previous firefighter's gear and checked the battery levels in both, switching them out if needed. I checked the EMS blue bag for an oxygen tank psi level, and the AED (automated external defibrillator) for a functional battery level. Then I walked around the truck and confirmed the location of all the tools in every compartment. So that I wouldn't have to run around looking for shit while someone was in the process of dying later that day.

I told the engineer when I saw them, what the EMS O_2 levels were, and that the battery levels in my radio, Streamlight, and AED were ready to rock. Then and only then, could I get coffee from the kitchen. If it wasn't made yet, I made two pots for the incoming crews.

As I carried that cup of coffee from the kitchen to the dining room table, I'd better not *dare* sit down in the captain's seat. His was the closest to the phone—always—at every station in the city. Engineers sat at the next closest seat, and the firefighters sat the farthest from the phones, opposite from the officers.

This made for some exciting phone races between the new kids, who were expected to answer it on the first ring. Sometimes an engineer or officer would be standing right next to the phone and would wait until the sprinting new kids were almost there, before picking up the receiver and saying, "Station 4, should've been Firefighter Lilly."

I'd meet up with the person I'd just relieved before they left the station for the day, and they'd relay any pertinent information from the previous shift. Things like missing or damaged equipment, food supplies that were running low, or crazy calls and juicy gossip that developed over the past twenty-four hours were usually the headliners for the day.

At 07:30 hours, the new kids would grab the flag and raise it up the pole. Then the entire station would dive headlong into the daily chores, cleaning the toilets and sinks, making the beds, mopping the floors, doing the laundry, checking the trucks and equipment, and filling out the employee attendance records so everyone got paid.

If we were on the ambulance for the shift, we went straight to our rig and began the daily inventory and cleaning procedures for the sleds. When we were done, we checked in with the Floor Boss, or the senior engineer, and asked if they needed help with anything. Only after everyone's chores were finished would the crews meet back in the kitchen for breakfast.

As a new kid, it was expected we'd be the first person up when there was work to be done, and the last to sit down after it was finished. If we were downtown at Station 1, there'd be a call over the PA system, after the previous shift had exited the belowground parking ramp, for "cars in the basement." All the incoming shifts would then move their personal cars from the front apron down to the basement parking ramp. Ones was an enormous quad company with a battalion chief, ladder truck, engine, two sleds, and two ATV jump rigs—one brush truck with a boat and an ATV for the river trails and concerts in the parks.

Some of the smaller substations (the single and double companies) played poker in the mornings for dishes. One of my captains, Matt Mardigan, once wrote in my probationary blue book how I was bad at poker and good at the dishes. That was always fun. Sort of like skipping school and getting away with it. While the rest of the city was checking their rigs and performing station duties, we were gambling for the post-dinner chores.

Every station had its own list of specialty chores in addition to the dailies. Universally, department wide, Monday was rig day. Off-site training on Mondays was kept to a minimum to help facilitate a thorough cleaning and check of our assigned vehicle. If the captain was a jerk, we might be scrubbing the rig's undercarriage with toothbrushes, or polishing ladder rungs, or any number of mindless acts of tediousness to make our thirty-year-old firetruck showroom quality again. We could always count on, at the very least, a wash, vacuum, and inventory of our rig every Monday, guaranteed.

The other daily duties varied by station, with typical chores like dormitory and bathroom deep cleaning on Tuesdays. Wednesday was kitchen day, when we threw out all the leftovers that were too hideous and awful to be eaten as midnight snacks, wiped down the fridge and cupboards (inside and out), and completely disassembled the stove tops to get every kernel of rice, popcorn, and burned pasta noodle properly disposed of.

Thursday was lawn day, and there were some seriously big-ass lawns we had to push mow; I'm talking acres here. Friday was window cleaning day or EMS room inventory day. Saturday was apparatus floor day—when we scrubbed the oil leaks from the garage floors and flushed out the floor drains that smelled like a backed up septic tank. On Sunday there were no extra chores for religious reasons. That was our free day to sit back and reflect upon the benevolent mercy of the fire gods and how they'd blessed us with no chores.

The daily lineup of personnel across the department was produced by the poor cats up in Operations. Poor because they didn't get paid anything extra for their efforts. Just the personal satisfaction of knowing they were the central information hub of the department, and had the power to assign the fates and destinies of staffing, training, and public relations events.

All information filtered through them first and foremost. If somebody called in sick to their home station, the captain called Ops for a replacement. If there was a school scheduled for the day, Ops made the list of attendees. Between three and six officers ran the phones at shift change in Ops, and it got pretty crazy at times.

Firefighter Christina Robertson (aka "C-Rob" and later Assistant Chief Robertson) called up Operations one morning and, believing she was talking to her confidential lover, Lieutenant Mark Taylor, proceeded to explain how he'd really stretched her out last night with his big fat kielbasa. The thing was, she was talking to BJ, not Mark Taylor.

BJ put her on speakerphone over the station PA, right at shift change, then continued to play along and coax more intimate details from C-Rob, asking, "What was your favorite part?" and "Tell me how that felt." Then he explained to a confused C-Rob that he wasn't sure she was talking to the right person, and he'd go ahead and put Mark on the line now.

"Mark, it's for you," BJ yelled. "It's your girlfriend." Then he proceeded to call up every station in town and tell them C-Rob's new name was "Stretch" and here's why.

Located at Station 1, Ops was a hub of activity in the early morning hours of shift change. Most of the smart officers did their mandatory time there, and then got as far away from Ones as they could. With five rigs stationed there, including two ambulances, the lights hardly ever shut off. It was like a disco dance floor with the strobe lights directly over our beds.

Each time an alarm came in, every light in the station turned on, a shrill tone sounded, the dispatcher called out the rigs that were going, gave an address, and a brief description of the situation. Then, after about thirty seconds, the lights would turn back off. It's damn near impossible to sleep when that happened every couple of minutes. It was like Chinese water torture or nails on a chalkboard after a few hours of trying to sleep through it all.

Ops was also the home of the BDD (back-door deal). If someone needed something to happen in their favor, they greased the palms of the guys in Ops. They had access to the chiefs, controlled the vacation and personal leave days, created the schedules, handled the payroll distribution, made the overtime and callback calls, and generally ran the whole she-bang. Need a tip on the check pool poker hand? Call Ops. Need a good square in the Super Bowl pool, or that first pick in the Fantasy Football draft? Call the boys in Ops. Want a better station assignment, or that pesky, annoying firefighter transferred? A favor for a favor—that's just how it went.

There was an old, mentally challenged, civilian named Tommy Tumenello who showed up downtown every afternoon and stayed through dinner. He'd done more time in the station than any of the captains and had been coming to Station 1 since before they were all new kids. He mumbled when he talked and gave the new kids a hard time, much to the chagrin of the station officers. He sat at the table next to the captains and battalion chiefs every day and ate dinner with us. After supper, the BC would drive him home just a few blocks away.

As time passed and Tommy grew older, his personal hygiene began to lapse, and his odor became offensive to the men in Ops. They hatched a plan to offer ambulance hours to any of the firefighters stationed at Ones if they would take Tommy to the dormitory showers and use a mop bucket and rig brush to clean him. The plan worked for a while and no one was the wiser, as the secret was kept in house. And for a twelve-hour reprieve from pecker-checking, new kids were all too eager to trade ten minutes of hell scrubbing a fat, naked old man with a truck brush.

Tommy didn't mind either since he got a free bath, had pretty young ladies (and men) washing his balls for the first time in his life, and could thoroughly embarrass and humiliate the new kids with lewd comments and gestures. As with all good things, this was not to last. Some of the senior firefighters noticed they were riding the bone box more often than their colleagues from Ones. Questions were asked, inquiries were made, and loose lips sank ships.

Bruce Allen was the first rover to get the full scoop from Eric Fisher and then relayed the details of the BDD to his officer Hector Garcia, the captain of Station 2. Garcia was a massive Mexican American who commanded respect everywhere he went. He was from the north side of town and knew every gangster, drug dealer, hooker, loan shark, heavy, and purveyor of all things criminal, from Canada to Mexico and they all feared and respected him. He called up the boys in Ops and had them spilling their guts and begging for forgiveness with just a few choice phrases. That was the end of the ambulance-hours-for-Tommy back door deal.

Hector taught me a lot about the seedy underbelly of the fire service. He introduced me to the players there. Advising who was OK to confide in and who the prudes, narcs, and snitches were. He taught me how to manipulate the system to my advantage. How blackmail worked in the fire department. How one should always party with the battalion chiefs because we'd get dirt on them, and sooner or later we'd need them to go to bat for us. "Have a BC in your back pocket," was the exact phrase. Nobody fucked with Hector. He was a god.

There were other stations that had their own drop-in civilians, like Tommy, who showed up on the daily. Station 3 had a postal worker named Russ, who'd stop in on his mail route and eat his lunch with us. Then he'd slide over to the brown chairs and crank out a short cat nap until it was time to get back to work and finish his route.

There was Ryan Nellis, a police officer that showed up at either Station 3 or Station 5 every day and hung out with the crews until mid-afternoon. He'd talk about union politics, crazy calls, and generally just shot the shit until a call came in and he, or we, or both of us had to go. Sometimes he too ended up snoozing in the brown chairs for a while.

He caught the ol' oxygen tubing in the urinal ports prank one day and didn't come back for a while after that. We heard he'd joined the undercover team at the local PD and couldn't have the same acquaintances he'd known in the past anymore. Not as long as he was undercover on the narcotics team.

Station 8 had an old, retired firefighter named Joe Palatinski. Every Saturday, Joe would show up and sit at the breakfast table with us, sipping coffee. Then at 07:30 he'd help with the apparatus floor cleaning duties. Apparently, it was one of his favorite chores when he was active duty, and he still enjoyed coming in and helping the boys, even at eighty years of age.

With the new kids expected to answer phones within the first ring, epic races were incurred between two probies battling it out for phone supremacy. One day at old Station 6, Chris "Pants" Meyer—we called him "Meyer, Meyer Pants on Fire" or just "Pants," because he always had to one-up everyone's story—and I were studying streets in the brown chairs when the Signal 1 rang. We both jumped up and sprinted to the dining room phone.

I arrived first and snagged it. "Station 6, Lil—"

Pants body checked me across the room and as I flew through the air, the phone cord snapped clean in two and I landed in a heap in the corner, with the receiver still in my hand. We laughed and argued over who'd really *beat* who, as the captain answered the incoming call at the front desk.

The lowest seniority person stationed at each firehouse was also expected to cook the meals. Which resulted in some god-awful culinary disasters. Having a new kid, who's extensive body of culinary knowledge included only hot dogs and mac n' cheese, or a frozen pizza and tater tots, was not who we wanted at the helm of the firehouse kitchen. The old-timers knew this and were like crocodiles waiting in the reeds. Ready to devour a young probie for their terrible cuisine.

Each day, after the morning chores were done, the crew met to break bread at the breakfast table, and the meals for the day were planned. Newspaper ads were consulted, sales were considered, and mess money was collected. Then the cook's rig would roll to the grocery store.

We were in service by radio and did our grocery shopping while on duty. We parked in the supermarket's fire lane because it was quicker to get back to our truck if we caught a run, than if we'd parked at the next available space from the door that could fit a fire truck, which was usually across the entire parking lot.

When irate citizens would approach us in the store and ask why we'd parked in the fire lane simply for mere grocery shopping, Lieutenant Benny O'Brien would ask them to take a deep breath and hold it. Then he'd make a pretend phone call to the 9-1-1 dispatcher and request a response for a person choking. As he walked in circles around the citizen, pretending to go to his fire truck, they'd usually run out of breath, and he would have clearly made his point.

If we did catch a run while grocery shopping, we ran our cart to the front of the store and left it with a cashier. The store manager would make sure it was put in the cooler, until we returned from our run. Sometimes this happened two, or even three times, while we were attempting to get groceries, so speed and efficiency at the supermarket was important.

We had to make a list of ingredients and grab everything in a strategic pattern throughout the store. Don't roll down the same aisle multiple times. Know the products and where they're located so we could efficiently plan the route and minimize our time there. This was highly technical stuff for the new kid to comprehend. We had to act professional—like we knew what we were doing—even though we didn't have a clue.

Back at the station we unloaded the groceries from the cab, or from whatever tool compartments they were shoved into, or from up on top of the pumper with the deck gun and booster reel. Then we began the food prep. At the double company stations there were always plenty of hands on deck to help cook and plenty of money to shop with. However, at the single companies, it was usually just me—cooking for two other people—who all had better things to do. Making two full meals on $21 can be difficult, so we had to be frugal.

To make things even harder, some of that money went to the station half bill and contingent funds. The half bill bought the staples like rice, sugar, saltines, cereal, and other things crews used the most each day. It was usually managed by a senior member of the crew that was stationed there most often. The contingent paid for the firehouse creature comforts—things like the newspaper delivery, cable TV, and the personal phone line. This was usually handled by the same poor schmuck as the half bill.

God forbid some idiot called a few 900 numbers (which happened) or ordered either porn or the big fight on Pay-per-view (which happened) and failed to pay up for their actions. It wasn't hard to find out whodunit—there were only so many people stationed there that day. So that $21 we thought we had to buy groceries with was now $18 after the bills were paid. And if Mean Dean threw a pack of chicken tits and a bottle of Zesty Italian in the shopping cart, our budget was royally fucked. The old-timers would tell me: don't even think about short-changing the whole station by not paying the half bill and contingent because my dumb ass went over on the mess and didn't have enough money to cover the overage. I'd better put those dollar bills in the lock box and sign the deposit register *before* we left for the grocery store, or I'd be getting a call from the half bill manager later on, doubling as a heavy. Shaking me down for two dollars like the obsessed paperboy in the movie *Better Off Dead*.

After the meal, the whole crew pitched in to help clean the kitchen. Except for the cook. They'd just busted their tail preparing the meal and were expressly forbidden from stepping one foot in the kitchen during the clean-up process. The officers did the dishes: one washing, one rinsing. Unless they'd lost the morning poker game; then it was just them in the suds.

The washer was required to get at least 90 percent of the food off and the rinser was expected to get the rest. Engineers packed up the leftovers in the refrigerator and fed the dishwashers with the scraped dirty plates, pots, and pans. Glasses were washed first, then flatware, followed by utensils and, finally, the cookware. There was a method to the madness.

Sometimes as a prank they'd recycle dishes back around to the dirty pile to see how long it would take for the bosses to notice. Three times through was about the industry average before they'd get wise to the fact they'd repeatedly washed the same spoon or pan. New kids had to grab a broom and dustpan to sweep the kitchen and dining areas. Then a bucket and mop to finish the job. Probies emptied the trash and took it out to the dumpster. It was a symphony of cleaning coordination with a finely tuned hierarchy.

Next, there was a school or some sort of training on the docket for the shift. If Ops hadn't called in the morning and assigned us a class or PR gig to attend, then it was left up to the station captain to determine the subject matter of the day's tutelage. Often, it was passed to the engineer, and the captain would go sleep off his hangover from the night before. Sometimes, the engineer was hungover, too, and would leave the training task to the senior firefighter.

The most convenient and frequent in-house training to do was street school. It's kind of important to know where we're going in a hurry, so we can get there faster. As a new kid, we were expected to use any available down time by studying our map book. It wasn't uncommon to find an exhausted rookie lying face down, asleep on his map book at the dinner table.

In every station, there were ancient Sanka coffee cans filled with tiny cut pieces of paper with local street names printed on them. The old-timers would pull out dozens of them and quiz the probies, adding chores as consequences if we failed to know the location or how to get there within a specified time frame, say, fifteen to twenty seconds to respond.

Street school was important for other reasons. Occasionally, Dispatch would throw us a curve ball, like sending us to a street called Westbury. One had to be aware there were, in our city, a Westbury, an Eastbury, a West Berry, and an East Berry. Hundred blocks or address numbers were crucial in determining exactly what the dispatcher had just said. Westbury went from 2900 to 1300, while West Berry was 1100 to 100, then East Berry picked up at 100 to 1200.

In our city, the hundred blocks spread out from the exact center of town, on an x and y axis much like a graph in algebra. If we were heading away from the center, in any direction, the address numbers would climb higher, with the even numbers on our right side and the odd on our left. If we were heading toward the middle of town, it was precisely the opposite.

This information was crucial in determining the fastest route to our destination. Other factors played into the route decision as well, like time of day, train crossings, number of stop lights, construction, and traffic flow. Certain neighborhoods had cut-throughs and back doors that people who weren't from our city knew nothing about. It was critical to beating other stations into their own areas to know about these time savers.

This was all before GPS and navigation systems were installed in the rigs, and smartphones were still years off. Sometimes we had to make a call to Dispatch for clarification before rushing out to the wrong part of town. Every city has their own little idiosyncrasies and it paid to put time into studying our maps and hundred block splits, so we could find the backdoor routes and beat everyone there. All the glory on the fireground goes to the first due companies.

Captain Larry Simmons had some of the hairiest eyebrows I've ever seen on a human being. Like Billy Crystal's character in *The Princess Bride*. As the black shift captain of Station 3, he tried to teach me his street school methods early on in my career and had a peculiar way of remembering them. He said to group them together in threes and repeat them over and over all day for one shift.

Then he demonstrated: "Madison, Kenwood, Rose… Madison, Kenwood, Rose." He must have said it a dozen times. Then every time he saw me for a month afterward, he'd say Madison, Kenwood, Rose. Not hi Brad, or good morning. I honestly think those were the only three streets he knew. It worked, though; I still know exactly where those three streets are.

Prior to the invention of the PA system, we used alarm bells to tell the station crew something needed to be done. The first group of dings was the station personnel by seniority, with the captain as one ding, lieutenant as two dings, and so on. The second set of dings was the task they needed to do: Signals 1, 2, 3, 4, and 5. Things could get pretty dingy if the number nine seniority firefighter had a signal four. The PA system helped eliminate the confusing ringy ding dings.

Now, we just called a name and a number. Signal one was the official department business phone line. Signal 2 was the personal phone line. Signal 3 was a holdover from the earlier days on our department and no one alive could even remember what it once had been. Signal 4 meant we had a visitor and needed to report to a designated area. Signal 5 meant a civilian was in the station and so we needed to mind our language and behavior.

When a BC arrived at the station, it was the lowest seniority person's responsibility to greet them and offer to help with anything they needed. Sometimes they had equipment to drop off from maintenance, mail, subpoenas, retirement helmets to sign, full Scott bottles to replace our empty ones, or any number of tasks beneath their pay grade.

It was also the lowest seniority person's job to handle tours of the stations. Sometimes school groups or civilians would request a tour and it was customary for the new kid to act as their guide. We'd get on the PA and advise the crews of a Signal 5. Then call Dispatch and have them put out test tones for the station, so folks would know what an alarm sounded like and what to do if one came in during the tour.

Points of interest included the living quarters, fire trucks, ambulances, turning the emergency lights on, showing the tools and turnout gear, dormitories, and sliding the fire poles. We'd answer any questions they had, round up the kiddies, hand them a plastic fire helmet and a sticker, and send them on their merry way.

We'd do public relations events almost daily, to stay involved and relevant in the community. Ops would call the station in the morning and say, "The mayor needs you for a press conference here," or "The chief wants you to pass out food at the rescue mission," or "The medic needs to do a standby at the local varsity football game," or "They're taking donations for hurricane victims here and we need you to help." Always with the media outlets taking pics for press releases and positive PR. They were generally a pain in the ass; however, some were quite entertaining to attend and occasionally for a worthy cause.

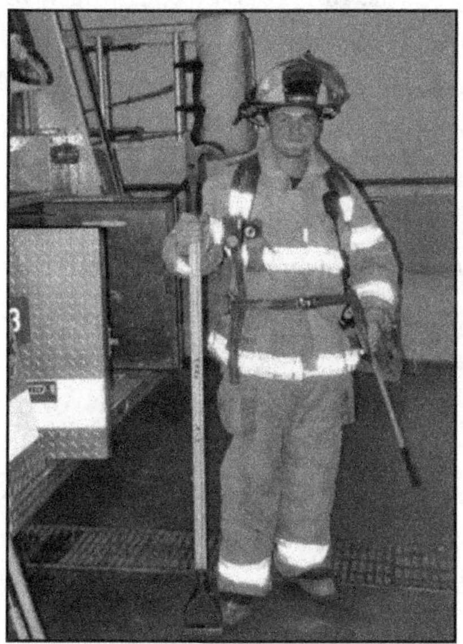

The author during a station tour at Eights

The best gigs were the summer festivals and concerts in the parks. We had two really big ones that drew in thousands of people: Riverfest, where there were things like Bluesfest and the Chili Cook-Off; and Summer Soundfest where they brought in dozens of popular bands and music groups over seven days. Both were held kitty-corner from Station 1, so we could bring our family down and watch from the roof of the fire station for free.

Being on duty, we'd staff an ATV and cruise the park during the concerts, posing for photo ops and mingling with the crowds. Occasionally, there'd be a medical emergency and we'd zip in, grab the patient, and dip out to a waiting ambulance. The best event staffing was backstage, though. We got all access passes to some of the hottest entertainment in the country.

The local minor league baseball team was directly across the river from Station 1. Every home game, there were fireworks that popped off at precisely 20:00 hours. Our city garage and fuel pumps were located just past the outfield where they shot them off, so we sent a couple of rigs over each night to standby in case any embers touched down near the pumps.

Once a year we'd participate in the MDA fill the boot campaign, helping to raise money for muscular dystrophy. Fire trucks would post up at the grocery stores, movie theaters or busy intersections and civilians would drop coins or bills into the old firefighting boots we'd hold out. Hence, "Fill the Boot." We'd get to see and meet some great people, and these were generally good times. As good as panhandling can be anyway.

There were 5K run/walks at the Riverfront and Swan Island parks, where one could meet and fraternize with the event staff and participants. The Insane Inflatables, Mud Runs, and Chalk Walks were always my favorites. Hearty participants would race through inflatable obstacle courses, crawl through mud pits, or get blasted by colorful chalk tossed at them, and they'd wind up looking like otherworldly creatures covered in goo.

In late Spring, during Fire Prevention Week, the whole department would travel to the elementary and middle schools in their first due areas and give school presentations. I remembered this from my days as a young child growing up in the city and was excited to carry on the tradition. The kids absolutely loved it and we tried to make it fun and informative.

We'd park our rigs, usually a ladder truck and an engine, outside the auditoriums or gymnasiums. The lowest seniority guys would dress in full turnouts and grab various hand tools for the show and tell. We'd meet with the principal and be ushered in, either to the stage or front of the gym, while classrooms poured in, one after another, single file, and took a seat.

We'd go over different types of emergencies, help them know how to talk to dispatchers on the phone and give their names and addresses. We'd talk about how lighters and matches are tools, not toys. We'd talk about smoke detectors and changing the batteries in them like their toys at home need battery changes. We'd talk about stop, drop, and roll if their clothing caught on fire. We talked about how the bad air in a fire is up high and the good, breathable air is down low to the ground so they could crawl under the smoke to safely escape a structure fire.

We'd emphasize the importance of knowing two ways out of their house in case one was blocked by smoke and fire. How they shouldn't hide in closets or under beds, that we'd be coming in to rescue them, and they needed to make a lot of noise to let us know where they were.

They loved this next part. "You all know how to be loud, right?" I'd ask. "On the count of three, I want you to yell for help as loud as you can. Ready. One. Two. Three."

They'd all scream, and the teachers would cover their ears. Of course, it wasn't loud enough for me.

"That's OK, but I think you can do better. Guys, what do you think?" The other firefighters would wave their outstretched hands in the universal language for pump up the volume and get louder. "I think you can do better. Everybody on three. Ready? One. Two. Three!" The earth would shake, and everyone was really into it now.

"All right, all right, you guys got it! That's what I need to hear when we come in to save you. It's important to make an escape plan and practice it. Have a parent hold the smoke detector test button down at random times and practice what you would do. You need to have a meeting place, so everyone knows who's out and who's trapped when the fire department shows up. It's important to have a plan."

Kids that age have about a five-minute attention span, so don't just sit there and ramble. Get up and get the blood flowing with some excitement. We'd invite everyone out to our fire trucks to see the equipment, hands-on. We'd let them hold fire axes and explain the difference between the flat heads and the pick heads. They'd hold pike poles and nozzles, and sometimes we'd flow water from the deck guns or hoses. They'd sit in the trucks and try on our gear. They were heroes for a day.

There were occasionally some pretty teachers that would make googly eyes at us. Sometimes we'd pass numbers and notes, like we were kids in class once again. No shit, I had one teacher at an elementary school, smokin' hot, give me her number. On the note it said her name was Miss Frisky, swear to God. I even confirmed it with one of her students to make sure it was real. I looked back at her, and she just smiled and winked as she walked away with her class. I loved school presentations.

There were some amazing places we toured and had access to that no ordinary civilian could go. The National Guard headquarters and armory were some of my personal faves. We'd tour these places to know the proper entry procedures and where they kept the really bad stuff. Munitions stockpiles, radioactive equipment, and such.

One day, my crew of Chuck Sanders and Carl Yankovic,

toured the State Capital Building with the Property Manager, who escorted us to the pinnacle up on top of the dome. We could see for fifty miles in every direction. There was an old logbook up there with signatures of every soul who'd been up there since it was built. Governors, mayors, dignitaries, and us.

The company that made the Anthrax vaccine for our soldiers was in town and they had live cultures for testing purposes. We'd take annual tours at the facility and ones like it, to know how to respond within proper protocols and not make the situation potentially worse than it already was. We were allowed everywhere and had keys to the city.

On paydays, the battalion chiefs collected the employee's paychecks, sealed in envelopes, and delivered them to the stations. Before direct deposit, we received actual paper paychecks. At the payday breakfast table, the crews on duty would bet on what their check numbers would be. The best poker hand would take the pot. This was called the check pool.

Sometimes a guy would have a friend in Ops call him up and tip him off to a great check pool number. A pair, or trips of a number, maybe a straight, or even four of a kind. The guy would get so excited he'd want everyone to bet $10 on the game. We'd all fold until the bet was a more manageable $1 or so. That would still cover our mess money for the day if we won.

Then the BC would drop off the checks and the winner would get the check pool money. Off duty firefighters would often call up to the station to ask if the checks had been delivered yet. Some of the wives would be up at the station waiting for the BC's red car to pull up. The poor guy wouldn't even get to see his own paycheck and his ol' lady would be out the door with it and off to the bank.

Dinner was to be served promptly at 17:00 hours, and after the cleaning rituals were completed, we were on our own time. We could relax in the brown chairs, watch some TV, work on a personal project, or grab a workout. So long as there weren't any night evolution training activities of course, which always sucked, and everyone was less than enthused for.

There's a phenomenon that occurs as the sun goes down at fire stations across the nation. Most call it affectionately, *Pong*. The old-timers would religiously meet at the table, from after dinner until bedtime. The entire station would often get in on the action and doubles tournaments would pop off for bragging rights. Some of those crazy old-timers would pull out a freakin' cast iron skillet from the kitchen, use it as a paddle, and absolutely destroy a new kid on the table with it. It was *Pong-Life*, and some firefighters lived it to the fullest. It was always a fun team building exercise and a welcome respite from the trauma and chaos going on in the streets.

In the evenings at dusk, we'd lower the flag and either fold or hang it up for the night. If we ever forgot the flag, someone would eventually call on the Signal 1 in a high-pitched voice like a Muppet, claiming to be the flag, and whining about how cold, and dark, and lonely it was out there on the pole, and could we please come take it down.

The lowest seniority person made sure the kitchen was cleaned, the trash was emptied, and all the doors were closed and locked before heading off to bed for the night. One time we found a bum sleeping in the mechanical room at Station 6. When he was discovered and promptly evicted from his new home, he revealed he'd been there for five days and was using the showers and bathrooms at night and eating the food from the kitchen when the rigs would roll out on alarms. It was important to make a thorough sweep of the station at night to ensure things were locked down and secured properly.

The lowest seniority firefighter would also be assigned to night watch. In a closet near the front door of every fire house in town was an old fold-out bed, where the new kid was required to sleep.

If the phone rang, or a citizen showed up at the front door with a cry alarm, or an alarm came into the station from Dispatch, the newbie up front was required to get up, acknowledge, and handle the situation accordingly. They were the night watchman.

Some guys had a difficult time getting up for calls and would sleep right through them. If we were at Ones and a fire alarm came in, and we weren't on the rig by the time the engineer and captain were, they were leaving our ass in the dust. There'd be a parade of shame for us when they got back, and we'd be disciplined accordingly in front of the whole crew.

This happened to my buddy RP several times, and he was almost fired because of it. He slept through three alarms as a probationary firefighter. His ambulance partners would be waiting with the rig running inside the station, then the station alarm lights would eventually turn off, and still no RP at the sled.

The night watchman was in charge of making sure all the troops made it to their rigs and if they didn't show, the PA announcement tone would sound and an angry voice would shout through the station, "Firefighter Powers, you have a run. Signal 4 to your rig, I repeat, Firefighter Powers, Signal 4 to your rig. You have an alarm." The captains, having just been woken up twice for an alarm that wasn't for them, would be especially motivated to make sure it never happened again. Transfers were made, derogatory marks in probationary blue books were written, and other firefighters were assigned to monitor calls for the sleeping beauty. Problem solved.

The night watchman was also in charge of closing the garage doors for the outgoing rigs and securing the station properly. Later, all the trucks would get garage door openers and the night watchman's position was rendered obsolete as doorbells and remote openers were installed in the antiquated fire stations. Ahh progress, it's a beautiful thing.

There were some great one-liners the old-timers would say in the firehouses. Some of the more famous quotes I can recall were:

When they were angry at someone, they'd tell them to "go shit in your hat."

If they had to go poop, "the old brown turtle is poking his head out," or "my baby just dropped, and I'm crowning," or they'd say they were going to either "make a statue of a chief," "take the Browns to the Super Bowl," or they had to "drop the kids off at the pool."

If someone asked where something was, they'd say, "If it was up your ass, you'd know."

If someone asked for directions, they'd answer, "You can't get there from here."

If someone was upset over something, they'd ask, "Who pissed in *your* cheerios?"

If someone went on a rant, they'd say, "Why don't you tell us how you *really* feel?"

If someone was extremely lucky, they'd say, "You live in a tree."

Then there was the ever popular, "I'd rather have a sister in a whorehouse than a brother on the black shift."

Chapter 5

This One's for the Ladies

Speaking of whorehouses, there were so many opportunities to have sex as a firefighter, it was ridiculous. The city was simply teeming with innumerable women (and men) who were trying everything they could to bang a man in uniform. If we were even remotely good-looking, offers to get between the sheets literally came knocking at our door and fell right into our laps. It was so difficult to say no when it was so damn easy to say yes instead.

The hospital emergency rooms were like brothels. One could make eye contact with a doctor or nurse and be screwing twenty minutes later in the linen closet. I knew one nurse who was banging at least three different firefighters, all on different shifts, and they all thought they were in love. When one of them started talking marriage, it was time to spill the beans. They were all devastated, and she just moved on to the next. We called her the Black Widow because she'd caused so many divorces on our department.

The fire department Christmas parties would kick off each year with the Old Newsboys fundraiser. Our local newspaper would create a spoof edition of the local celebrities and major events that occurred over the past year. The local firefighters were the newsboys—the criers—hollering out headlines and collecting donations to purchase winter clothing for the city's less fortunate children. After volunteering for the worthy cause at local supermarkets and malls, the weary newsboys gathered at the closest pubs and threw back a few drinks to celebrate.

Invariably, the group would eventually flock to the closest strip club, where more firefighters would arrive, and a huge party would pop off. I can remember at least fifty firefighters surrounding the stage at Omar's one year. Remember Tommy Tumenello? Spike Young and I paid the ladies to bring him up on the stage and they all danced on him together at the same time. It was crazy. I understood why the spouses weren't invited to the holiday events.

Now that everyone was all worked up and covered in stripper glitter, the party moved to the closest hotel, where we'd booked a block of rooms. The department Christmas poem would be read, copious amounts of drugs and alcohol were consumed, and we'd crash the hotel pool and bar before retiring to our rooms for a long winter's nap.

Speaking of strippers, we'd occasionally make emergency runs to the strip clubs. Every time an alarm came in for some poor bastard with chest pain, or one of the girls fell off the stage or had overdosed at Omar's or Déjà vu or Centerfolds, there was a mad dash to the rigs. It wasn't uncommon for two ambulances to race each other to the scene, or for officers to self-dispatch on the call, just so they could walk in and get a glimpse of boobies or stripper ass.

One time on Medic 11, we were the only rig dispatched for a woman feeling lightheaded at Omar's, and all of Station 1 emptied out. The other medic, the BC, the engine, even the fucking ladder truck came with us for *moral* support. The Omar's staff were surprised when fourteen dudes piled into the club to help assist with patient care.

Another time, on a call to Centerfolds, the same thing happened for a guy with chest pain. Ambulance, engine, and ladder truck were all initially very concerned for the gentleman's safety. Once inside, they could've cared less if the guy was dead on the floor with a knife in his back. It's doubtful they would've even noticed.

There were some major perverts working for our department—in case you haven't already figured that out. Ron Finkle, our union secretary, and later vice president, would routinely say while watching a woman on TV, "My god, I'd love to drink her bath water," or, "I'd lay in the sewer for a week just to see one of her turds float by." Then his wife would swing by the station to visit after dinner and all his lewd comments would cease. We wondered if he was living a double life or if Mrs. Finkle just wasn't into his dirty conversation starters.

When I hired on, my buddy Chase's father, Gary—who was a firefighter before him—had certain generalized and stereotypical truths he clung to, based upon his years of experience. Gary had sayings like "Just cuz you're poor doesn't mean you've gotta be dirty," and "Women in the fire service are either sluts or dykes." Having spent significant time with the fire service, as well as with sluts and dykes, I'd generally agree. Although there were a few faithful and straight anomalies. Like five out of the fifty or so women I worked with over the years, so the odds certainly weren't in their favor.

I've seen two (allegedly) hetero female firefighters (Gretchen Olsen and Ginger McEntire) screwing each other on the bed in a hotel room full of drunk firefighters and a whole orgy pop off. Married battalion chiefs were fucking probationary firefighters. This was at my very first red shift Christmas party, when I had just two months on.

Incidentally, as a twenty-one-year-old new kid, unskilled yet in the ways of the world, I got way too drunk and high at that event and ended up hugging the porcelain throne for four hours before sobering up enough to drive home to my *very* angry first wife. Afterward, Hector Garcia would instruct me in the fine art of riding the wave. Like a surfer—never getting too high on the wave, or too low, but finding that perfect buzz and riding it all the way in to shore—thus avoiding a wipeout. Words of wisdom from a true master of the craft.

The lesbians in the fire service were simply amazing, most of them tough as nails and stronger than many of the men on the job. As long as they could pull *my* unconscious ass out of a structure fire, they got my vote of approval, regardless of sexual orientation. I appreciated the straight talk we got from them, too. Some of my best friends on the department were loud and proud lesbians. They worked just as hard in the stations and on firegrounds, if not harder than their male colleagues.

The sluts, God bless their souls, were a wonder to behold. It doesn't take much to entice a man who's away from his family for the night, to stray waywardly into the arms of a seasoned vixen. I can't count how many times I've witnessed fucking in the firehouse. Or at Christmas parties. Or golf outings. Or at damn near any fire department function other than a funeral, although I'm sure it's probably happened. Hell, in Akron they made real pornos on duty.

After the majority of the station crews headed off to their dorm rooms to hit the rack for the night, the players would stay up, pretending to watch the late show or work on a personal project. Soon, a pair of headlights would pull into the parking lot and a young lady would arrive for a personal and intimate tour of the firehouse at night.

Sometimes, we'd just look over at the person next to us in the brown chair and ask them if they wanted to fool around. If yes, a short trip to a quiet corner of the station and we were getting busy. If no, just don't push the issue and harass them and everything was fine. No meant no. It hardly ever was no, though. When things got slow in the station, sex was the perfect cure for boredom. And who would ever know? Or even care for that matter?

One of our female firefighters, we'll call her Bubbles, was an extraordinarily ditsy bleach blonde, who slept her way through paramedic school and the fire academy. She fit the stereotype of Gary's slut category quite nicely. When I hired on the department, every battalion chief on both shifts had, at one time or another, been balls deep in Bubbles.

Her husband Rusty was a massive man who, in his travels as an interstate commercial plumber, had run through more bar whores than Bubbles had firemen. But that only seemed to fuel the flames of her fiery passion and it was fairly commonplace to walk into the public men's restroom at a fire department function and find her on her knees giving head to some random guy or bent over a countertop getting railed from behind.

Rusty helped me install my bathroom fixtures at home, and I always had too much respect for the guy to bang his wife, regardless of opportunity. Bros before hoes; that's how I rolled through much of my life, and this was always the case with Bubbles, no matter how drunk or readily available she often was.

One day at Station 6 during shift change, Gretchen Olsen was excited to show off her new set of triple D fake tits she'd just installed. The black shift employees had all seen them the day before, and with hardly any encouragement, she lifted her shirt right at the head of the breakfast table and revealed them to the incoming red shifters.

"Wow!"

"Those are nice."

"Holy shit!"

And they were spectacularly nice store-bought tatas. She was extremely proud of them and offered to give the guys—and girls—full motorboats in the captain's office. I politely declined, while most of the officers exited, along with her, stage left. Her face, however, resembled one of those troll dolls. In fact, her fire department nickname was Gretchen *Trollsen*.

There was another stereotypical category of women, the ones who washed out. Women who gave firefighting their best shot, but in the end the job was just too much for them. For certain, there were a lot of guys in this category, too. Don't get me wrong. If one could do the job, that was all that mattered to me, regardless of gender. They'd have earned my respect. It's not an easy profession.

Sherry Horton was a probationary firefighter who caught a bucket prank at Station 8. She was upset the water had ruined her new $150 hair weave and demanded to be placed on "stress leave." She left on a disability shortly after, filing a harassment and discrimination lawsuit against the city, which was all too happy to cut her a settlement check and wave goodbye.

Many women and men followed similar paths, leaving shortly after realizing the job was a bit more than they'd anticipated or wanted to continue doing. Some quit. Some faked injuries. Some really were injured. But they all walked away, never to return.

Occasionally, the guys in Operations thought it would be fun to create entire rigs fully staffed with women. On ambulances, it was particularly cruel when they'd assign two petite ladies to the same sled. When the next day's running charts came out, everyone department-wide knew the engine companies would be running with them, often on ambulance assists.

On engine and ladder companies, Operations would sometimes do the same thing with the ladies. We referred to these as "triple chick days." It wasn't uncommon, especially at Fours, to have both rigs completely staffed with women. Depending on their personality traits, this could make for an awesome shift. Or it could make for an awkwardly long day that made us seriously contemplate going home early on sick leave.

To be fair, it wasn't just women the fellas in Ops would fuck with. They enjoyed sticking men together on ambulance crews that created awkward dichotomies. Like the 6'7" Keith Michaels, who looked like Lurch from *The Adams Family*, and the 5'4" Billy Engler, who—minus the orange skin—resembled an Oompa Loompa from *Willy Wonka's Chocolate Factory*. They rode together constantly on the black shift. We thought it must've made it exceedingly difficult, carrying a loaded cot up and down stairs. There had to be strategy sessions about this at the breakfast table before their shift began.

It was always a shame when one firefighter married the former throwdown of another. For instance, when RP's previous call girl Crystal from our Sin Bin days, became engaged to, and then married Seaboy, it made for some awkward moments whenever the two firefighters were in the room together. Gretchen Olsen married not one, but two firefighters from our department—at different times of course—then promptly divorced both.

Some lucky couples found their soulmates in the firehouses around town. Brett Davis and Monica Lewis began dating and before long, were married with children. The same happened for my classmate and high school friend Tim Carver and his wife Lena Small; it was love, marriage, then the baby carriage. Engineer Mike Hilton married Barb Baker, a dispatcher. Firefighter Mary Rosenthal and Captain Mick Foster found love and marriage in the fire stations, too. Tragically, he died from a heart attack shortly after retirement, and then she burnt up in a fire and dutied out.

Ginger McEntire and Cain Long hooked up together, after she'd run through BJ, Russ Jackson, Jake Potter, and God only knows who else, all while married to a local cop. This happened so frequently at Station 6, that one night when she knocked on what she thought was Cain's dorm, a nonchalant reply of "wrong room," was delivered through the closed door. The crews had fun with that one at the breakfast table the next morning.

Let's talk next about the cheaters. The fire service is full of them. Like I said earlier, it's tough to leave your family, stay the night in a firehouse, and be a straight shooter. It takes a boatload of commitment. There were cheaters everywhere. The station doorbell would ring, and we'd see a captain escorting a young hottie off to his bedroom in the middle of the day. They'd emerge a short time later and kiss goodbye. Then his wife and kids would show up after dinner and be running around the station.

I witnessed my first captain (who was married) at my first fire department Christmas party screwing a new kid, who afterward became a devout lesbian and then, much later, became the first female battalion chief in the history of our department. First impressions are everything and seeing this was one of mine. Nearly *everybody* was cheating.

Matthew Hawk was cheating at Sevens with a pretty young thing in cowboy boots and skintight Wranglers. Mark Taylor had a different girl every week at Fours. Russ Jackson was cheating on his wife with Ginger McEntire. Hector Garcia was cheating, and it caused his divorce. Dan Martinez was cheating. So was Chase Powers. Everyone was fucking around.

And it wasn't just the firefighters; even spouses were getting in on it. Dave Austin's girlfriend was cheating on him with another local firefighter while he was at work. Jeff Fentin's wife was cheating on him with a firefighter on the other shift. Carlyle Luciano's wife was cheating, and he ended up quitting the profession and moving out of state to save his marriage. Dave Ramos's wife was cheating on him, and he hung himself over it. Ray "Fergie" Ferguson's wife was cheating on him while he was in the station, and when he came home early from work one day and caught her, he dove headfirst into the bottle and never climbed out.

I think back to JT's locker full of porn and Paul Wilson, Rudy Alsdorf, and Tom Riddell, the swingers who had open relationships and would go to orgies and tell crazy stories at the breakfast tables the next day. It's no wonder I made the terrible choices I did. And so it was, when I was faced with the proposition of cheating, I gave in to the primal urges and fell headlong into sin and temptation.

Pam Stokes was a cougar in every sense of the word. A female black shift captain, a devout nudist, body builder, and a sultry, experienced woman who knew exactly what to do to get her way every time. She asked me, when I was a probationary firefighter, to install new carpet in her town home. Too naïve still, and unaware of her intention to take advantage of a young man, I agreed.

While installing the carpet in her upstairs bathroom, she came into the room and sat down on the toilet completely naked. She tinkled away inches from my head while I continued to work on the flooring around the bathroom cabinet, respectfully pretending not to notice.

"Well," she said, when she finished, "are you gonna fuck me or what?"

Let me just say it's exceedingly difficult to remain faithful to your spouse in a situation like that. It's also very hard to go back to work and finish your flooring job. It's also very awkward to sit across from your captain at work as she sips her coffee, winks, and blows you a kiss right in front of the whole crew at the breakfast table. But I digress.

Chapter 6

Fightin' Fives—Year Two

Everything I've related so far happened in my first year on the fire department. It's difficult for one to fully comprehend the massive impact the fire service can have on the human psyche. Progressing into my sophomore year on the department, I became desensitized to trauma. The adrenaline highs of emergency response turned me into a different person. It's like there's a chemical response inside of us and if we don't maintain that dopamine high, we start going through withdrawals. I began to seek the rush of danger off duty as well. My late-night extracurricular activities increased in frequency, and the prior commitments I'd made of being a parent and a faithful husband became mundane. I craved more excitement, more adventure, more danger. This chapter chronicles my highlights—and lowlights—in year two as I faded away from my former self and transformed into an adrenaline junkie.

Chuck Sanders made the battalion chief rank and left Station 3 in July 1999. The extrication tools left Threes around the same time and were sent to Station 5, a more centrally located firehouse. In September, I wrote a letter to the chiefs requesting to follow the tools and remain at a vehicle extrication focus station. My transfer request was granted in January 2000, no doubt at the recommendation of BC Chuck Sanders, and it was off to Fightin' Fives for me.

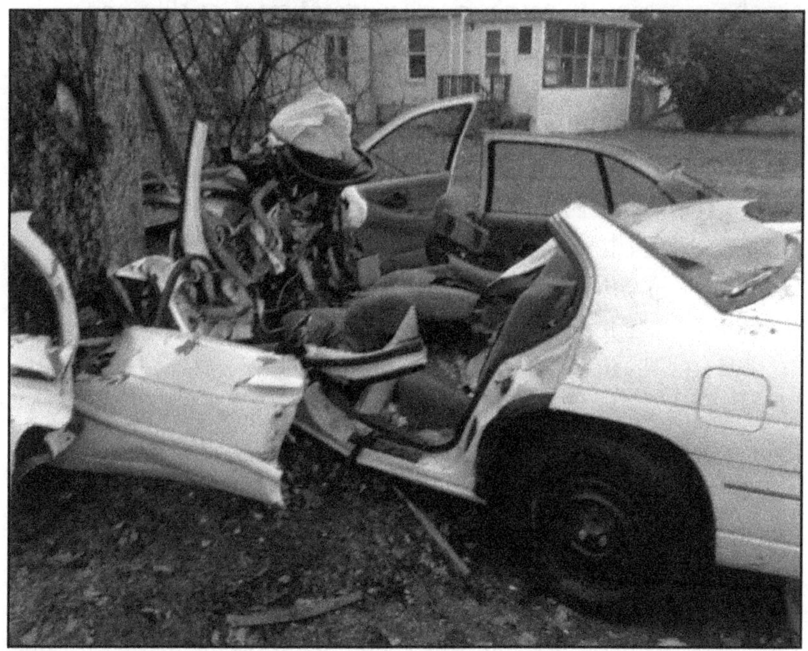

Vehicle extrication; door pop, roof removal, dash roll

I arrived at the center of the vehicle extrication universe—for our department at least—and made myself at home with one of the best crews in the city at the time. The station captain was Craig "Mumbles" Henderson, Hector Garcia was the engineer, and Chase Powers, Dan Martinez, and I rounded out the firefighters on the red shift.

Mumbles said the most important piece of equipment on the fire truck were the people who staffed it. That's probably why he was so great a firefighter—because he valued human beings over things. We answered to no one except each other and raised hell every day, all shift long. As long as we were ready to respond when the alarms came in and gave him 100 percent effort on the scenes, Mumbles didn't care what we did with our time in between calls.

There were no rules, and the world was our playground. It was absolute anarchy. It was the single wildest time in my life, and to this day, I wish it could have continued that way, with that crew, for my entire career. However, the only constant in life is change, and we were all destined to make rank and transfer to other stations around the city. For the moment, though, it was our turn to have outrageously good times and party like there was no tomorrow.

Fives was located on a sleepy little neighborhood street in the center of town. It was a single company engine house with a medic unit. As long as I was there, I never had to rove to another station to ride the sled. Our crew hung out together on our days off and we were closer than any other group of firefighters I've ever worked with.

Chase and I were virtually inseparable. We spent many of our days off out at Mumbles' house with his family, and our nights partying with Hector and Dan out on the town. We played sports together all year long and vacationed together. They were my "band of brothers," and we knew each other inside and out, backwards and forwards. We were comrades in arms, and we ruled the firegrounds. We'd beat other stations into their first due fires, pull up to their scenes, and take over the best jobs, and were completely unstoppable together.

On February 17, 2000, Sonya delivered our second daughter, and we welcomed her into the family. After the delivery, I went home to get some sleep while Sonya stayed with our newborn baby in the hospital. Sonya's younger sister—we'll call her Porsche—showed up at my home unannounced, knocking at the front door. I invited her in and asked: "What's up?"

She said she just wanted to check in on me to see how I was doing.

"Fine," I replied as she removed her coat, her shoes, then her shirt and pants, until she was standing in my living room in her underwear, just staring at me.

I was absolutely certain Hell was going to have a special place for me when I arrived there in the afterlife. She was nineteen, and in between kisses she explained she'd had a crush on me since junior high. We screwed on the marital sofa, right there in the living room. It was a horrible thing to do, and I knew right then I had some major fucking problems.

Sonya and the kids would visit at me at the station occasionally and enjoyed sitting in the fire trucks and watching their dad slide down the fire poles. We were one big happy family on the surface, but on the inside, I was struggling with my misdeeds and the very same vices my own father had fallen victim to. I was becoming everything I despised about my old man. My self-discipline was severely lacking when it came to the black-hole pull and Death Star tractor beam vortex of ready-and-willing-to-screw females.

With my porn and sex addictions proving too much for me to overcome, Porsche and I would meet up occasionally when my wife was out of town, or I'd head off to cover a shift at work for a friend, or get a friend to cover the last half of my shift. She worked at one of the local strip clubs as a waitress and in the Love Boutique, where they sold sex toys and pornos. It was always an exciting time with her, with new tricks and party favors awaiting the young firefighter.

Cocaine was always spread on the tables at her place when I'd show up. Her roommates were all strippers from the club, and if they weren't high and conscious, they were passed out naked on the floor or collapsed comatose across various pieces of furniture from the previous night's debauchery. One time on the dining room table, another time on the kitchen counter, another time half in/half out of the bathtub. Never asleep in bed like normal human beings.

Porsche would swing by Fives occasionally, late into the evenings, and we'd smoke cigarettes, maybe a joint, and hang out with the crew. We'd talk about life and the latest interesting pop culture events. It was no different than what any of my other station mates were doing. We all covered for each other whenever our throwdowns came by for some quality time, never letting on to the spouses what we knew about or had witnessed. Always living and abiding, first and foremost, by the bro code.

My all-time favorite person to ride the sled with was Chase Powers. We had a routine where we'd try to make it within five minutes from alarm to hospital. Everybody was a load and go. See, a patient is either "stay and play," or "load and go." That means, based on the severity of the situation, we either treat them on scene and transport once they're stabilized, or haul balls and treat them en route to the hospital. We always did everything en route, on every call, every time. There was no such thing as a stay-and-play patient for us.

We'd walk in and say, "Hey, wanna go to the hospital?"

If they answered yes, then "Let's go!" If they couldn't walk, we'd carry them. Fast. We'd get a set of basic vitals en route, start IVs en route, write our reports en route, transfer the patient over to the hospital bed, wink at the nurses, and we were ghost.

Life's too short and we had way better things to do with our time. Plus, most of the homes we went into were absolute shitholes. Why get bed bugs or roaches in our gear when we can grab the patient and move them outside to our office. That way, we stayed fresh instead of absorbing the eau de chain-smokers-delight in the patient's house and then smelling like we'd rolled around in a dirty ash tray.

When a shooting came in one sunny, summer afternoon at the zoo, Chase and I on Medic 5, along with Jonesy, Agent, and Kevin Norwood on Engine 3, rushed into action. We arrived so fast we beat the police there. We flew through the park entrance gates and zipped down the roads that bordered the parking lots. Halfway between the parking lot and the ticket booths was a woman lying motionless on the concrete.

Park staff and civilians were waving us in, so I jumped the curb and drove right up the wide sidewalk approach to the woman lying on the sidewalk in a pool of blood. Her two children were screaming and crying beside her, being unsuccessfully consoled by the park staff, as I whipped the sled around and stopped near the body on the ground. We hopped out and Chase threw the monitor and jump kit onto the cot, then I yanked it from the back doors, placing it on the ground next to the unconscious woman.

She had a gunshot entrance wound on her right side near her right breast and an exit wound on the left torso that passed through her left arm as well.

"GSW, torso, through and through," I said to Chase as he knelt beside her.

Bystanders advised that the woman was walking out of the zoo with her two young kids, holding their hands, when a gunshot rang out from the train tracks a hundred yards away. Chase put her on the heart monitor, and I checked for a pulse. There was none, and she wasn't breathing.

"Load and go," Chase said.

Captain Jonesy from Engine 3 walked up and remarked at the faint rhythm on the cardiac monitor. "PEA," he said, referring to the heart rhythm known as pulseless electrical activity.

We rolled her onto a backboard, lifted her onto the cot, and loaded her in the bone box. Chase dropped an ET tube with precision, and I hooked a BVM up to it. It was hard as a football when I tried to squeeze it. Chase listened with the stethoscope for lung sounds as I used two hands to compress the BVM. Finally, it gave way and air flowed into her lungs. At the same time a fine red mist sprayed from both sides of the holes in her chest coating the ambulance cabinets on one side, and Chase on the other.

Kevin Norwood hopped up front and began to drive us to Saint Mary's Hospital, as Agent slapped Vaseline gauze onto the holes in her torso. Chase hooked up an IV while I squeezed the BVM, and Agent began chest compressions. Chase called the ER and we rolled up less than a minute later. We had an on-scene time of under three minutes and our total time from dispatch alarm to arrival at the ER was 5:47. It was an epic response time.

After a while of doing CPR and administering shocks to restart her heart at the ER, they pronounced her dead at the hospital. We discovered she was married to a state police trooper. One week earlier, the man she was having an affair with was murdered at a party store on the north side of town. Now, apparently it was her turn.

Both homicides were never solved. We all had our theories and conjectures about who did it, or, at the very least, who'd arranged it. That was a cold, calculated, professional hit. The bullet passed through both lungs and her heart, killing her instantly as she held the hands of her two children at the zoo. Her husband had dropped them off at the park just an hour earlier. Then she was sniped in broad daylight. My first murder victim always reminds me of the Filter song "Hey Man, Nice Shot."

There was a metal heat treating factory across the street from Station 5. Every now and again, the temperature in the chemical vats would get too high and ignite. When we responded to the occasional alarms, we only needed to stand by while the equipment was turned off and cooled itself down, because it was self-contained. Initially, we didn't know that, and Dispatch scrambled a full alarm.

Chase and I arrived on Medic 5, and our engine crew with Mumbles and Dan Martinez made entry into the factory. Nines showed up next and we helped them set their aerial ladder up to access the roof. Captain Charlie Peters headed up to the turntable and waited for his firefighter to follow. On the ground, Firefighter Wendy Simpson was having trouble finding a ladder belt that fit around her waist. Charlie was yelling for her to hurry up, but she couldn't fit any of the belts, so Chase and I decided to help.

We each grabbed an end of the largest belt and wrapped it around her.

"Suck it in!" Chase told her as we pushed our ends together.

"I am!" Wendy said, as we still came up short.

Chase put his foot on Wendy's thigh and, exchanging ends of the belt with him, I did the same. We pulled with all our might, practically standing off the ground on Wendy's hips as she screamed in pain.

"It's no use!" Chase yelled. "You're just too fat!"

"Thanks, Captain Obvious!" Wendy said. "You don't gotta be an asshole about it."

Charlie was sick of waiting for his heavyset firefighter and headed up the ladder toward the roof without her.

"Just go," I said, giving up on the ladder belt and sending her up to the turntable without it. She didn't really need it anyway for a climb to the roof. The fire went out on its own after a while, and Chase and I laughed for days about Wendy's FUPA (fat upper pubic area) and the ladder belt incident. Later, she managed to get down to, and stay at her fighting weight.

Ginger McEntire had a friend named Lisa who was interested in becoming a nurse. Lisa was doing a ride-along on the ambulance with Ginger at Station 5, and after lunch asked if I'd give her a tour of the firehouse. Sure, no problem. I showed her the trucks, the equipment, the office, the lounge, the kitchen, and the upstairs dormitory.

"That's about it," I said.

She closed the door of the captain's room and grabbed my uniform, pulling me close, as she blocked the door with her backside.

"Want to fool around with me?" she asked, looking at me with bedroom eyes.

"I'm married," I replied.

"So am I. And what they don't know won't hurt them," Lisa retorted.

Just for the record, I'd like to be clear: that statement is absolutely false. This is the kind of shit that happens to firefighters. How's a young man supposed to stay faithful when a beautiful woman drops her pants and grabs her ankles right in front of him. I'd have to be Clark Kent, Superman, and the Reverend Jimmy Graham all rolled into one to stand up and say no to that shit when it's staring me right in the face. I couldn't resist.

We both agreed to keep it a secret. She was in her early twenties, and I found out later she had five goddamn kids. She was a sex fiend and I'd bet dollars to doughnuts a paternity test would prove they weren't all from her husband. Every week, for the next several months, we'd meet after dark at the firehouse and bang.

At Station 5 one night, Marv Holcomb was the roving captain and Pat Duncan was the engineer. We woke to the loud "Ka-chunk!" when the alarm system opened up and the station lights kicked on above our beds. Steve "Showtime" Hitchcock, downtown at Dispatch, "hit 'er two" for a first due full alarm fire. We slid the pole, jumped in the open cab rig, and raced into the night. Rolling down Kindle Avenue, through a neighborhood of turn-of-the-century two-story homes, I stood up, looking over the open cab roof at the scene unfolding ahead of us.

We were still blocks away when the glow of a large fire began to light up the night sky. As it came into view, I could see a one-story bungalow made of cinder block walls, with bars on the windows and doors. Fire was showing from every opening and had already made its way through the roof. Marv radioed in the fully involved structure fire as I pulled the pre-connect and advanced it to the front door. Pat put the rig in pump and charged the hose line. We had 250 gallons of water in our tank, and, being the first ones there, I went hard from the yard while waiting for my officer to return from his walk-around.

When he arrived at the front door, Marv informed me we were going defensive and would *not* be making entry.

"WHAT?!" I asked in disbelief.

"There's no reason to risk anything on this one. Everyone's out, and the place is a total loss," he explained. Then he said he'd be at the curb if I needed anything and walked away, leaving me alone with the nozzle at the front door. Other trucks began arriving, Matthew Hawk and Juan Ortiz from Engine 9 stretched the second pre-connect from my engine and met me at the door.

"Where's your boss?" Hawk asked.

"There." I pointed to the road where Marv was standing talking to the BC.

"Well, grab your shit and stick with us if you want," he offered.

I looked at Marv and couldn't believe he'd do that on a first due fire. No balls. We had a chance to be on the nozzle and battle the beast and he was standing in the goddamn road.

Fuck *that*.

"Let's go," I said to Hawk as we forced the door and made entry.

Ortiz and I opened our nozzles and together we pushed into the flames. As the fire yielded to our streams, we could see through the smoke this was an old garage converted into living quarters. We advanced into the middle of the structure and suddenly lost all our water pressure. Ortiz likes to say his line went flaccid, but I say mine went limp. Tomayto, Tomahto.

Hawk leaned in close, looked down at our barely trickling nozzles, then back at us, then jokingly advised us to "put your thumb over the end of it," like a garden hose.

Then something wonderful happened. Hawk told us to close the bales and drop our nozzles. He produced an axe and began smashing anything and everything that was on fire.

"That's how you fight fire with no water!" he yelled.

We followed suit, taking our axes and pike poles, and destroying anything still glowing with flames. Once it was in pieces and on the ground, we stomped out the embers. The fire was just a smoldering ashtray when we exited minutes later, with our hose lines still flat.

As we approached the BC, we could hear him yelling at Pat, "You dumbass! You hooked the water supply into the front discharge, you moron!"

"Hey, uh, Pat, we ran out of water in there, bro," I said, adding fuel to his humiliation. "It's all good, though, we put it out with axes," I offered, winking at Hawk and Ortiz as they cleared the scene for another full alarm fire across town.

Marv was being interviewed by a reporter and camera crew at the curb. I walked past them and went back inside the structure to put out hot spots and overhaul the joint. Duncan got the hydrant supply line connected to the engine's intake proper and we finished the job. I didn't realize it then, but a seed was planted that day. As the years went by, it grew into an obsession. The lawn, the curb, the battalion chief's car; that was *not* the place for me. No sir.

Chase and I were on the medic out of Fives when we caught a run for a police standby. A woman had doused herself with gasoline at the corner fueling station and was standing in the middle of the intersection holding a lighter in the air. The police eventually talked her down and escorted her to our ambulance for transport to CMH (Community Mental Health) for a psychiatric evaluation.

The fumes alone! When she entered the ambulance and took a seat on the cot, Chase and I became instantly lightheaded. I wrapped her up in a disposable blanket. Chase asked if I was all set and we drove the two blocks or so over to CMH. They refused to take her because of the gasoline contamination, and we transported to the hospital for decon instead. She and I had a nice long conversation as we rode to the ER. Jadine was a former volunteer firefighter and convicted arsonist. She was going through a rough patch and was crying out for help.

We dropped her off at the closest hospital, and she stunk the whole ER up for hours.

Several days later, there was a knock at the fire station door. It was Jadine asking the captain if I was working that day. He told her to wait outside and advised Chase and me.

"Dude, you got a stalker!" Chase said.

"No way, I'll go see what she wants," I replied casually.

I went out and sat down on the bench with Jadine. She just wanted to thank me for being so kind and listening to her. That was really all she'd needed that day. Then she left. I estimated around 75 percent of our EMS calls could've been solved by just being a street therapist—someone who listens and gives sound advice—in my humble opinion.

After being up all night on Medic 5 during a major snowstorm, Chase and I caught an alarm at shift change for a young man with back pain. We headed out to a tiny bungalow on Washington Avenue. Inside, a young man named Gene explained he'd been snowmobiling through the city three days ago and hurt his back when he jumped a snowbank.

Chase asked if he could walk and he said no. Looking at the young mother holding her baby and standing in the doorway of the trash-strewn home, Chase was disgusted at the man's lack of gumption. He threw Gene over his shoulder and carried him from the house. He slammed the man onto the cot outside the door and we rolled to the hospital, only a block away.

"Just cuz you're poor, don't mean ya gotta be dirty," he told the man as we dropped him off in the hospital waiting room. We never even wrote a run report and returned for shift change.

Chase was a wild child. We partied everywhere we went, and work was no different. When we were together, life flew by with raucous laughter and 100 percent adrenaline overload. We banged women, got in bar brawls, rode motorcycles, went to concerts, and had both saved each other's lives more times than we could count.

One day after eating one of Dan's Mexican dinners, Hector and I were at the back of the fire trucks on the apparatus floor, when Chase ran around the front of the ambulance and yelled, "Hey, *fuckers*!"

As Garcia and I turned to look, Chase dropped his pants, bent over, and smacked his own ass. Our eyes now seared with Chase's brown eye reveal, we burst into laughter. He had shreds of that cheap-ass city toilet paper stuck to the hair in his crack. Hector said between belly laughs, "Dude, you've got toilet paper dingleberries!" We died laughing as Chase ran off, embarrassed.

The Squid Band was playing the Silver Dollar Night Club one evening. Chase and I were stuck on the ambulance together at Station 5 in midtown, and the Dollar was on the northeast side of the city near the border. We decided to go anyway, on duty, and in uniform. We told Dispatch we were in radio service and neglected to mention where we were headed. Easier to apologize and beg for forgiveness, than to ask for permission, Chase always said.

We ended up catching a run to the opposite corner of the city and made it from the Dollar to the scene in under three minutes. Which was probably faster than if we'd been in our own fire station. I flew down the highways at 80 miles per hour and took the off ramps and turns on two wheels while Chase worked the air horns and the Federal Q like a madman. The proverbial traffic waters parted for us, and we cruised our way across the city like the Israelites crossing the Red Sea. We called it the Squid gig ambalancin' event, and it was goddamn biblical.

My second murder victim was an elderly man who was the unfortunate recipient of a stabbing in a downtown park. We were called by police for a possible DOA. A group of children playing snow football, had found what appeared to be a frozen man. We parked our sled and trudged the blue bag and cardiac monitor across the snowy, frozen tundra to the back of the park, near a tree.

The man was stabbed twice in the chest through his coat. Probably the night before, because he was frozen stiff in the thirteen-degree temperatures of the new day. We confirmed the victim was deceased, then headed back across the park to call the hospital for a time of death from the warmth of the meat wagon.

This proved to be more commonplace than I'd anticipated as I progressed through my career. I responded to another DOA in a different park months later. Same thing, only now it was summertime. Kids found a man the next morning, stabbed through the heart, rigored in the agonal throes of his death. The cops just needed confirmation and we obliged.

Back at Fives that afternoon, Chase and I put paper bags over our heads with holes cut out for our eyes, and went streaking through the station naked. Chase led the way and I followed him at full sprint. Krishna was a new kid studying streets in the lounge and couldn't believe his eyes when we ran by.

We ran past Mumbles at the front desk doing his report writing, then through the kitchen past the cook, across the apparatus floor, between the trucks, and past the engineer checking his rig. When they all came looking for us, we were back in uniform, in our ambulance, checking the equipment. We played it off like we didn't know what they were talking about. Good times.

Another time Chase and I were on the medic we were called to Edwards Street for a possible suicide. We rolled with the engine company and arrived to find a twenty-six-year-old woman on the floor at the base of the stairs. She was lying in a pool of blood, had a hole in the top of her head, and a long rifle at her feet. There was a man crying and sitting on the steps a few feet above her. He said he was her husband and she'd shot herself.

Something just felt off about the whole scene. The lady was stunningly gorgeous and as I checked for a pulse, I noticed there was no entry wound to the front of her head or neck area. Finding no pulse, we loaded her immediately for transport and hit the road, taking the engine's firefighter Spoons with us in the back, while the engineer drove the sled. Spoons hired on with me and earned the nickname after the *Silver Spoons* TV show character Ricky Schroeder. Spoons had drawn first in seniority for our class, made it off the ambulance rotation in seven years while I put in fourteen, never got demoted when *everyone* else did, and always had his uncle Willy P pulling strings up in Ops for him. Born with a silver spoon in his mouth, Spoons seemed fitting.

"How'd she shoot herself in the top of the head with a rifle?" I asked, hopping on chest compressions, as Chase looked for an airway.

Spoons just stood at the back doors of the ambulance staring at the woman.

"Spoons! Look for a line dammit!" Chase yelled, snapping him back to reality.

"She's so beautiful," Spoons said.

"She's so *dead* right now, so get your ass in gear," Chase shouted as he placed the ET tube into her trachea and inflated the cuff.

I passed Chase the BVM, he hooked it to the ET tube and squeezed, while I listened for lung sounds with the stethoscope.

"Positive lung sounds, apexes and bases, negative on gastric," I advised.

Spoons clicked the Protect IV catheter into its sheath and I handed him the IV tubing. He secured it and I continued chest compressions. Chase called the hospital to alert them to our arrival time. Spoons cracked the drug box and pushed the first-round of meds into the IV port.

We paused CPR to check for a heart rhythm. It was asystole with no shock advised, so we quickly resumed CPR. As he squeezed the BVM and breathed for the woman, Chase checked her head for another hole. There was none. The only one was on the top of her head, near the back. Right about where someone would catch a bullet if they were walking away from the shooter, down the stairs, and someone above them pulled the trigger. There was no way this was a suicide. Not with a rifle. It was physically impossible to pull off.

"Maybe she had the barrel in her mouth," I suggested, "and the entrance wound is really an exit wound."

"No holes in her throat except the God-given ones," Chase replied.

We transferred patient care to the trauma room staff at the hospital, then washed up and wrote our report. On calls like these, we knew we'd be coming into work and finding a subpoena taped to our floor locker. We had to write a good report, because inevitably some defense attorney would be grilling us on cross examination six months from now, asking us shit like, "Mr. Lilly, I see you used the CHART method as opposed to the SOAPE method when writing your report, can you explain to the court why you chose to do that?" Or "hmm, it says here your IV was established right antecubital, but the Emergency Department report says it was left antecubital. Which was it, exactly?"

She didn't make it, and a husband lost his wife that day. We poked fun at Spoons for being caught up in the siren's call and standing there motionless in the sled. We never did find out how it turned out or have to go to court. It just went away, like a lot of our calls did. I'll never forget it, though. She was beautiful, and it was tragic. Beautifully tragic.

At 20:00 hours we'd typically kill the lights in the common dormitories for the night. Chase and Jughead were already in their racks when I hit the lights and climbed in bed.

After a few minutes, Chase whispered, "Hey, watch this."

As I waited, the dark dormitory lit up with a giant fireball from Chase's bed. He was on his back with his knees pulled to his chest, his hand holding a lighter to his naked ass. The fireball disappeared and Chase began yelling and smacking the fire in his butt hair out. Jughead and I busted out laughing and the dorm smelled like burnt booty hair for the next hour or so.

We had some *really* old fire trucks at our department. Some of them had open cabs, meaning the engineer and officer were inside, but the firefighters rode outside, backward, right next to the engine cowling. There was a small section of roof—more like an awning—that covered our heads, but our legs got absolutely soaked if it was raining out. In the winter, we'd arrive at our destination frozen and snow covered, having hugged the engine cowling for a degree or two of heat along the way.

Those old trucks smoked horribly when the driver mashed the accelerator. We'd be riding dirty, or backward, in the firefighter's seat, stopped at a red light, and some poor soul would be in the lane beside us. They'd be directly across from the exhaust pipe that stuck out midship, with their window down and elbow hanging out, enjoying the cool breeze.

If we had half a heart, we'd get their attention and tell them to roll up their window. If we were a sick bastard, we'd sit back and watch as the light turned green and our rig belched a cloud of black diesel exhaust into their car so thick, we couldn't see the driver anymore as we pulled away. They'd roll by hacking, coughing, and cursing, with black flecks of diesel soot stuck to their car and face, as they passed the captain calling him motherfucker, cocksucker, and other various and assorted terms of endearment.

We ate so much diesel smoke in those things. At Sevens, they were parked right in the living room. So when backing in, the driver had to kill the engine outside and hope he had enough momentum left to roll in quietly or the firehouse would smell awful for the next few hours and us along with it. On scenes, backing into stations, stopped at red lights, every day, everywhere we went, we were eating diesel fumes. It's one of those smells that triggers bad memories for me even now. We fucking choked on that shit all shift, every day.

Some of the rookies would throw their turnout coat or helmet up onto the open cab engine cowlings if there weren't any hooks to hang them on. Many a firefighter had their jackets, or helmets, or bags of groceries slide off the engine and across the intersections when the truck made a sharp turn, or hit a set of railroad tracks too fast and bounced everyone's heads off the roof. Shit would go flying everywhere.

Hector Garcia routinely had his fire engines up on two wheels trying to get us first-in to other station's fires. If we weren't being tossed around like a rag doll, we weren't driving it right he'd say. Sometimes a cabinet door would fly open, and the contents would dump out onto the streets. A motorist would call Dispatch and they'd alert us, or they'd just collect it and follow us to the scene, or leave it on the doorstep of the fire station for us when we returned.

The absolute best and most rewarding part about open cab rigs was standing up just before arrival at a scene and looking over the roof as we rolled up on an address. I felt like one of the old-timers in hip boots and rubber coats, hanging off the running boards and tail boards, gripping a handle tight as we rounded corners with the Dalmatian barking in the seat next to me and the boss clanging the bell to clear the traffic. That's what made riding outside worth it.

I purchased a fire engine red, two-door 1992 Jeep Wrangler while I was stationed at Fives. My roving captain, who filled in for Mumbles on his day off, was Hank "Hammer" Schmidt. He convinced me a lift kit and some bigger tires was just what the old girl needed, and for $3,500 he could do the whole thing, over the weekend, in his garage. I agreed and the Barbie Malibu Jeep was born. Only it was red—not pink like hers.

With a set of 33-inch BFG Radial All-Terrains, some Rancho adjustable shocks and a three-inch BDS suspension lift, she was ready for the trails. We tore up the deer camp two-tracks, rock crawled over boulders, shredded the PPP mud holes and fields, made it to the top of test hill at the sand dunes, and partied all over the state in that old girl.

When I took the top off one day to drive to the Burn Center Softball Tourney, Jughead wanted to ride along. He asked and I immediately knew I'd regret it. Awkward moments followed that boy around like a lost puppy. My roommate for the weekend ended up standing me up at the last minute and Jughead offered to step in and pay for half of the hotel suite. Nobody else wanted to share a room with him, so reluctantly I agreed.

As we cruised down the freeway with our shirts off and the top down, the other guys in the caravan dubbed us a couple of Ken dolls in the Barbie Malibu Jeep. *Hah, hah, very funny.* Right out of the gate, this was proving to be a crazy trip. When we arrived, we checked into our suite at the Marriott Residence Inn to drop our gear off, then we headed to Hector Garcia and Jimmy Knight's suite to toss back a few cold ones before our first game.

As the boys rolled in, the place got rowdy, and pretty soon there were thirty or so drunk firemen, all yelling over each other, in a two-bedroom suite. It was a damn sausage fest in there and I stepped outside to smoke a joint. As I finished it off with a cigarette, Seaboy and BJ exited the room yelling about fighting and beating each other's asses.

"You might damn well end my life," Seaboy slurred, "but you're a bully and I'm not gonna take your shit anymore."

"Your drunk and stupid," BJ said through a mouthful of Kodiak dip as he took a drink of beer from his can and tossed it onto the lawn. "but if that's what you want, I'll kick your ass for you," BJ kindly offered. He spit to the side as they postured for battle on a small patch of grass.

They started shoving each other and BJ landed a right hook to Seaboy's face. Seaboy spun back around and tackled BJ to the ground, right before Jimmy and Hector stepped in to break it up.

"What the hell guys," Hector said disappointed, "I've got a great weekend planned and you want to start it off like this? The fuck is wrong with you?" He finished shaming them both and everyone went back to partying. There was a softball game in an hour, so I headed back to my suite to get ready. We ended up winning our first-round game of the tournament, then the after party started.

We showered back at the hotel, dressed up in our club attire, and all piled into Battalion Chiefs James Farnum and Amir Zarka's conversion van for a night on the town. We bar hopped, stopping at a five-story club that had different themes on each floor and was open from floor to roof in the middle. We lost Jughead in there—he just disappeared. We left the bar and hit several different strip clubs. Some of the guys brought hookers and strippers back to their hotel rooms, and the party carried on until the sun peeked over the horizon.

James Farnum was a red shift battalion chief, a PPP regular attendee, and a founding member of *The Corporation*, a group of four firefighters who decided, as new kids, to pool their money and purchase commercial and residential investment properties. He was the cousin of WWF superstar The Iron Sheik. We smoked a lot of ganja together over the years, and James was definitely one of my favorite BCs. His son supplied several of the local medical marijuana dispensaries with his crops, so there were always high-quality supplies to go around at parties when James was in attendance.

Amir Zarka was a cool as a cucumber, black shift battalion chief. A charter member of *The Corporation* and the PPP crew, he was probably my personal favorite BC I'd worked with. Nothing rattled him—ever. He could pull up in a red car and be the only one there at a raging inferno of three houses in a row, all fully involved with flames through their roofs, with men, women, and children dangling from their balconies, and in a calm, slow, and monotone voice, size it up over the radio, like, "Dispatch, Battalion 1 on scene, three two-story homes fully involved with fire showing through the roofs, life safety issues on all three. Send me a second alarm and two additional medics, first-in engine and truck companies handle the rescues, second and third-due handle the fire attack; Battalion 1 has command."

The next morning, we had an early ball game, so most of us just grabbed our gear and headed off to the park. Aspirin and coffee were available at the concessions stands because all the firefighters running them knew exactly what we'd been up to all night. It was par for the course. A couple of pretty local cops waved and laughed as we stumbled on to the fields, looking like hell and smelling worse.

We won our morning game and had about six hours to kill before the next one, so I headed back to the hotel to get cleaned up and sleep by the pool. Most of the other guys just passed out at the fields. We won the evening games and were done for the night. Back at the hotel, the guys were buzzing, talking about what was going on at Hector's room later. Jimmy Knight had lined up a woman that was into gang bangs, and everyone was supposed to meet at their room around 21:00 hours.

"I don't know guys," I confessed. "That doesn't really sound like my kind of thing."

"It'll be a blast," Hector advised, "You've gotta at least check it out."

I agreed to swing by and immediately knew I'd regret it. When the time rolled around, we all made our way over to Hector's room. There was an RV parked out in front and the guys were milling around on the porch.

I cracked a beer and headed inside. It was, yet again, a fucking sausage fest. About 40 men stood and sat around the perimeter of the room and there was an old man and a woman dressed in black leather over in the back corner. Jimmy Knight shouted for everyone's attention and introduced the unfamiliar man as the husband of the woman.

The old man said Jimmy was so kind to invite them up for the night, and he wanted everyone there to have a good time with his wife, that she was into gang bangs, and the more dick she could get, the happier she'd be when it was all over. Happy wife, happy life he added.

He laid down the ground rules: be gentle until she asked for it harder, the more the merrier, and if all holes and hands were occupied at the time, to just touch her gently until one became available. Everyone had to wear condoms from the giant party bowl of rubbers he held up, and the safe word was *bananas*. Everything immediately stopped if that word was said. He mentioned he'd be right there taking still photos of his wife and her Johns, and if things got out of control, he'd end it, and Hector and Jimmy would become the enforcers.

Like a strip club DJ, he introduced his wife as Vegas, and the stereo kicked on. A woman only slightly younger than my dead grandmother began to striptease the guys in the room. When the song finished, she was on her back on an ottoman, and her husband was calling for Hector.

"Mr. Garcia, Vegas enjoys starting her shows off with this," He pulled a sixteen-inch stark white strap on dildo from behind his back and helped Hector put it on over his clothes.

Now, Hector was a dark-skinned Mexican, and he had what appeared to be an albino python hanging from his loins. He stepped in between Vegas's skyward legs with a grin from ear to ear. The music blared and the drunk guys howled with excitement. I headed outside for a cigarette.

As my retinas burned from my eye sockets, I walked past the bathroom just in time to see Chase throw open the door butt naked, raise his hands in the air, and gesture at his loins yelling, "I've got nothing!" Apparently, he'd been trying to get his friend to stand at attention. That was definitely my cue to leave. I headed back across the parking lot to my suite. I had something better planned, and she was right on time.

My sister-in-law Porsche pulled into the lot just as I was walking up.

"Hey there, aren't you a sight for sore eyes," I said as she grabbed her things and joined me in the suite.

We rolled a fat Bob Marley joint and smoked it down to the roach. She cut a few lines of coke and we snorted them. We banged in the loft of the hotel suite, then smoked another joint. We were lying in bed laughing at imaginary animals in the ceiling stucco patterns when her car alarm started going off. We got dressed and went outside to check on it.

Someone had opened her passenger door and been rifling through the glove box.

I heard a twig snap in the bushes behind me, and in the street lamplight, could just make out a human figure.

"Jughead?" I asked. "Is that you?"

Jughead rolled out of the bushes and fell onto the sidewalk.

"What the fuck, dude? Where've you been? No one's seen you in two days, and you look like hell," I said.

"Ecstasy, bro," was his reply. It turned out Jughead had taken some mystery pills—that ended up being Ecstasy—at the club the night before, and he'd been trippin' balls ever since.

His phone and wallet had been stolen and he'd been wandering around the city like a vagabond for the past thirty-six hours. How he made it back to the hotel, I have no clue. He was in rough shape.

"Why the fuck were you in my car, asshole?" Porsche chimed in.

"Ecstasy, bro," was his reply again. We sent Jughead inside to get cleaned up and eat some food, and I said good night to Porsche.

"I'll see you later," I said as she drove off.

"Only if you're lucky," she hollered back.

PPP, the Private Party Paradise, was an annual firefighter getaway to the Squid Band guitarist Jeff Lundo's property up north. Jeff invited his favorite people to party with and we all crashed his property for the weekend. Massive bonfires, extreme off-roading, sleeping under the stars, and consuming enormous amounts of weed, coke, shrooms, acid, booze, and tobacco were on the agenda for the weekend. When we returned home, everyone had difficulty breathing from what came to be known affectionately as the PPP wheezies.

Jeff had a small cabin on the property, where he slept. Others brought campers or tents. We ate well from a Coleman camp stove that always seemed to have a delicious spread being prepared on it. All the fire department ranks were represented and only the players were allowed. We dealt cards into the night, then Jeff would bust out his guitar and play requests. *Night Moves* by Bob Segar was one of my faves, and Jeff taught me how to play it there, around the bonfire. It was surreal—and perfect.

We burned whole trees for logs. Stoking the fire was an endeavor—a feat of honor and strength. When it was time, the whole camp would select a stoker, then everyone would chant, "Stoke, Stoke, Stoke," while the chosen intoxicated fool had to lift a tree and properly place it into the pit. Cheers of nice stoke would ring out for the successful stokers, and boos for the misses and fails.

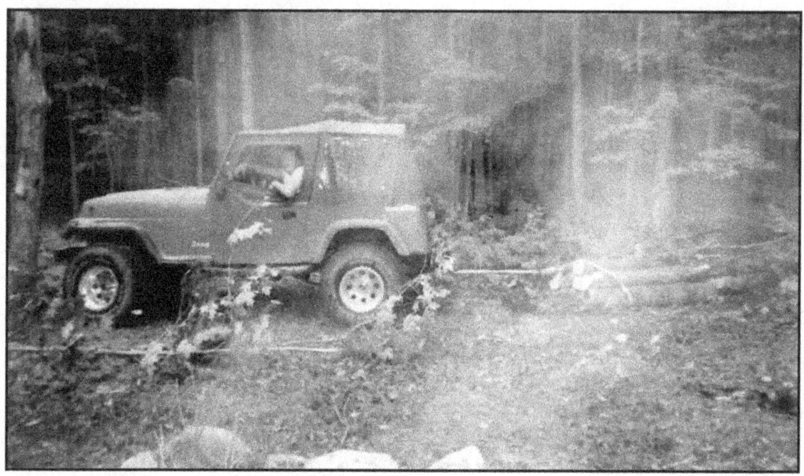

PPP firewood run with the Malibu Jeep

One night Steve Pagano went out for a walk and when he didn't come back, we went looking for him in the dark. We found him hours later, half naked—the top half thank God—drunk, and trippin' balls on mushrooms in the enchanted forest. There were forty acres of 60-foot-tall pine trees, all planted in rows, rolling over hills and valleys and stretching seemingly forever in all directions. When the moon was full, it was a magical place, hence the name. Steve could barely talk and I'm pretty sure he was hypothermic, but he otherwise appeared to be enjoying himself. We helped him back to camp and partied on deep into the night.

The next morning, as Jeff was sleeping in his cabin, Hector and I snuck in and lit up a Bob Marley, one of the four-paper joints he rolled that looked like a miniature baseball bat. I snapped a pic as Hector exhaled a massive hit into the intake port of Jeff's CPAP machine while he slept. Jeff awoke coughing and trying to figure out what the hell had just happened.

"You fuckers!" he said, when he was finally able to breathe again.

"Rise and shine," Hector said, "That's how we start our PPP day off right!"

We loaded our bellies with breakfast from the camp stove and hit the two-tracks with our four-wheel drive trucks. Climbing sand dunes, plowing through water holes on flooded trails, and shredding soybean fields playing tag in our trucks. It was an epic time of friends and fun.

If our frontline fire rig ever broke down or needed to visit the garage for maintenance, we had to transfer the equipment onto a reserve fire truck. This was an enormous pain in the ass. There are hundreds of pieces of firefighting equipment on a fire truck and most of them had to be transferred to the backup rig. A list was created of the crew who'd made the transfer, all the equipment moved, and the date it was done.

Some of the frontline fire trucks were custom built to house specialty equipment like Engine 5 with its vehicle extrication tools. The older, reserve trucks were smaller and had less space, so it was often a jigsaw puzzle trying to fit our current equipment into a tighter space. Twelve pounds of shit in a ten-pound bag, as the saying goes.

It always seemed to happen at an awful time, too. Not that there's ever a good time for our truck to break down, but it generally occurred while we were either on a call, grocery shopping, cooking a meal, or getting ready for bed. Sometimes, it happened multiple times over the course of the same shift. Like switching into a reserve in the morning while cooking lunch, then getting a call on the Signal 1 from the city garage while cooking dinner, saying our frontline rig was fixed and to come pick it up before they closed at 4pm. Which was usually closer to 3:30, or 3 p.m. if it was a Friday.

The medics were in the same boat. Old reserve ambulances were rarely, if ever, stocked with a full complement of equipment, ready to roll out the doors. AEDs (automated external defibrillators) were expensive and so were the majority of the transferable items the department refused to purchase duplicates of. Rig transfers at 02:00 hours always seemed to drag on and on since it was just two people doing the moving and cataloging of items.

Regardless of fire truck or medic unit, transferring rigs was a nightmare. It ate up huge chunks of our day, being out of service until it was completed. Sometimes, even the reserve truck would break down and we'd have to move into a third rig in twenty-four hours.

If we were on a ladder truck when our rig broke, the city only had six of those total and four of them were in service at the same time. The odds were pretty good that two of them would already be in the garage for ladder testing or mechanical issues and none would be available to switch into.

Enter the Trungine.

Many times, we either borrowed a reserve ladder truck from a neighboring department through a mutual aid, short-term lease, or switched into the dreaded Trungine. A reserve engine—most likely a smaller open cab engine—that the truck company had to use to transport all their truckie equipment on.

This was a hybrid of a truck crew and their equipment, riding on a reserve engine, because there was no aerial device available, and the union contract stated the city had to provide four ladder trucks fully staffed at all times. Hence, the Trungine—ladder truck crews and equipment placed onto an old reserve engine.

It was embarrassing to roll through the city with another municipality's name on our truck doors. But it was even worse to be a truckie on a Trungine. We felt less than men, like our giant aerial ladder had been castrated and we just couldn't handle the loss of our manhood.

It sucked, no doubt about it. We couldn't rescue people from high-rise balconies anymore or do a Rollgliss pick from a roof for the injured construction worker. No, we had to respond to the scene, then request another truck company that had a working aerial ladder to come handle our responsibilities. We were second-rate rescuers, and it was shameful.

When the garage called to say our frontline rig was done, that was the one time we were actually excited to go transfer rigs. I'd drop the spoon in the pot and shut off the stove, saying, "Fuck dinner. I'd rather starve than ride a Trungine for one more minute of my miserable existence."

The equipment transfer down at the city garage was a happy time of reunion and jubilation. With the whole crew delighted to be a fully functioning ladder truck company once again. Never mind half of the hose appliances and hand tools were missing. We had a goddamn aerial stick, a chain saw, and a pike pole. That's all a truckie really needs. Life was good again.

As my two-year hiring anniversary was approaching, I began second driver's training. I was the first person in my class to break in on all the apparatus the department owned. I passed the training division's heavy equipment operator course and was cleared to drive.

A short time later, Hector and Mumbles took me to a huge, flooded parking lot at a warehouse on Mt Hope and Washington. It'd been raining all night and there was standing water on the surface. Hector explained the same thing Dolph had earlier; that a good driver needed to know the capabilities of their rig. Then he floored it and at around 50 miles per hour he hit the water, hydroplaned, cut the steering wheel hard to the left, and we spun the fire truck in a 360-degree turn, then straightened it back out. It was awesome!

They let me cruise around the parking lot for a few minutes, just to get the hang of handling the fire truck with the pedal to the metal, then we headed down the road to the grocery store. On the way back, Hector was driving us again, when saw a pedestrian walking down the sidewalk, and a huge puddle of standing water in the road beside him.

"Watch this," Hector said, as he veered close to the curb and plowed through the puddle, drenching the pedestrian in a towering wave of filthy street curb water.

We laughed our asses off like a bunch of hooligans as we headed back to the station. It absolutely blew my mind how they could get away with the things they did.

Out of Fives again, we were called to a house a few blocks away from the station by a hysterical young lady who'd found her father dead in the bathroom. We arrived to find a home completely covered in blood spatter, with a man lying half in the bathtub and half out. The daughter explained he had DNR (do not resuscitate) orders and produced the paperwork for us.

As the medics looked the papers over, I examined the scene. The daughter revealed that her father had stage-four lung cancer and they were watching a television program on the sofa when he began coughing up blood. A pink, frothy mist was sprayed over every surface from the living room to the bathroom. Of course, the bathroom was painted white, with a white sink, white toilet, and white bathtub, only serving to accent the copious amounts of bright-red blood coating every surface, including the ceiling. We called this one, the lung cancer blood-splosion.

Occasionally, with multiple rivers converging at our city, we'd be called to perform body removals from said rivers. Such was the case one morning, when a jogger on the river trail spotted a body floating along the banks. The water rescue teams were called in. We deployed our boats at a nearby launch site and zipped off downstream in search of the victim.

Crews and civilians were gathered at the shore, near the body, and directed us right to it. The floating corpse was stuck in a tangle of dead branches about twenty feet off the shore. It was obviously bloated, with rigor and mottled skin, and had clearly passed away some time ago. We hooked the victim's belt with a pike pole and motored slowly upstream toward the shore. Where police and ambulance crews were staged in a small clearing between the brush.

The victim appeared to be a middle-aged man with no obvious signs of trauma. The CSI team wrapped the body in a tarp to preserve any physical evidence and hauled him ashore while we cruised back to the boat launch upstream. The wallet, still in his back pocket, provided a positive ID of a homeless man who'd been reported missing by his peers a week earlier.

Lisa and I continued to meet occasionally. She was a wild and untamed creature. When she called my house one day and my wife answered the phone, saying it was some girl named Lisa for me, that was it. She was just way too much crazy for me to handle. We were finished.

Speaking of done, my first marriage was a joke. It was falling apart due to my inability to say no to the constant sexual advances of women who wanted to bang, no strings attached. There are always strings my friends, always. When your spouse visits the family doctor and he tells your faithful bride she has a case of chlamydia, that's a tough one to explain away. After a few rounds of antibiotics for the both of us, we agreed to work on our (and by our, I mean *my*) commitment issues and to make things work for the sake of our daughters.

With Lisa out of the picture now and Porsche not returning my booty calls—most likely because her older sister had relayed the chlamydia story to her—the prospect of remaining committed to my marriage seemed somewhat achievable now. That was, until Sonya called one afternoon and explained she was with her sister Porsche, who'd just confessed to having an affair with me. Confused, angry, blindsided, and betrayed (probably the same way Sonya felt), I denied it all and told her to put her sister on the phone.

"It's over Brad," Porsche said, "I told her everything."

I attempted to lie and connive my way out of it, but the damage was done, and it was irreparable. Sonya and I separated and filed for divorce. I took a few days off from work and moved in with two firefighter buddies. It wasn't the best of choices looking back on it, but I didn't have many other options at the time. It was the beginning of the legendary Sin Bin. A house of ill repute where inhibitions were checked at the door and fantasies became reality.

Mumbles made the battalion chief rank soon afterward and on his last day with us, during his midday nap in the brown chair, Chase, Dan, Hector, and I duct taped his ass to the brown chair and left him there for about twenty minutes after he woke up. We explained how much we loved him, and we didn't ever want him to go. When he started to get pissed off, Chase duct taped his mouth shut. A few minutes later, Hector cut him loose and we all ran, while he chased us around the station. I could've sworn I saw a single tear fall from his eye that night.

Chapter 7

Hammer Time—Year Three

In two short years I'd managed to destroy my marriage and had fallen so far from grace my own parents questioned my sanity. I was corrupted beyond recognition or redemption. The fire service tempted me with its forbidden fruit, and I'd fallen headlong into its fiery pit of depravity. I craved action. Something—anything—to make me feel again. I was numb to everything but the most shocking endeavors and nothing seemed to quench my thirst for danger and adventure.

Year three saw the collapse of everything I'd built in my life. I lost all that was good. I learned what true heartache was. I buried my brothers. I suffered addictions. What had once been a dream of a better life became a constant nightmare. I traded my entire family for a moment's pleasure. The next morning it became a deep and enduring pain as I sought the next high.

After Mumbles left Fives for the BC rank, Hammer became our new red shift station captain. Hammer was a hillbilly, who'd been hired in a fire academy class of one. At the time, he was engaged to the fire chief's daughter, and the chief needed to know his little girl had a husband with future financial stability. Incidentally, they broke up a short time later.

"Fuckface" Johnson was the new roving captain on Hammer's day off. A few years earlier he'd been caught screwing a city council woman by her husband, and it caused a real stink for the department. Hence the nickname. He ran an HVAC business on his days off, openly hated anyone with a skin color darker than his own, and would set up his ammunition reloading equipment and repack spent rifle rounds all day at the fire station.

It's debatable whether it was our karma or theirs, but either way, we had a beneficiary of nepotism and an ignorant racist as our new bosses. Things were really going downhill fast in the officer's department for the crew at Fightin' Fives. It was a big ol' steaming shit sandwich, and we all had to take a bite.

One evening at Fives, I was having an awful phone conversation with Sonya, who'd finally had enough and left me. I don't blame her. Any rational person would've done it long before. As I sat in the lounge, emotionally exhausted and distraught over the ramifications of my life choices and actions, Hector slapped me on the shoulder and said to follow him. So, I did.

We went out to the parking lot and Hector pulled out a small pipe that looked like a cigarette. He packed the tiny bowl at the tip with weed and took a drag. After clearing the pipe with a hard rap on the side of the one-hitter's wooden well, he repacked it and handed it to me along with a lighter. I took a long pull and coughed my lungs out as Hector laughed.

"You don't get off 'til you cough," he said.

He took another hit, passed it back to me, and I followed suit. He lit two cigarettes and handed one to me. As we stood in the darkness, the marijuana taking hold of my worries and washing them away, he said something profound. He explained how a friend had consoled him during his divorce. His buddy simply told him that if something was meant to be, it would be. And if it wasn't, there wasn't a damn thing anyone could do about it. So I should stop trying to wrap my head around the situation and let it go. Just let fate take care of it.

I felt woozy and crouched down between the cars. I was all fucked up from Hector's one hitter and could barely stand up.

Hector laughed and said in a Guido accent, "Hey, Tommy Two-Hits, maybe you should just stick to one, ya lightweight."

Just then an alarm came in.

"Come on, big guy, time to go," he said, pulling me to my feet.

We took one last drag on our smokes and entered the station. I was high as fuck now and had to respond on an emergency run. We jumped into the engine and drove for a short time to an apartment on Alpha Street. I helped the medic crew carry their gear in and stood back while they assessed the patient. He was high on blotter acid and mushrooms and was having a bad trip.

I looked at Hector and he gave me a wink and a smile. I was certain he was trying to figure out which of us was higher, me or the patient. We helped the young man down the stairs and into the sled. The medics cleared us, and I was never so relieved to be done with a call. We headed back to the station, and I fell into bed.

What the *fuck* was I doing?

Somehow, though, I felt more at peace and able to cope with the difficult circumstances, and had just functioned through a run, high as balls. I remembered Hector telling me how damn near everyone is high, all the time. Maybe he was right.

From that day on, every day I worked with Hector, we were blazing weed whenever the opportunity presented itself. The basements and boiler room closets were ideal spots because we could blow our smoke into the vents. We packed small cardboard tubes with dryer sheets and exhaled through them. We couldn't smell the cannabis, just the dryer sheets.

I picked up a one hitter from the local smoke shop and packed the well full of ground ganja. Cigarettes provided cover smoke and a nice finish to our buzz. A breath mint or chewing gum, some cologne to mask the scent, and we were golden. We blazed in hose towers, rooftops, back porches, side porches, laundry rooms, decon rooms, parking lots, cars, captain's rooms with fans blowing out the open windows—nowhere was off limits. Aside of course, from sitting down right at the dinner table and lighting up. If we were smart about it, and were still functional, no one knew or even cared.

I got to know the down boys, too. Working with Hector, all the stoners would appear when the signal was given, and the boys would blaze. People I never would have imagined showed up to hit the peace pipe and bum a ciggy. Chiefs, captains, lieutenants, engineers, and firefighters, pretty much everyone was high. Hector was right. As I made friends and in-roads into the stoner clique, doors began to open, and things I never thought possible, came to life.

Pretty much every day I came to work, from 2000 to 2018, I was high as fuck. So was at least half our fire department. For me it was weed; for others it was pills, or coke, or porn, or alcohol, or sex, or shrooms, or acid trips, but everyone was getting their fix. It was mind blowing. On the medic? High as balls. Truckie for the shift? Even better. Sometimes we'd have to sneak, other times we did it right in the open with the whole crew. It all depended on the risk factors of the situation at the time.

We banged chicks, snorted coke, smoked weed, sold drugs, and partied nonstop, all while on duty. If someone caught us, we either bribed them with their known vice of choice or threatened to blackmail and expose their intimate secrets to their most prized and beloved relationships. It was a lawless time of unbridled recklessness, and there were no rules. Even the cops were in on it and partied like rock stars with us. The BCs at the time were all PPP attendees and most likely just dropped by the station for a quick pick-me-up before the staff meeting, or for a nice cool down afterward. People simply did whatever the hell they wanted. Speaking of that…

Freelancing was a big problem for the fire service in the past. Fire companies used to just show up and do whatever they felt needed to be done to put the fire out. The Incident Command System was developed to fix the lack of accountability on the fireground and provide a chain of command structure that assigned crews to tasks based on priority and risk assessment. Breaking ranks and freelancing to get the job done, while increasingly frowned upon as the years went on, was sometimes necessary to win the battle on the fireground.

I know every firefighter wearing a white shirt just gasped in horror and disbelief at my last statement, but anyone who's been neck deep in shit before knows I'm right. I'd trust my gut feeling over a guy in a white shirt any day. You know who wears white shirts? People who don't get dirty anymore. Well, I do. When I'm done on a fireground, I'm usually the filthiest motherfucker on the scene. Because I do whatever it takes to win there, and leaders in white shirts with true wisdom respect that shit from their ass-kicking task level troops.

There were times on fire scenes where things were getting out of control, shit was hitting the fan, and the only way we were gonna turn it around was to kick the fucking door in, yell say hello to my little friend, and spray the place down with lead. Yes, I know Tony Montana died in that *Scarface* scene, but he looked cool as fuck doing it. I suppose that's the risk we take when we freelance, so it had better be worth it.

Chase and I were assigned to Medic 5 and had just finished eating lunch when a full alarm fire came blaring through the station speakers. It was a structure fire in our first due and the table cleared in a rush of bodies and flying chairs. Medic 11 from downtown had just cleared the mid-town hospital and decided to jump the run.

"Medic 11, clear, we'll take that call." Dispatch acknowledged them; oblivious that we were still closer to the scene than they were.

"Nah, *fuck* that shit!" Chase cried. "We're going!" As we pulled out of the station, Medic 11 raced by.

"Go, go, go!" Chase yelled.

We pulled up just behind Engine 5, because on fire runs the ambulances had to let the engines go first. Agent Mulder on Medic 11 gave the initial scene size-up report, having barely beaten both crews from Fives to the scene by a mere truck length.

Engine 5's Hammer and Dan Martinez pulled pre-connect and made entry on the 3-story house, with smoke and fire showing from the charlie side of the upstairs apartment. They advanced to the fire floor and attacked the fire. On Truck 9, Lt. Fuckface and Connie Wagner went to the roof to vent the fire. They cut a two-foot by two-foot hole with a chainsaw over the opposite end of the building from the fire and did *not* bring a pike pole with them to break through the ceiling.

See, a vent hole is supposed to be big, and at the highest point, directly over the seat of the fire. This lets the heat and deadly smoke follow a natural path of exit, since the heat rises. After they cut the roof decking, they needed to break through the interior ceiling drywall and plaster with a long pike pole so the smoke could escape. Our engine crew was screaming over the radio for a vent, and we could see none was forthcoming.

The safety officer on the scene was Mumbles, one of the best damn firefighters around, anywhere. This guy had his vocal cords *seared* in a structure fire as a child—that's why they called him Mumbles—and had dedicated his whole life to the craft of firefighting. He gave us the green light to go up on the roof and re-cut the vent hole proper.

We sprinted to our ambulance and donned firefighting gear. We lugged the chainsaw and twelve-foot-long pike pole up to the roof and repositioned the roof ladder directly over the seat of the fire. I held tight to the rung of the ladder with one hand,

and Chase's Scott Pak harness with the other. So that if he fell, I'd pull hard and swing him back onto the roof ladder below me.

Chase deftly cut through the roof decking, carefully backing the saw blade up and over the trusses so he didn't weaken the roof by cutting through them. He zipped off an eight-foot by eight-foot hole, with louver cuts in the roof decking to help the air flow. When he stepped back onto the ladder, I popped open the louvers with the pike pole, then drove its spike hard through the attic space and into the ceiling. An entire four by eight-foot sheet of drywall fell loose and dropped to the second story floor. Through the thick black smoke, I could see Dan Martinez and Hammer looking up at us.

That's where I popped my firefighting-on-the-ambulance cherry. The first of many dangerously awesome freelancing adventures. The battalion chiefs knew when a hero broke ranks and saved the whole goddamn scene. We got the obligatory, freelancing-the-fireground, ass-chewing from BC Chuck Sanders afterward, but the good officers like Mumbles always stuck up for their boys. Usually ending said ass-chewing with a "Helluva job guys!"

Out of Fours one day, Pants and I were on the medic. While returning home from the hospital, we noticed a plume of smoke coming from the road up ahead of us. Just as we were about to call Dispatch, a full alarm came across the airwaves for a fire at Tony's party store, in our first due, just blocks away. Having a tremendous jump on everyone, we pulled into the parking lot before Dispatch even finished their broadcast.

Heavy smoke was rolling from the front double doors of the store. Pants gave a first-in size-up over the radio and we changed into our fire gear. We approached the front doors and crouched low as we entered the structure. Pants went one way down the aisles, and I went the other, looking for victims. We met at the back of the store and hadn't found anyone.

Bud Adams was at the front door, and we could hear him say, "They went where?!"

Pants looked at me and asked if I could breathe.

"Not really," I replied, "You?"

"No. Let's get out of here," Pants suggested.

We headed toward the exit, down the cooler aisle, opposite from the entry path that the nozzle crew had taken. We could hear them breathing through their Scott Paks like Darth Vader walking past us through the smoke. We made it back to the front doors and exited the store.

Outside, we were certain the BC would have our ass for making entry on the sled. We passed Engine 4 as Bobby Franklin stood at the pump panel and advised we were, "in a heap of trouble." As we crossed the parking lot and approached our ambulance, Battalion Chief Larry Simmons made his way over.

"Aw shit, were fucked," Pants said, as we removed our gear and turned to face the firing squad.

Larry quickly dispelled any fears we may have had with a "Great job boys!"

Pants and I just stared with raised eyebrows as he went on about how we really saved the day, and we could be out of service until we got back to the station, took a shower, and changed.

"Holy shit," Pants said as Larry walked away. "Didn't see that one coming."

Bud and his crew put the fire out and then a whole slew of recruits from the next fire academy class showed up to help with overhaul activities. We cleared the scene and headed back to Fours. After a hot shower, we were back in service. Over dinner that evening, Bud just laughed at our story and advised we should've waited for a hose line before going in.

"You guys live in a tree," Bobby said, in reference to us being lucky and avoiding getting in trouble with the brass. She was right.

After an elementary school fire safety presentation, I was on the sled with Bubbles out of Station 5. The presentation was over, and the engine was still hooked to a hydrant, flowing water from the deck gun onto the playground field where kids were playing in it. The ground had turned to mud when Captain Fuckface turned to me and said, "I'll give you twenty bucks if you throw Bubbles in that mud."

I looked at Bubbles and she gave me the "Don't you dare" look, shaking her head no.

Chase Powers said he'd double it to $40.

I looked back at Bubbles and shrugged my shoulders. I fireman carried her, kicking and screaming, into the mist and mud, setting her down gently on her back in a puddle. The kids ran over and joined in, tackling us both. As we struggled to stand up a mud wrestling match broke out. We laughed as we made our way back to the engine crew, covered in mud.

I collected the winnings and handed Bubbles $20, saying, "Here, don't be mad at me."

Another time on 5 Engine we were called to a home for a decomposing body. This guy was *really* dead, though. The mailman called 9-1-1 after his letters hadn't been collected for a week. He peeked through the front porch window and discovered the resident's body in the recliner, bloated, and being defiled by hundreds of flies.

It was mid-summer, and we could smell the decomp from the road when we pulled up. We needed to Scott up with our air tanks to avoid ralphing all over the scene. Hammer said he'd open the windows while I placed the medic's three lead on the man and ran a strip of asystole. That, my friends, was harder than it sounded.

On a bloated corpse with the skin slipping off, EKG patches don't exactly like to stay on. We got the job done, though, with some minor retching, and left the ambulance Scott Paks at the scene at the request of the Medical Examiner, who'd just eaten a big lunch.

New Year's Eve in 2000 was a crazy night. There was all this concern about how the computer programming wouldn't be able to handle the coding change when the clocks kicked over to 2000. People speculated the electrical grid could go down, black outs might happen, chaos would erupt, and electrical appliances would go haywire, but none of that ever happened.

Incidentally, there was a lot of chaos, but it was from the usual suspects, not a computer glitch. At 00:30 hours on 5 Engine, we were called out for a brawl at the old Greyhound bus station, which had recently been turned into a bar. Medic 5 came with us for an injured patient in the back. Hammer, Chase Powers, and I were on the engine. Dan Martinez and Vince "Big Daddy" Garlitz (nicknamed after the WWF wrestler Big Daddy Don Garlitz) were on the sled.

When we pulled up, there were people fighting everywhere. Hundreds of them. We could barely pull the truck off the street. We grabbed axes and Halligan tools and escorted the medics to the entrance. Cops were randomly showing up, one at a time, and trying to break up the combatants. When a group of police saw us, they came over to help escort, with guns drawn.

We approached the front door and made our way inside, dodging thrown bodies and people tackling each other to the ground. It was like an old western movie with a bar fight in a saloon—everybody was going at it. On the other side of the bar, about a hundred feet away, a police officer was waving both hands in the air to get our attention.

"There!" said one of the cops, pointing across the bar.

We moved in with our pick head axes and spiked Halligans sparkling in the dance floor strobe lights. People stopped mid punch and stared as we made our way through the crowds. Once we'd passed by with our firefighting gear and ambulance stretcher, they went right back at it again. We made it to the patient who was lying on a high-backed bench seat. The police formed a perimeter with our engine crew, while the medics assessed the injured man.

He had a nasty laceration to his face and scalp from a broken bottle. The medics wrapped a trauma dressing around his split melon, slapped a C-collar on his neck and loaded him on the cot. When they were ready, we pushed back into the fray, which was amazingly, still going on. The cops went first to clear the path. The engine crew surrounded the patient, being wheeled on the cot by the medics.

Outside, it was a full-blown riot. More police had shown up, and so had more people. A bottle whizzed over the cot and hit one of the cops in the back of the head. His colleagues stopped to help him, and we pressed on without our escort. Making it back to the rigs, we loaded the patient and immediately drove to a safe distance a few blocks away. We helped the medics treat the patient, then cleared when they went to the hospital.

Later that night, Medic 5 was T-boned in an intersection by a drunk driver as they were heading to a call. We responded to the scene and discovered their rig was totaled, and the guy who'd hit them had fled the scene. He didn't get very far after crashing his sedan into an ambulance, though. The car was nearby, disabled in the road, a trail of oil and antifreeze drawing a line on the pavement between it and the sled. The driver had bailed and fled on foot.

Those poor guys had been running all day and night, and now they had to transfer rigs at 03:00. That task sucked at midday. The BC gave them a ride to Ones to switch into a reserve while we waited at the scene for police and a wrecker. It took a while, since most of the cops in the city were either still at the bar brawl, or in the hospital from the brawl.

When I hired on, there was a sense of brotherhood that slowly evaporated as the years went on. Guys would hang out on their days off and take vacations together. The wives would go places together and hang out while their husbands were in the firehouse. There was an event, gathering, or party every month. Some of them, like sports leagues, lasted for several months.

There were Squid Band gigs on the weekends, group vacations to Canada and Mexico, PPP, deer camp, day trips to local lakes, concerts, ski trips, the Borderline Funfest, the red and black shift Christmas parties, the Firefighter's Ball, groups chartering busses to professional and minor league sporting events. There were local leagues for softball, bowling, racquetball, soccer, pickup games of basketball at the police precinct gym, snow bowl football games, and a semi-pro football team in a league of police and fire departments. There was *always* somewhere to go and something fun to do. That all faded away toward the end of my time there.

Chase and I went out one evening to the Silver Dollar night club to see the Squid Band play. Some of our coworkers had shown up in tuxedos from a wedding party, and their wives were dressed up, too. Everyone was having a great time. Then some drunk asshole and his friends pushed their way right through the center of our group and shoved one of the firefighters' wives.

It was one of the dumbest things I'd ever seen. In an instant, forty firefighters were beating the shit out of this guy. His friends all jumped in next and before we knew it, even the ladies were throwing blows and breaking bottles over heads. To my left, Benny O'Brien had a guy by the throat and was using his face as a speed bag. To my right, Chase was repeatedly kicking a man on the floor in the head. Right in front of me, a guy lifted a bottle in the air to hit Chase from behind. I threw a right hook, landing it squarely on his nose. His face imploded and he fell to the ground. I grabbed Chase and we made a break for the door.

A few minutes later, outside the bar, the guy I'd hit was walking around with ice on his head. He didn't recognize us from the brawl and struck up a conversation. Come to find out, he was the son of a Fire Commissioner for our department. Even better, he'd just been hired in the latest recruit class. Later, Chase would often joke right in front of him, about me denting his face that night.

I remember when a married Fuckface told us in the morning we were having a guest over for lunch and he was kicking in a couple extra bucks for their mess money. When we asked who was coming, he pulled a picture of Tina Price, a classmate of mine, from his wallet. She later reported him for stalking because he'd randomly show up at her house unannounced and mow her lawn, or shovel snow from her sidewalks, after she'd told him to leave her alone. HR busted him down to lieutenant for life for sexual harassment. Everybody knew Tina was already banging the red shift Battalion Chief Barry Wahlberg. Why would she ever sully herself with him? He was delusional. That, right there, is why you never fuck with a BC's throwdown.

Barry Wahlberg was an amazing man. A battalion chief when I hired on, he was one fourth of *The Corporation*. All four were independently wealthy by the time they'd hit retirement age. As a new kid firefighter, I'd helped them with the flooring in several of their properties. Barry was a member of the PPP crew, and we smoked a metric shit-ton of weed together over the years. He was the connection that brought my wife, Lee, and me together, and we still talk occasionally to this day.

Racism was unfortunately still rearing its ugly head when I hired on. Most of our staff saw sexism and racism for what it really was: ignorant stereotypes that have no place on the battleground of life. Our partner was our partner. We shared a foxhole, and it didn't matter what color or gender they were as long as they performed and could be counted on when needed.

I recall a time at Station 5 when Fuckface had us doing rope school all day long because he disliked Marky Mark, who happened to have darker colored skin. He sent us to the roof to work on hauling tools up over the edge. Marky Mark had a difficult time tying the clove hitch properly, and Fuckface wanted him to work on it—all day, in the summer heat, on the roof.

I asked Marky Mark if this happened to him often, because Fuckface had never done this to me when I worked with him.

"Every day I work, everywhere I go," Marky Mark replied.

I asked if he ever thought about filing paperwork for discrimination, and he said no, he just wanted to do his job the best he could and endure the hard times. It made him stronger, he said. I thought it was terrible.

Sometimes, the lineup comes out for the shift, and before we even get started, we just know it's going to be a long day. Such was the case when Fuckface was the boss and Jack Goff was the engineer on 5 Engine. Jack was perpetually giving me shit. He was one of those people who just had to make people look bad, to help him feel good about himself. A real egomaniac, he was my sole nemesis on the department.

Jack's older brother Dick—also a jerk, perhaps it was genetic—worked at the department, too. Dick Goff was a mortician on his days off, which was just plain creepy. As if this job didn't expose us to enough death already. I pictured him with his Crypt Keeper hands, sliding grieving family members a business card for his side gig after a patient of his passed away. When the two brothers made the officer ranks, we called them collectively the Gofficers. Sometimes they were the captain and lieutenant at the same station, on the same day. Then we were double fucked.

Back to Jack and Fuckface.

We caught a mid-afternoon full alarm fire on Kindle Avenue at the old Bread Factory. I could see the plume of smoke when we were halfway there and readied for a first-in attack line stretch. To my surprise, Jack blew right past Kindle, and continued up to the next main street. *OK, no big deal,* I thought, *maybe his way is faster*. He is the engineer after all.

As we approached the factory, smoke was billowing from the eaves of the building, and this dumb motherfucker turned the wrong way. He went the opposite direction from the building right on the corner that was on fire. I lost it!

"What the *fuck*, Jack, you just drove right past it!" I yelled from the back as he continued to drive farther down West Kindle. "Didn't you see the smoke pouring out of it!?"

I was disgusted these two idiots had just cost me a first-in fire, and now I was going to have to hear it from some other nut-sack new kid about how he beat me into my own area and stole my nozzle time. I saw Jack look into his rearview mirror and see the dark smoke rising from the end of the street behind him.

5 Engine was the extrication engine because it was located in the center of town. It was considerably longer than the other two extrication rigs because it carried twice as much gear as the others for all the specialty equipment. Kindle was narrower than most other neighborhood streets in the city, with only enough width for three cars to fit shoulder to shoulder, instead of the usual four car widths.

Jack decided halfway down the block that he was going to twelve-point turn the rig around right there, instead of circling the block and heading back to the fire. He told me to jump out and back him up, and I suggested just going up to the next cross street—that the road's too narrow.

"Get the fuck out and back me up," he said. So I do.

Fuckface just sat there in the boss's seat because he's too lazy to get out, and I circled around back to the driver's side and started to back this idiot up. On about the sixth cycle of back-and-forths, he's almost perpendicular across the road and the second-due rig just gave a first-in scene size-up over the radio and pulled their pre-connect.

I gave Jack the two-handed signal for stop and he kept coming.

I yelled "STOP!" with both hands in the air and he kept coming.

I yelled and waved both arms as he smashed into a tree, breaking off one of the rear lights and denting the diamond-plated tailboard.

Both morons got out to inspect the damage, and I knew then I wasn't even going to make the scene, let alone be first-in. We straightened the truck back out and called for a battalion chief and police for an accident report. The BC was busy commanding the fire scene, which had just been extinguished and was currently being overhauled, and the police were tied up as well. So with a rear floodlight swinging from its wiring and a crinkled-up tailboard, we limped back to the station and waited for them to meet us there.

As I finished preparing the noon meal, Fuckface and Jack sat at the dinner table discussing how best to handle the situation.

"I have to write you up, Jack," Fuckface confessed.

"Well, then you have to write Brad up, too, because he was backing me up," Jack said.

Hearing the ignorance ooze from Jack's mouth, I lost it again.

"Then he'd have to write himself up too for not getting out of the rig like the protocol says. And what the fuck are you gonna write me up for, huh? I did my job. I told you to fucking stop three times asshole. YOU, missed the goddamn fire, YOU blew the first-in attack, and YOU wrecked the truck!"

"I don't have to take this shit from you, new kid," Jack said, turning back to Fuckface.

"Put me on sick leave, Cap," I said, unbuttoning my uniform shirt and slamming it on the table. "You and me, apparatus floor, NOW!" I said, looking Jack dead in his eyes from a foot away. "I don't have to take this shit from YOU, and it ends right here, right now," I yelled angrily as I kicked the swinging door open and waited outside for Jack to follow.

When he did, he was apologetic. Coming at me with a "Hey, ol' buddy, what's wrong?"

"Fuck you. I'm not putting up with your shit anymore. That's what," I replied.

"What do you mean?" he asked, his open hands outstretched as I readied my fists to rearrange his face.

"You're always dumping shit on me to make yourself look better, instead of owning up to your mistakes!" I yelled. "And I'm sick of it. It ends now."

"You're right," Jack said, "I'm sorry."

"What?" I asked, perplexed at the sudden turn of events.

"You're right," he repeated, "I have been doing that and I'm sorry. Can we get past this and go back inside?"

Surprised I wouldn't need a union steward, a BC, and an attorney to keep my job, I agreed to give him a second chance. It actually worked, and though I could tell it pained him greatly, he never openly fucked with me again. Although I'm sure he secretly wanted to. I could see it in his beady little eyes.

The battalion chief finally arrived and so did the police for the accident report, and Jack received his write up for crashing the rig. I suppose all's well, that ends well. Sometimes the details aren't exactly the way we'd like it to have played out, but variety is the spice of life, and I believe everything happens for a reason—however unclear that reason may be at the time.

Jack did fuck with Bubbles, though, and various other firefighters he perceived as weaker and less intelligent than himself. One day at Sixes, Jack was the lieutenant and Bubbles was his engineer on Engine 6. Bubbles had worn a long-sleeve T-shirt she'd recently purchased from the fire department clothing store run by DanHanna, the partnership of Lieutenants Dan Cooper and Joe Hanna that provided alternative clothing choices with the fire department's logo on them.

Jack contended to the station captain that because it wasn't officially issued department clothing, Bubbles needed to change out of it, and into official gear. It was balls ass cold out that day, like 6 degrees, and I'd been wearing my DanHanna winter cap all day on the medic.

Bubbles, when confronted by Captain Ginger McEntire about the complaint levied against her attire, promptly claimed discrimination because, well, Brad was wearing his hat, which wasn't department issued, and if she had to change, then so did he. When I returned from being gone from ten in the morning until seven at night running ambulance calls, Ginger called me into the office and explained the situation: that, in all fairness to Bubbles, I needed to remove my winter hat.

So I did. Revealing a fucked up, matted down, head of hair. "OK, but you're going to have to look at me like this for the rest of the shift," I said. "Just out of curiosity, does Jack still have that giant-ass belt buckle on his waist? Because that shit is not the department-issued belt buckle we all have on ours. Just sayin'."

"Go comb your hair, Brad," Ginger replied, "and don't give me anymore shit about this; it's been a long day."

This is yet another reason I considered freezing my rank at firefighter. Petty-ass morons making an officer's life more difficult than it already was. Like little children finding all the tiny chinks in their parents' armor until they give in and give them what they want. Why would I want to be the boss of a bunch of idiots?

I went to the gear cabinet on the ambulance and dug out my Nomex hood. I pulled it down over my head, so only my face stuck out like a ski mask and went to get some food. While I ate, Ginger came into the dining room and saw me.

"Oh no," she said, "You can't run around here like that either."

"It's like minus thirteen degrees wind chill out there, Cappy. Its department issued and if you have problem with it, you can call me a BC and a union steward. It's your call.

She backed down and I switched in and out of the Nomex hood and the winter hat, depending on whose company I was in, for the rest of the shift. Making sure to let Bubbles and Jack know at the breakfast table the next morning to keep my fucking name out of their mouths and to grow the fuck up and treat each other with some human decency and respect.

One day at Fives, as evening fell, I received a phone call from Amy Goodyear. Amy was a local police officer and the sister of Chris "Wheels" Goodyear, a probationary firefighter on the department at the time. She mentioned she was getting off from work around 01:00 and was wondering if she could swing by the station and hang out. I agreed and when she arrived, I let her in the back door. Backdoor guests are always the best.

I offered her food and drink from the leftovers of the day, and we engaged in rhetorical conversation until she finally asked, "So, where's a good spot to bang around here?"

I smiled, took her by the hand, walked to the downstairs bathroom, and closed the door. Her gun belt hit the ceramic tile floor with a heavy clunk and her pants fell with it. Afterward, she promptly dressed and bid me adieu, turning to wink at me as she left the station.

Chase had been listening outside the door and the next morning told Willy P (the notorious mouth of the east side) who wrote the incident into the next Christmas poem. Chris Goodyear and I were standing next to each other during the reading of it. When the part about gun belts on the floor of Station 5's bathroom was read, I tried to say something consoling.

"Stop," he interrupted, "She's a big girl, and she makes her own choices."

True enough, my man. True enough.

I was three years into my career and had gone from bible studies to bar brawls. From church choirs to gang bangs and strippers. Perhaps I'd been living a lie all along. Maybe I was living one now. I was losing my identity. Tossed around like a rudderless ship on the open sea. My emotions and attitudes swung wildly from one end of the spectrum to the other. There was no meaning or purpose to my life anymore. Just extreme highs and abysmal lows.

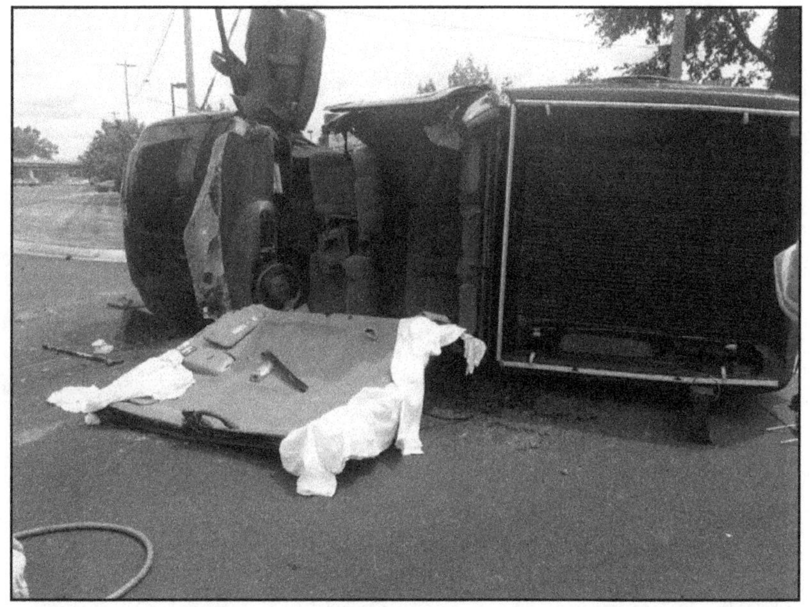

Vehicle extrication; door pop and roof flop

Chapter 8

The Sin Bin

The Sin Bin was named by Squid Band bassist Brent Gillette after he'd attended a few parties there. Some described it as a sort of Playboy Mansion, without the mansion part. It was my high school buddy RP's former grandparents' home, which he'd rented from them when they'd moved to Florida for retirement. Steve Burnworth from EMT school had just been hired at the fire department and rounded out our tenant list. It was a wild and crazy time.

Steve worked on the black shift and RP and I were red shifters with different schedules. So there were only two days a week when everybody was home. Those were the party days. Typically, for twenty-four hours straight, we were drunk, high, and fucking everything that moved. It was glorious and terrible, raucous and sublime. A living, breathing, dichotomy.

One day I arrived home from work to find Steve greeting me in the garage. "Dude, RP brought a chick home, and she wants you," he said excitedly.

"Aw, thanks, but I'm not really in the mood right now," I said, heading inside. RP was in the kitchen and repeated what Steve had just said. They followed me to my room and explained how RP had brought home a married bank teller from the credit union and she was in the upstairs bathroom.

She'd been promised a gang bang and was screwing anyone who wanted to. RP and Steve had already taken their turns, and RP's little brother Cory was in there at the moment. I politely declined again. Steve continued on about how she was going to be disappointed if I didn't, and that I should at least go in and get some head, then slapped a string of condoms against my chest. "C'mon, bro, for the Sin Bin," he pleaded.

"All right," I reluctantly agreed, and headed upstairs.

Cory was walking out of the bathroom and said, "She's all yours," with a smile.

I entered the dimly lit room, and a woman was standing there in front of me, naked.

"So, you're next," she said, looking me up and down. "I do like a man in a uniform," she admitted as I closed the door.

"What's your name," I asked as she stepped closer and began to unbutton my work shirt.

"Does it matter?" was the sultry reply.

"Not really," I responded as she yanked my pants to the floor and went downtown. Afterward, I felt dirty all over, inside and out, and headed off to shower. Twice.

We ran through so much ass at the Sin Bin, it soon became known throughout the city as *the* place to party for nurses, cops, or firefighters. There were always people there, never sober, always partying, crashing for the night, ready to hook up whether guy or girl, straight or lesbo. Cars were constantly parked in the front, side, and back. Sometimes folks stayed for days at a time, going on benders, and completely abandoning their families and jobs. A regular *House of the Rising Sun*. There were different women there every night, and we slept with them all. Some we knew, some we didn't. Everyone came there for a good time, and always left satisfied.

One night, Chase's friend, we'll call him Casa Nova, stopped by. Nova had a penchant for the booger sugar and was a guy who could get some if we needed it. He explained to us how, earlier that night, he'd hooked up with a young lady he'd met on an adult website. She turned out to be a local county sheriff's deputy who was into bondage.

He said he drove to her house, they role played, and had a great time. He told us he'd duct taped her to the dining room chair and they played all kinds of kinky games.

"In fact, she's still there," he mentioned.

"Oh, and she was on duty when all this went down," he continued.

"And she's still on duty," he went on.

"Oh, and I took her police cruiser for a little joyride, and it's parked in your front yard… and I have her gun, too."

He pulled a Glock 9mm from the back of his jeans and showed us all right there in our kitchen. I looked out the window and sure enough, there was a County Sheriff's police cruiser in the middle of our front yard.

"What the *fuck* Nova!" we all yelled at him. "What are you thinking? Get the fuck out of here man!" we advised, as he just laughed at the folly of his misdeeds.

He told us to chill out and then calmly agreed to head back over to the officer's house, release her, and return the stolen property.

"You were never here!" RP yelled as Nova left and drove off into the night in the Sheriff's car.

Dispatch had been trying to get the deputy on the radio to respond to emergency calls for hours when Nova showed back up at her place and was promptly arrested. Apparently, he had answered several of the calls over the radio and told the dispatchers where they could find their deputy. She was subsequently fired for her compromising role, and Nova received a nice prison sentence for kidnapping and stealing a Sheriff's patrol car for his epic joyride.

On one of our days off, Brent Gillette, Chase Powers, Steve Burnworth, RP, and I headed over to Duck Lake to enjoy some water sports and sunshine. We hooked an inner tube to the back of Gillette's boat and took turns cruising around the lake. More people showed up than we could safely fit on the boat, so we set up our lawn chairs on a sand bar near the shore and posted up there with coolers of refreshments.

As the sun sank low in the sky, we made our way back to the public access boat launch and carried our gear to the cars. A conservation officer was checking the fishing boats for limits and licenses, and we waved as we passed by. After loading the gear, everyone needed to empty their bladders; however, the public restroom was padlocked shut. RP and I walked a few yards into the tree line, just ahead of our cars, and stood behind trees, watering the earth. Steve was less discreet and stood right at the tree line, with his back to the parking lot.

"Hey!" came a yell from the CO as he walked past. "Stay right there. I'll be back to talk with you," he told Steve. Then he headed back down to the boat launch with a stack of tickets fluttering in his hand.

"C'mon, Steve, let's go!" RP said as he and I hopped into my Jeep. Steve drunkenly declined and said he'd rather just wait and talk it out with the guy.

We headed back to the Sin Bin, and Steve arrived home a short time later with a ticket in his hand. He explained how the "motherfuckin' C.O." had written him a fine for public indecency and advised Steve he was now on the state sex offender list for whipping out his johnson in public and pissing in the woods. Steve had to get an attorney and go to court to get the charges reduced. Thousands of dollars later, he was removed from the naughty list and only had to pay a fine and check in with his probation officer once a month for the next year.

I'm just gonna end this chapter here. Believe me, the less said about this part of my life, the better. Things began to change for me. And I knew then, this rock star life was going to be my downfall. If I didn't pull up or bail out of the tailspin I was in, soon, I was going to crash and burn. I'd ruined my relationship with my first wife, Sonya, and the Sin Bin was not the place to have my two young daughters come and stay for a family visitation. I needed to make amends and began to plan my return home.

I gave Steve and RP notice I was moving out and reconciled with Sonya. I moved back home and tried hard to make things work again. It was a difficult proposition to juggle a marriage, parenting two young children, a career that took me away for days at a time, addictions to sex/porn/drugs, and a compounding case of PTSD from all the traumatic calls at the fire department. But I was hopeful and determined to give it my best shot.

CHAPTER 9

Dad and Lad—The Yankovic Years

When Fuckface got busted back down to lieutenant for stalking Tina, Carl Yankovic showed up as the new roving captain at Fives. It was still Hammer's station, but Carl filled in on his day off. Carl took an instant liking to me because I gave him exactly what he asked for and was willing to do damn near anything on the firegrounds. We had met at deer camp with Chuck Sanders, and I'd roved into Station 2 several times where Carl was the lieutenant. We got along famously.

One morning he asked me to tidy up the front office while he finished his morning paperwork duties. As I followed orders, my ambulance partner Pants started giving me shit from the breakfast table about how I was "Stokes-ing" them (a reference to Pam Stokes, who would get stoned on duty, then go around the station doing busy work on her own, making the rest of her crew appear lazy). By continuing to work while they ate breakfast, they felt like I was making them look bad in the eyes of the captain.

I ignored Pants and continued to work, straightening the papers on the desk, and organizing the items on the office windowsills, recalling the personal time I'd spent with Captain Stokes at her townhome. Pants yelled from the breakfast table how I was sucking Carl's dick and licking his balls to gain favor, unaware the captain was right next to me, out of sight.

Carl came around the corner and lost it on Pants, charging into the kitchen and shaming him for mocking me while I was following a direct order. Questioning his own laziness for just sitting there while work still needed to be done, and basically ripping him a new asshole for what seemed like several minutes.

When I joined the group at the breakfast table, the legend of Dad and Lad had been born, and Pants told everyone who had ears about it. If they ever did before, nobody fucked with me now. Carl was my bodyguard and headed everything off at the pass. If anyone ever tried to come between us, they met with his full fury, which was significantly brutal. Later in his career, as a BC, he'd be given the nickname "The Iron Fist."

Assigned to a medic unit downtown one night, while relaxing in a brown chair and watching TV, a voice began yelling unintelligibly over the fire department radio. The dispatcher requested the voice to repeat—that they were unreadable. It was Stan Cosgrove on Medic 4. He screamed they'd just hit a pedestrian while en route to their emergency call and needed another medic to respond in their place, another medic for their victim, the police, an engine, and a BC.

Dispatch quickly confirmed and scrambled the response on what turned out to be a horrible and successful suicide attempt involving one of our ambulances. We listened in shock as details began to trickle in through various informants and eyewitnesses.

Medic 4 had just turned onto westbound Liberty Road. They were heading lights and sirens to a medical call they'd just been toned out on. Two blocks later, while passing the Community Mental Health facility at around 40 miles per hour, a patient ran out in front of them and chose to end their life. The young man had been allowed to step out back to smoke a cigarette between therapy sessions, in an area not fenced in for the patients.

Natalia Popovich was driving the sled. Stan Cosgrove was riding shotgun. He recalls the belt pulling him back in the seat as Natalia slammed on the brakes and swerved into eastbound traffic to avoid hitting the man. Cosgrove said he heard a loud bang and what appeared to be a "bag of fur" launch off the passenger side fender and fly through the air, landing motionless in the road ahead. Natalia recalls doing a 180-degree turn and coming to rest facing eastbound.

"Oh my god," were her first words.

Stan jumped out and raced to the patient, screaming into his radio handset. He was nearly struck himself by three cars that swerved and screeched trying to miss him. Natalia quickly moved the rig to protect them from the oncoming traffic.

Stan recalls the patient was about twenty years old, lying on his side, with his right leg twisted around his back and his left leg folded up and tucked under his left arm. The patient was unresponsive and moaning, with blood coming from his nose and right ear. His facial bones were crushed and moved freely upon palpation, as Stan took C-spine control.

As Stan assessed the patient, a security guard ran out of CMH and explained he was trying to hold him back. That the young man had a history of trying to do that, and he'd pulled free in an attempt to commit suicide. Natalia and Stan worked feverishly to establish an airway, secure C-spine, and package the patient until help arrived. The patient was transported to the hospital, where he was later pronounced dead from his injuries.

After being sued by the patient's family and found innocent by a jury twice, in criminal and civil court, Natalia had a tough row to hoe. She continued along her career path, albeit somewhat jaded. When a person takes their own life, there are always unintended consequences, and a trail of destruction is left in their wake. That man stole a piece of Natalia when he chose to end his life with her ambulance.

As I wrote this story, I recalled an incident that I'd completely forgotten. It happens often with the thousands of calls I've been through, but this one was different. I have difficulty remembering when it happened. I know it was early in my career; however, I don't remember what rig I was on, or what station I was out of, or the crew that was with me that day. It could've even been during a ride-along from way back in EMT school.

It was a warm, sunny afternoon. The children at the elementary school had just been released from class and were heading home for the day. A crossing guard was helping the kids navigate the busy street in front of the school when a motorist plowed right through them and sped away. As they drove off, a child lay dying in the road, and we were called to the scene to try to save him.

I remember the sun beaming off the nine-year-old boy's face as I approached him. He was on his back in the road just beyond the painted school crosswalk. As I took C-spine, the sunlight shone brightly on his right eye, which was protruding from its socket. The pupil was blown.

I'd never seen a blown pupil before, only read about it in textbooks. It was oddly mis-shaped, the black center of it no longer a perfect circle, more oblong, and it seemed to ooze blackness onto the light blue color of his iris. The colors were so vivid. Life around me seemed to freeze. There were no cars, no people, no sounds, just me and this little boy. I remembered from EMT school, a blown pupil was a sign of serious head trauma, and I kicked it into gear.

As I took C-spine control and started checking him over for injuries, I noticed he had clear fluid draining from his ears and nose. Cerebral spinal fluid, or CSF, was another indication of the massive head trauma this young boy had sustained. His right leg was twisted back under him, and the distal end of his broken femur was poking, jagged and bloody, through his torn blue jeans. His blond hair was matted with blood to his scalp and forehead, and it covered my gloves as I spoke to the unconscious boy and told him that it was OK, that we were going to help him.

We packaged him with a C-collar and backboard, then loaded him into the ambulance. An airway was established, two IVs were started, and a traction splint was applied to his broken leg. CPR was begun en route and continued long after patient care was transferred to the hospital staff. The boy didn't make it, and I questioned God why. He didn't answer.

On Engine 5 near midnight, we were called out on a full alarm to a state office building fire with Chase and Captain Carl. When we arrived, it was eerily quiet. We could see Lenny Smith yelling wide-eyed down to the BC's car from a balcony, about how it was really smoky, but they couldn't find any fire yet. Joe Hanna was with him, and as we grabbed the high-rise tools and made our way up to the building, we could sense fear from them like I'd never seen before. This was the first time I'd seen these heroes from Ones scared. It was in their eyes.

A still alarm had been called in by the alarm monitoring company for a smoke detector activation on the fourth floor. The *real* problem was the third floor was almost fully involved with fire below them, and they didn't know it yet. They were right to be scared. We never want to have the fire right below us, because fire burns up and out. If it burns through the floor below, we risk falling straight into the fire. We discovered it on our way up the stairs and radioed the guys above us to bring their hose lines back down to the third floor.

With two 2 ½" lines deployed, the fire went out a short time later, and we began overhaul activities. I'd never seen so many cubicles in my life. One room was like a whole football field of them. The drop ceiling frame and support wires had melted and collapsed on top of the filing cabinets and cubicles, which made moving around extremely difficult.

Nobody had their Scott masks on as we put out the hot spots. So when "Moose" Morgan yelled at me about my Scott mask being off, I just ignored him. He hollered at me again from the stairwell doors—even though there were seven other people between us who didn't have their masks on, either.

Apparently, Moose was on a medic crew and, since there were no patients, the BC had sent him up as a staging officer on the floor below to coordinate equipment and change out air bottles. Nobody was using their air, so he didn't have much to do other than pick on new kids. After he said it a third time, Chase let Carl know what was going on. Carl was instantly pissed off. He walked over to Moose and began ripping him a new one.

"Are you talking to *my* firefighter? What the *fuck* rig are you on? Do you have any idea how chain of command works around here? If your dumbass wants to say hello to my firefighter, it comes through me! You got that? What, you want him to wear his Scott mask? You don't even have a Scott Pak on your own goddamn self, and you're bothering *my* hardworking firefighter with your dumbass bullshit? Get the *fuck* out of here! You *fucking* pecker checker! Don't you *ever* come at me with some bullshit like that again or I'll have your *ass*!" Carl screamed.

Moose had backed slowly down the stairs as Carl was wrapping up his tirade and turned to run when he was done. Chase and I just laughed and went back to work as Carl returned with a calm "It's cool, were good." We finished hosing down the smoldering papers in the filing cabinets and were soon cleared by the BC. On the way home, I thanked Carl for sticking up for me, and he told me a good crew always stayed together—nothing ever came between them.

When I hired on, my captain at Threes, Chuck Sanders, was also the captain of the Honor Guard of our department. An ex-82nd Airborne soldier, he felt he was duty bound to ensure active and retired firefighters received a proper sendoff at their funerals. He recruited me, and for the next three years we performed graveside funeral proceedings.

We attended around thirty or so funerals for our fallen comrades, some for other fire department and police line-of-duty deaths around the Midwest. We performed ceremonies on Memorial Day and Veterans Day at local cemeteries, always with full regalia, dressed in our Class A uniforms, marching together as a unit in step.

Chuck carried on until he retired, then passed the torch to Wayne "Smoothbore" Pizzo. After a while, the constant connection to death in the fire service began to wear on me, and I resigned, hoping to avoid the added heartache of funeral parlors and graveside services. We volunteered out of the kindness of our hearts and weren't paid anything for our time. My home life was suffering from a lack of attendance, and it was best for me to hang it up.

Chase and I made a call out of Fives on the medic for a heroin overdose on a twenty-two-year-old female on Palmer Street, at around ten o'clock in the morning. She was unconscious in the house, lying on the sofa in her underwear, and a tourniquet was still draped over her arm. Chase threw her over his shoulder, and I helped him place her on the cot that was waiting at the porch steps. We loaded her into the sled, and I got a set of vitals as Chase drew up the Narcan.

He started an IV and pushed the meds. To my surprise, Chase took a pair of trauma shears and cut the center piece of material on the patient's purple Victoria's Secret bra while we waited for the drugs to take effect. I remember the morning sun shining in through the back windows of the ambulance and illuminating her breasts. For a moment, we were both silent and staring at the unconscious beauty that lay before us.

After a few seconds, she began to stir on the cot.

Chase yelled, "Hey! What's your name?"

As the woman opened her eyes, she looked at Chase, then at me, then down at her body. "What the hell?" were the first words she spoke, grabbing the blanket around her waist and pulling it to her chin.

"OK... what the hell... Do you know where you're at?" Chase continued.

She answered, "In an ambulance?"

"That's right, and do you know what happened today?" he asked.

"Yeah, I shot up some fucking heroin," the woman replied.

"Ding, ding, we've got a winner!" Chase joked.

The woman didn't find it very funny and hit Chase with a litany of cuss words for cutting her favorite and expensive bra. Chase explained how she was dead to the world a few minutes ago and she should be grateful that he'd saved her life.

"You cut my bra, you *fucking* asshole!" was the reply.

Chase did his best impression of Rodney Dangerfield's "I get no respect."

Riding with Bubbles out of Station 5 on the medic, we caught a run for a suicide and possible DOA on Forest Road. When we pulled up, her best friend was standing out front crying. Her father had shot himself after being diagnosed with cancer. Inside, I'll never forget it: the man was dressed all in white, sitting in a white chair, in front of a white wall. A bright red V-pattern of blood started just behind his head and continued up the wall to the white ceiling.

We stuck around for a while, after confirming the man was deceased for the cops, while Bubbles comforted her friend. He'd taken a pistol to the chin and sprayed his brains on the wall for his own daughter to find. Suicide seemed like a horribly selfish way to skip out on life. Some people went out like they lived, though, and I suppose they had their reasons.

I rode Medic 5 with Dave Ramos three days before he committed suicide on February 20, 2002. He just hadn't been himself; he didn't smile or laugh at any of my dirty jokes. He just sat there, stone faced and dejected, all shift long. Later, I'd be able to recognize the deep ruts of depression like I was looking at my own child. I'd just thought he was really bummed about something.

He went on Kelly the next morning and never came back. He'd mentioned when we rode together that his wife said she wanted a divorce, and he thought she was cheating on him. In the throes of my own affairs at the time, I advised Dave to cheer up, look at it as an opportunity to live his best life, get a hooker or have his own throwdown on the side. He was a family guy, though, dedicated to his wife and kids, and didn't appreciate the idiot new kid's advice.

Three days later, his father, a retired fire department captain named Randy Ramos, found Dave's body swinging from a rope in his garage. He cut his own son down, started CPR, and called 9-1-1, but it was too late. Dave told his wife and kids goodbye, that he loved them, then went outside and hung himself. This was my first colleague to commit suicide.

There was a call one night for a man trapped beneath a car. It was at a residence in Station 2's first due, and we were toned out for a vehicle extrication response from Station 5, at the request of first-in Engine 2's Captain Charlie Peters. The man was pinned under the car from his waist down, with the upper half of his torso free, lying on his back on the driveway concrete. The lower half of his body was completely crushed by the vehicle. Rather than lift the car up and find that his crew needed to operate beneath it for an extended period of time to retrieve the man's lower extremities, he called for Engine 5 to utilize our heavy lifting air bags.

When we arrived, the medics had already started two large bore IV lines and administered morphine to the patient. We positioned our two sets of airbags, one at the front and one at the rear, and prepared to build box cribs at the four corners of the car while slowly raising it up. The medics anticipated the patient's vital signs would crash when the vehicle was lifted and alerted the hospital staff to be on standby.

We had a crew at each air bag and another at each box crib location ready for the operation. The bags were hooked to the regulators, and we began the process of lifting the car. The command and safety officers supervised and coordinated the front and rear lifting operations accordingly.

When the vehicle came up off the patient, his pelvis was flattened like a pancake and his legs were nearly severed clean through. It took two people on each leg to hold them together as they slid a backboard under him. He was loaded into the sled and transported to the hospital. Though he had a long road to recovery and faced the terrible possibility of never being able to walk again, he still survived the incident thanks to the teamwork and skill of his rescuers.

Out of Station 5 one night, Chase and I were on the medic when an alarm came in for a shooting at Lucky's Bar. We responded with the engine and police, and made our way in. There was a man in the driver's seat of a pickup truck, parked behind the bar. The windshield was riddled with bullet holes and the man was slumped over with five holes in his chest and two in his face. He sat there motionless and not breathing as we put the cardiac monitor on him and officially pronounced him deceased. Chase called the hospital for a time of death, and I packed up the equipment and stowed it away on the ambulance.

Then Chris Goodyear shouted from the driver's side door of the bullet-ridden truck, "He's alive!"

We knew he wasn't, but when someone does that, and the whole scene hears it, we have to get to work, or it looks bad on the department. We hauled the man's body out of the truck and loaded the cot into the ambulance.

"What the *fuck*, Wheels?" Chase asked as we put the corpse on the monitor, and it read asystole again.

Chris stared, dumbfounded, at the flatline on the monitor's screen. "I checked a carotid and felt a pulse," he explained.

"You felt your *own* goddamn pulse. This guy's dead as a doornail, with seven bullet holes in him," Chase replied. "Now what? We've got a dead body in our sled that we already have a time of death for. We can't transport because it's a crime scene, and the hospital doesn't want him." We were stuck.

Chris apologized as he and the engine cleared and returned to the station. We ended up sitting on scene for two hours, out of service, in the middle of the night. Waiting for the coroner to show up and take possession of the dead man in our ambulance. It's a surreal feeling, sitting in the cab, shootin' the shit with your partner for hours, with a dead body just chillin' in the back.

Chase and I were good friends through dozens of throwdowns, eight steady girlfriends and three wives, combined, between us. Sometimes, on duty, we'd take the ambulance over to our throwdown's places and one of us would sit in the sled while the other took a handset radio inside and made a booty call. The person on the booty call would acknowledge Dispatch if they called us for an emergency run so the guy waiting outside would know they'd heard it and were on their way.

Chase ended up marrying an ER doctor, and promotional transfers took us to opposite ends of the city. After that our interests turned to family and kids, and we just didn't party anymore the way we used to. We grew apart, and unfortunately, rarely even talk these days. As the French say, *C'est la vie*, or *tant pis*. Whichever fits best—they're both accurate.

In July 2001, I was driving Medic 5 in a thunderstorm. The rain was coming down in sheets as Cain Long and I were responding to the grocery store for a diabetic emergency. I was heading southbound on a five-lane road, going around 35 miles per hour due to the weather conditions, with lights and sirens. Approaching the intersection, our light was green. As I proceeded, in the left southbound lane, a minivan just ahead, came to a full stop in my lane, failing to yield right. To make matters worse, they angled the nose of their vehicle two feet into the left turn lane of oncoming traffic, effectively blocking the entire road.

I stood hard on the brakes, causing Medic 5 to hydroplane as we entered the intersection. Both lanes of northbound traffic were full of vehicles, and so was the right (and now the left) southbound lanes. Cain threw his foot up onto the dashboard and his hand pressed the ceiling as he braced for impact.

As we continued to slide sideways through the intersection, I let off the brakes and mashed the accelerator. I cranked the steering wheel hard to the right, attempting to regain control and steer between oncoming traffic and the minivan, via the left turn lane. I regained traction and righted the ambulance, narrowly squeezing between the stopped traffic. As I passed within inches of vehicles on both sides, my right fender hit the minivan's driver's side mirror.

I stopped the rig and called Dispatch, requesting another medic to take our call, and for police and a BC to respond to our accident. Cain went over to the minivan to check for injuries. Other than some cosmetic damage to the vehicles, everyone was fine. Truck 9, Safety 1, and a Fire Marshal responded as well, for traffic control and to take photos. The driver of the minivan was a refugee from Somalia and was cited for not having a driver's license, no insurance, and failure to yield right to an emergency vehicle.

We threaded the needle in our Big Red International ambulance, in the pouring rain, with 4.2 out of 5 lanes of traffic completely blocked. We fit that big-ass red semi-truck of an ambulance right between two vehicles with no room to spare. The BC gave us a "helluva job, guys," with no write-up. I felt like Ricky Bobby from *Talladega Nights*. "Shake 'n' bake, baby!"

We had an end of summer festival called the Borderline Fun Fest. All the area police, fire, and hospital agencies would come together and take over a city park for a weekend of barbecues and beers to commemorate one of the first major mutual aid fires from the past.

Softball tournaments and waterball were the games of choice. The later having two opposing patrons aiming fire hose streams at a giant beach ball on a rope, kind of the opposite of a tug of war, spraying water in every conceivable direction to the delight of soaked onlookers. There was booze, coke, weed, people screwing in public bathroom stalls, and no one called the cops because they were already there enjoying themselves. It was beautiful.

My own mother showed up to the festival after party and had three battalion chiefs trying to sleep with her.

"Hey, Brad, can I bang your mom," asked BC Jonny Parker as she stood right next to me.

"She's a grown woman, ask her," I replied.

The giggling couple ran off stumbling and tripping as they made their way through the park at night. Good times.

On September 11, 2001, I was mopping the floors at Station 8 having roved there for the day, when Willy P told everyone to come into the lounge and watch the news. CNN was reporting that a plane had flown into the World Trade Center in New York City. We watched as the fire burned out of control, knowing steel burns at a fixed rate and expands when heated, leading to an increased chance of structural collapse the longer it's exposed to flame.

We watched in disbelief as a second plane hit the other tower minutes later, and knew it was no coincidence. This was a terrorist attack on America. We knew the towers were coming down and discussed it amongst our crew. What would we do in that situation, we asked each other? We all agreed we'd go in and try to save as many people as we could, knowing we'd most likely die doing it. We watched in horror as the media broadcast people jumping out windows to their deaths below, rather than burn alive in the heat.

The towers fell a short time later, and the mood was somber. The fire service lost 343 FDNY firefighters that day. 343 of America's bravest made the ultimate sacrifice in service to their fellow men and women. The patriotism afterward was immediate and profound. I remember in the hours after the event, there was a rollover accident we responded on.

One of the vehicles was on its side and the back window had shattered onto the pavement. Lying in the road, there was a paper American flag taped to what used to be the rear window and was now framed by tiny broken pieces of tinted glass stuck to the tape around it. Everyone had seen the attack, and everyone was affected. There was an outpouring of support from the entire country to help aid in the recovery efforts.

We sent our department's FEMA and USAR firefighters to help with the search for survivors. Later, our city purchased a mangled steel girder from the tower wreckage and built a memorial park downtown. There was an article in the newspaper with a photo of me looking stoically at the twisted metal I-beam. "There is no greater honor than to lay down your life for your friend," was the quote they pulled from our interview and labeled the photo caption with. I'd remembered it from my father's bible thumping days from John 15:13.

One week later, there was the Amerithrax anthrax scare on September 18, 2001. It happened when letters containing anthrax spores were mailed to Democratic senators and media outlets in Washington D.C., New York City, and Boca Raton, Florida. Five people died and seventeen were injured in the attacks that garnered major press, just a week after 9/11.

People were calling our fire department every time they saw white powder on anything. Each of our nine stations was pulling an extra five calls a day for possible anthrax exposures, and double that in station phone calls. New kids would race to the phone, and we'd hear, "No Mrs. Johnson, if it's in your cupboard that's probably just baking soda." Or things like, "No, stripper lady, that's most likely cocaine, but we should probably head over, you know—just to be sure."

Or: "No, Mr. (or Mrs.) So-and-so, its sugar," or its salt, or its moldy bread. You get the picture. It was certifiably crazy. The Hazmat teams were running their asses off during that one, testing all kinds of bullshit. I mean c'mon people. Who's going to try to bump you off with anthrax spores? A senator in D.C.? Maybe. But freekin' Johnny Average Citizen, in Nowheresville, USA? I don't think so.

There was a time on Medic 5 when we responded to Maple Avenue for a crazed, combative guy. We pulled up with the engine to find a man on the sidewalk yelling at invisible people. When Pants tried to speak to the man, he took a swing. At that point, the poor guy didn't stand a chance. He was a pretty big dude, though, so we didn't mess around.

Pants tackled him and Carl, Chase, and I beat him up pretty good. If someone gives four guys with a metric fuck ton of PTSD the green light to legally fight their ass, they are going down, my friends. Fergie just stood there and wussed out. He did grab the cot, though, so I guess he wasn't entirely worthless.

We restrained the crazy guy who was trippin' balls on PCP and loaded him into the sled. We tied his arms and legs with cravats to the cot rails, so he wasn't going anywhere. I recall him spitting at Carl who was standing over him at the back doors of the ambulance and Carl stomping full bore on the guy's huevos and screaming, "You want a piece of me?!"

Fully restrained and with another cravat over his face now so he couldn't spit on us anymore, the man began to relax. Fergie, who'd stood in the corner and flat out refused to help, exited the sled, stating he didn't want any part of this, while Pants snapped the patient in the face with a nitrile glove repeatedly, before we left for the hospital.

Back at the station, Fergie got called multiple names from the female anatomy. We joked about the patient being potentially sterile now because of Carl's lingering size twelve boot print on his nut sack, and recalled all the other times throughout our careers when deadly force had been authorized. Pants got the last word on every one of them, of course. The machismo flowed like wine, and we all drank our fill.

Carl, Chase, and I worked together every shift. We learned each other's limits and motivating factors, how to coax more productivity and when to back off. We fought fires and saved lives on medicals and rescues. We partied on our days off at each other's houses and out on the town. We rode motorcycles, boated, fished, and hunted together. We were a family.

With Carl as my officer and Dolph as the engineer on Engine 5, we were refueling downtown at the city garage one day. As I was pumping diesel, they were bullshitting about the latest gossip, when Dolph looked up and saw a column of smoke rising in the east.

"You boys hear a fire get called in over the radio?" he asked, pointing in its direction.

We hadn't.

As we were discussing plans to head over when the refueling was done, Dispatch lit up the airwaves and toned out a full alarm. I hung up the pump, capped the tank, then jumped onto the truck as we raced out of the garage. This is exactly why we always positioned our rig backed in, ready to roll out. If we have to turn around or back up multiple times, we're shaving seconds off our arrival time. If we wanted the first-in jobs, we always had to be ready for takeoff.

Carl had a gut feeling we should hold off on this one. He stopped us at the road and made Dolph and I cool our heels while we sat in the rig and followed the radio. Then he said to head to the scene normal traffic.

Station 8 was on the same street as the fire address. Even being in the station, they were only five blocks away and we were still a few minutes out. Engine 8 and Truck 8 got the initial size-up, a multi-unit dwelling that was once a turn of the century mansion, converted to four separate apartments now. Fire and smoke were showing from the second story units upon arrival. Engine 1 hooked the hydrant and Engine 3 backed up 8 Engine on the fire attack line.

Guys started screaming over the radio and bailing out of the structure. BJ and Krishna had pulled a 2 ½" hose line to advance upstairs through the cut-up maze apartments when a flashover occurred. It blew all the windows out of the second story, raining glass onto the fireground below. There's an awesome photo of Krishna, taken shortly after, with his helmet practically melted to his body. Thinking back on it, if Carl hadn't followed his gut feeling back at the pumps, that would've been us caught in the flashover.

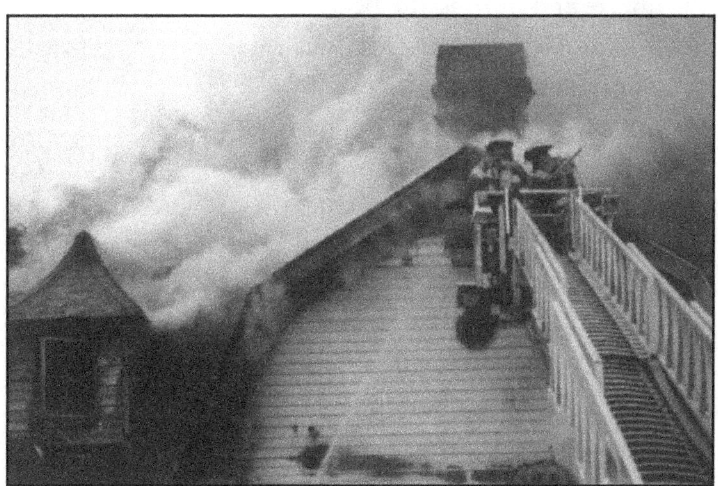

Magnolia Street fire post flashover

Hearing the trouble on the radio, we picked up the pace and upon arrival, Carl and I walked over to the BC's car to give him our passport tags. Dale Karnes was the BC and looked like he was literally having a heart attack. He was sitting in the front seat of his Suburban facing the fire, pale, sweaty, and shaking. I'd never seen the normally stoic man like this.

I remember when Carl walked up and said casually, "Howdy Dale, how can we help?" a wave of relief seemed to wash over him.

Dale knew Carl was an ass kicker on the fire ground. Seeing Dolph and I with him, just strengthened the odds we could make a positive impact and get back ahead of this thing. He gave us free reign to make entry and do whatever it took to turn the tide in our favor. We selected our favorite hand tools and made entry to the second floor.

With all the windows blown out, the smoke had cleared out nicely. There were pockets of rooms free burning and we commandeered an abandoned 1 ¾" pre-connect, extinguishing them easily. We pulled a large section of ceiling in a living room and found the fire rolling over itself in the attic. It was beautiful and we paused to watch it, like all good firefighters do, before opening the nozzle and putting the beast down.

As we sprayed the attic fire out, three long air horn blasts sounded from outside, and Dispatch sounded the evacuation tones over the fireground radio channel.

"God dammit," Carl said. "We've got it right here, keep going boys."

We kept spraying and Carl ignored the evacuation orders. When Dale called him personally over the fireground channel and advised him to exit the structure, we had to go. Back outside, Carl and Dale met at the red car and discussed the reasoning for pulling us out.

"It was clear as day in there Dale. What the fuck?" Carl said.

"The eaves started puking heavy smoke and I thought we might have another flashover," Dale replied.

Carl explained the heavy smoke from the eaves was because we were spraying a fog nozzle into the attic, forcing air and water in, so the smoke had to be pushed out somewhere. He promised Dale we could put this fire out in fifteen minutes if he'd let us back in. Dale agreed, and a few minutes later, it was done.

This is a prime example of why I detest 2½" hose lines for interior attack. They lack maneuverability and can exhaust the crew's trying to handle them. They're heavy, unwieldy, and I greatly prefer them for exterior operations like ground monitor supply lines, or exposure control. Any time we're advancing a charged 2 ½" hose up stairways, and around corners, we're just asking for fat, dry dick in our asshole, period. We can get plenty of water volume with lighter weight and better handling from a 1 ¾" hose line, in my opinion.

I met my current wife in the spring of 2002 while doing a flooring job for *The Corporation* group of battalion chiefs. They owned a large commercial building with businesses downstairs and apartments upstairs. I was contracted to install new flooring throughout the whole place. After working there every day off for a week or so, I was in a closet on my knees, when the most beautiful woman I've ever laid eyes on walked into the room.

She was a paralegal at a law firm on the first floor. When the other ladies at the office returned from lunch one day talking about the cute flooring installer working on the second floor, Lee told them she'd be the judge of that. She had no idea what she was getting herself into at the time. She returned to the law firm and confirmed to her colleagues that the rumors were true.

Lee told the girls, "Yes he is fine, and he will be mine."

"Too bad you're married," they replied.

I spent about two and a half years total at Fives, then in July 2002, Carl Yankovic made captain and was given his own single company firehouse. He was transferred to Station 7, the only one available at the time. He told the BCs that the only way he was going to that shithole of a firehouse was if he could bring a fireman he trusted along with him. Apparently, the current crew there was on his less-than-desirable-to-work-with personnel list.

No one bothered to let me know, and I came in to work one morning at Fives, as the senior firefighter on my shift, to find my lockers had been cleaned out. My gear and personal effects were in a pile on the floor by the back door of the station. What the *actual* fuck?

"Oh, nobody told you?" the new kid who'd recently taken over my lockers explained. "You were transferred to Sevens."

I stood there in disbelief. Station 7 was dubbed The Cottage by the other firefighters because being stationed there was like going on a vacation. They hardly made any runs at all. Why would they do this to me? I was the senior firefighter at Fives, and there were no extrication tools at Sevens. No, they had to reconsider. I packed my things and headed to Sevens, where Carl was waiting for me.

"Welcome home, ol' buddy!" he said as I walked through the back door.

He explained the situation. That he hadn't told me because he knew I'd refuse. That he knew it sucked, but it was only temporary, and he promised to take me with him when he received a double company. That motherfucker transferred out to Station 8 two weeks later, and I was stuck there for the next six months until the next round of transfers.

CHAPTER 10

Pranks

Few things are as synonymous with firefighting as pranking. Since time immemorial, the practical joke has been a cornerstone in its foundation. Hilarity is probably the best way we know of to deal with all the trauma and suffering that pervades our profession, and a good laugh is sometimes just what the doctor ordered. Just be sure to always follow the rules of engagement:

(1) Don't fuck with someone's gear. PPE (personal protective equipment) is vitally important for a firefighter's life safety; it's off limits. (2) Don't mess with their personal vehicle. That's their baby. It's right up there with their wife and their money, and a guaranteed way to start a fight. (3) Don't throw water when the temperature is below freezing (aka winter rules). And (4) for god's sake don't do something that's going to physically injure someone.

There would occasionally be notes taped to our ambulance windows saying things like "Hey, cute firefighters, call us for a good time." Don't ever call those by the way. It's either a surefire way to catch STDs (sexually transmitted diseases), or it's a prank from the guys on the other sleds, most likely, with the battalion chief's personal cell phone number. Which, by the way, is a much more sophisticated prank than the standard KY jelly on the door handle, gear shifter, steering wheel, or radio knobs.

Turning the sirens on full blast while the vehicle was off was always one of my favorites. When the driver hopped in and started their vehicle, they, and everyone around, would freak out. The BC would often leave his SUV running while parked outside the stations and we'd sneak in and turn the air conditioning on full blast in the wintertime. The same with the heater in the summer—along with setting the radio to a genre of music they despised at full volume.

Firefighters were masters of pranks and practical jokes, and buckets of water from the roof were the old standby. A drop's as good as a bucket some would say, if accidentally sprayed during the washing of the trucks and then mark the offender for retribution. Some would run and hide after throwing a bucket, others would just stand there stoic, looking you straight in the eyes.

Some, who'd just been douched, would walk calmly over to the hose rack, hook up a fifty-foot length and a nozzle, charge it, then march into the living or dining room areas where the culprit was, and open the bale point blank. They advised new kids coming out of training to put their phones in a Ziploc bag and bring at least three changes of clothes to work with them.

There was the ol' dollar bill taped to a fishing line. This was used in front of the stations, where there was heavy foot traffic walking by on a consistent basis. The firefighters would sit on the benches and cast it out toward the street. When a civilian would make a move for it, they'd holler "fish on," reel the bill in when the dupe tried to pick it up, and tease their unsuspecting victim until they finally became wise to the shenanigans.

Other classic pranks were the quarter superglued to the floor by the kitchen phones at Station 5 and Station 1. A heap of flour in a dish cloth on the kitchen counter, waiting for someone to dry their hands on it. A cup full of water, balanced just right inside the cupboard door, so it tips and falls out when the door is opened. The salt and pepper shaker lids—unscrewed and just sitting on top of the shakers—so they fall off and dump their entire contents onto the victim's plate of food when used was another old standby.

There was the box of cereal with the bottom cardboard removed and the bag placed in it upside down and open, so when someone grabbed it, the entire box dumped all over the floor. Clear tape over the sink's faucet opening, with the front of it slightly uncovered, to direct the spray up and at the operator. The faucet sprayer nozzle taped with clear tape and aimed forward at the operator. Coffee filters full of flour carefully hung above doorways with paper clips and trip wires that dumped them when the door was opened. These were just some of the easier and less complicated setups for the occasional episodes of firehouse tomfoolery.

The old-timers would have their new kids searching their fire trucks for nonexistent tools on rig days. Perhaps looking for a water hammer, which is actually the dangerous increase in hydraulic back pressure that occurs when a vehicle drives over the supply line coming from the fire hydrant. When the new kids would ask if they needed any help with the inventory, wily engineers would have them checking the slop room for a quart of blinker fluid to top off the reservoir on the rig. The designated carpenters on the Tech Rescue truck would have their newbies searching for a board stretcher to make their lumber the proper length, after they advised they'd cut it just shy of the mark.

There were, of course, no such things. But it was fun to watch the FNGs struggle to locate them. Timers were set and the veterans would gauge the general intelligence levels and worldly knowledge of the probies based on how long it took them to realize they'd been duped.

If we left our uniform shirt lying around for a few days, we'd return to work to find it encased in a block of ice in the freezer. If someone had to run to the bathroom to go number two, another firefighter might call up Dispatch a minute later and have them send some fire alarm test tones into the station. It was awful to be mid-poop when a fire alarm came in. There was the ol' cellophane over the toilet, shoe polish on the eye holes of binoculars, and so many, many more.

There were artists here. Some would take pranking to a whole new level. Oxygen tubing cut into two-inch strips, then melted at 90 degrees with a lighter. Make about ten of these and place them into the urinal flush ports. Remove the cap cover and turn the water pressure screw with a flathead screwdriver until it shot ten feet across the room. Clean it up, reset the area, then wait just outside the door for the screams and curses.

We'd take twenty feet of oxygen tubing and run it through the ceiling tiles, so it exited just above our partner's bed. Hook a syringe filled with water or an IV bag up to the other end in our own dorm room. We'd wait for our partner to hit the rack and give it a few minutes to make sure they were nice and cozy. Then squeeze the plunger or the bag and be ready to move fast when they came looking for us.

While we're up there in the ceiling tiles—Marv Holcomb would sometimes place an old alarm clock up there with the alarm set for 02:30 or something crazy like that. He'd always put it above a firefighter's room he didn't really like that much. When they'd bring it to his attention after finding it, he'd launch his "official investigation."

This consisted of the captain at the head of breakfast table, giving a Signal 4 to the dinner table for all personnel, explaining the situation, then asking everyone in clockwise order around the table if they knew anything about it. Of course, everyone said no, and when it got all the way back around to him, he'd say he didn't know anything about it either and state, "case closed, nobody knows anything about it." That was his firehouse justice system.

Then there were the masters. BJ once tied a ten-pound sack of potatoes to the corner of a guy's bed spread. When everyone was asleep, he kicked it down the pole hole. The blanket was ripped off the bed, shot across the dormitory floor, and disappeared down the hole. The poor guy shivered and wrapped up in his sheet. Then BJ kicked a second bag of potatoes he'd tied to the *sheet* corner down the pole. The guy was left lying there in his underwear wondering what the hell had just happened.

One day Krishna and Jeff Fenton were in the kitchen cooking at Station 9 when BJ informed them he'd be up on the roof doing some rope training. Earlier, he'd carried the 150-pound Rescue Randy mannequin up to the roof and dressed it in his spare uniforms. Minutes later, BJ carefully positioned Rescue Randy at the edge of the roof, just above the kitchen, and kicked it over the side. He screamed in terror from the roof as the dummy fell to the ground and landed in a heap, right outside the kitchen window.

Out of the corner of their eyes, the boys in the kitchen saw a body fall from the roof.

"Grab the blue bag, I'll call 9-1-1!" Fenton yelled in horror to Krishna, who sprinted out of the kitchen to grab medical supplies from the fire engine.

When the two new kids went to help the injured BJ, only to realize it was a mannequin, BJ jumped out from behind the corner and scared the pants off the bewildered responders.

BJ was a maniac. He was relentless in his persecution of new kids. He'd send them to the roof with a handset radio and make them sit in the rain for "Storm Watch." Or, in the blistering summer heat, send them to the roof for "Train Watch," instructing them to watch the nearby tracks, and if a train rolls by, to radio it in. People all over the city would know when BJ had a fish on the hook because a crackling voice would come across channel 1: "Ahhh, hey Engineer BJ, I see a train coming..." or "Yes, sir... it's still raining up here..."

He almost got me with the Scott bottle number prank. At the bottom of our Scott tanks are numbers etched into metal plates that identify them for testing purposes. BJ would call up every station and pretend to be Mumbles Henderson. Doing his best impersonation—and it was pretty good—he'd ask the new kid to get all the Scott bottle numbers off their rig and call up the Chief of Maintenance with the list.

He probably would've got me, except when he called pretending to be Mumbles, the real Mumbles was sitting at the desk right next to me.

"Yes sir, Captain Henderson, I'd love to get those Scott bottle numbers for you sir," I said, as Mumbles looked up from his paperwork.

"Gimme that phone," he mumbled. "BJ, quit fucking around and get back to work, you moron," Mumbles said, slamming the receiver down.

Apparently, Mumbles wasn't too fond of BJ's little charade.

The best pranks were the two-for-ones. Like when we caught a new kid with the water cup in the cupboard trick and then stashed a flour towel nearby for them to grab to dry off. That takes precise calculation and pre-planning the whole event through. Of course, there's always the off chance we'd forget about the towel we'd just prepared and flour ourselves before some unlucky sap came around to open the cupboard. That's always humbling and fun for others to watch. Or we could just walk up to our victim of choice with a cup of flour in one hand, a cup of water in the other and hit them with both. But that's just plain malicious.

Then there's the ol' double-double, where we set someone else up to take the blame for the prank. Feigning innocence while some other dupe takes the fall. Examples include putting on someone else's uniform when we're about to be bucketed so they end up with the wet clothing. Or bucketing ourselves then blaming our colleague after the captain has ordered all bucket throwing to cease for the day. The double-double took an immense measure of ingenuity and forethought not common in the average firefighter.

Mike Shaver was a black shift captain with a large afro hairstyle. Think Bob Ross only he's bald on top and the afro is gray. Kind of like an elderly Bozo the Clown. One day we found an Elmer Fudd Chia Pet at the grocery store and thought it'd be funny to spread the seeds around the base of his head, leaving the top bald, and fashion a pair of wire rimmed glasses from paper clips—just like the real Mike Shaver in his reading spectacles.

It was a perfect match. Chia Mike Shaver sat on the windowsill near the breakfast table. When the seeds had grown, we stopped watering it and they turned gray. Mike actually seemed to like our artistic impressionism and let the little guy stay around for a while.

Barry Clevenger was one of those old salty dog captains. The ones that wore handlebar mustaches, cussed like pirates, and looked like they'd survived a thousand structure fires without ever wearing a Scott mask. If he had a pair of hip boots and a rubber fire coat in his floor locker, I wouldn't have been surprised. He was the black shift boss of Twos when I hired on.

At the shift change breakfast table one day, Barry was on the Signal 2 phone, yelling and cussing up a storm.

"What the hell?…you stupid motherfucker…what's wrong with you?…You're a goddamn moron…how can you let someone just fuck you in the ass dry like that?…at least make 'em rub some Vaseline or KY on it first…you're gonna rip something…you took the whole thing?…all the way?…balls deep?...yeah…yeah…all right…love you too, Grandma…Bye.

Or sometimes it was his mom, but you get the picture. Dirty conversation, at elevated voice levels, in front of a room full of people, all stopping what they were doing to focus on Barry, talking to his loved one. The old-timers were an unscrupulous lot, full of tomfoolery.

Another classic prank was the phantom shitter. Someone would drop a deuce in the toilet, usually right before they left the station for the day, and walk away without flushing or wiping, leaving it for the new kids coming around to do their daily station duties. Barry would often line the toilet bowl with "shit rafts" of toilet paper, so no water was visible. He'd do his business, so it was suspended above the water, floating on the rafts. Then he'd waddle over to the next stall to finish cleaning up, and head home for the day, leaving it to hot box the bathroom.

At Station 4, later in my career, the phantom shitter struck again. Our team launched an official investigation. We knew it wasn't Barry because he'd since retired. We knew it wasn't someone from our shift, because it landed in the pot on the days we were arriving for duty. It had to be a senior member of the black shift. That only left 2 guys. Tommy Rush or "Singin" Stan Cosgrove.

Tommy was a hard-nosed captain. Strait laced and by the book, he demanded excellence and professionalism at all times, so we could pretty much rule him out. Stan was a portly, jolly old man who whistled often and sang old folk tunes while working around the station. He could be our guy, judging by the immense size of the floaters left in the toilet. Tommy was small in stature, and it'd be quite a task for him to brew a turd of that magnitude. No, it had to be Stan.

The stage was set, and on Stan's next work shift, we enlisted a few black shift spies to patrol the dormitory rest rooms during the early morning shift change. Getting a guy to roll over on his officer was difficult if they were respected, but if they had beef, guys were more than willing to spill the beans. We were all at the breakfast table sipping coffee, when an anonymous tip came in for a phantom shitter sighting. The table cleared and everyone headed over to the dormitory men's room. Outside, we waited for the phantom to exit.

As Stan opened the door, we all piled in and pushed him back inside. Two guys held Stan in place at the sink, while another two checked the stalls.

"What the fuck is this, Stan?" came the cry from behind me.

Holding the door open, we could see the phantom had struck again. Stan was cold busted and confessed on the spot. We made him flush his own dirty work and then clean the shitter to boot. Some people's children, I tell ya.

Joe Coddington was a black shift captain at Fours when I caught overtime there one day. He enjoyed making lewd comments and had a dirty old man mentality. So it was no surprise when he came skipping through the station singing the Beach Boys' "Wouldn't It Be Nice" and wearing only a bright yellow thong, which he affectionately called his "banana hammock." Guys or gals, it didn't matter: he wasn't ashamed to bear it all while on duty.

Paul Wilson was an engineer at Station 2. Tall and lanky, Paul liked to prank new kids by wearing only a hot pink thong and lying face down on his bed, pretending to read a book or a magazine when they unsuspectingly walked into the common dormitory. He would then raise his ass up off the bed for emphasis. He only tried this once with me because upon seeing him, I sprinted over and slapped the shit out of his bare ass cheek so hard it left a handprint for days. I damn near broke my hand on that piece of ass.

Out of Station 3 one morning, Sanders, Koz, and I were on the engine when Ops called. Station 8 had to go to a Technical Rescue class in the next town over, and we had to go cover their area while Eights was gone all day. We showed up just as they were getting ready to leave.

Captain Charlie Zamora handed Koz their mess money and told him specifically, "No fucking meatloaf!"

As the rigs rolled out of the station, Koz turned to me and said, "Guess what they're having for dinner."

"Meatloaf?" I answered.

"You're goddamn right!" Koz said, and we rolled off to the grocery store. Koz carefully prepared ten pounds of ground beef with spices and sauces, eggs, and crushed crackers, then shaped it on a large cookie sheet into a giant phallus and threw it in the oven. He even sprinkled some shredded cheddar cheese around the balls and base of the cock during the final ten minutes for added visual effect.

When the crews returned from their training, Engineer Bubbles ran into the kitchen, saying she was starving and how it smelled so good in the station. She didn't even notice the cock and balls shape of the meatloaf. We all winced and laughed as she pulled a giant knife from the drawer and chopped off the head of the cock with it. As she ate, she kept saying, "Mmmm," and how it was so good. Charlie just shook his head in disbelief as he tried to hold back the laughter, and Koz just shrugged and smiled. It *was* damn good meatloaf.

Sometimes it all goes south on us in a hurry though. Pranking is not for the faint of heart. At Fives one day, Smoothbore was having a particularly difficult day dealing with his significant other. He'd been yelling on the cordless Signal 2 phone with Jackie for the better part of a half hour, when Julian Burke leaned over to Dave Owens and stated bluntly, "You don't have a set of nuts if you don't go bucket Wayne right now."

Dave, being new and needing to prove himself to his more senior FTI colleague, went to the slop room and prepared a bucket. His first and last. He climbed up to the roof and peered over the edge. Smoothbore stood outside the back door arguing incessantly with his crazed girlfriend. Dave pulled back the five-gallon bucket and let it fly.

Direct hits make a loud slapping noise when they hit the back of the neck. As a victim of a plethora of buckets myself, I can attest, they shock the shit out of the mark and have a certain unexpected heft when falling from greater than one story. Hence the slapping sound when it hits the neck and shoulders of the intended target.

Now, as the thrower of the bucket, one has several choices to make in the immediate moments after the water has left the bucket. They can stand there and verify the enemy has, in fact, received a direct hit. However, that greatly increases the risk of detection and identification. Dave chose the run-and-hide approach. The victim usually looks up to the roof first. Then, seeing no offender, they make a beeline for the stairs to the roof, attempting to locate the culprit and cut off their escape route. Often, the victim would find the roof empty, and the whole station sitting calmly at the table, or in the brown chairs (La-Z-Boy recliner).

This is where the pulse check was key. The dripping wet firefighter had, within their rights, the ability to request a pulse check of all suspects, to identify the guilty party. Having just pulled off a daring escape, the idea was, the pulse of the person having just run down the stairs would be elevated, allowing the victim to successfully identify his assailant.

Dave knew Smoothbore was coming for him. He stopped at the second-floor bathrooms and crouched on a toilet holding his breath as Smoothbore rampaged through the station, kicking open doors and threatening to kill "whoever did it."

Julian and I were up front when Smoothbore kicked in the door and yelled, "Who the *fuck* just did that!" with water still dripping from his chin. I struggled not to laugh as he locked in on me and pointed. "Was it you?" he growled as he walked toward me.

"Swear to god, it wasn't me, bro." I offered my arm as an effigy to the pulse check clause.

"Was it you?" he asked, zeroing in on Julian.

"Not me, ol' buddy," Julian casually stated.

The "ol' buddy" was a wild card. One could say damn near anything they wanted if they threw an ol' buddy on the end of it. Ol' buddy was a calming, rational way to say we're still friends even though I just said something offensive. One had to add this phrase within a certain time period, say, within three to five seconds after the offending phrase, or it lost its validity, and the offense was thereby deemed legal and binding. Julian's ol' buddy was within fully acceptable parameters, so Smoothbore moved on with his list of suspects.

There were only two other potential bucketeers left: the captain and the new kid. As Smoothbore stormed off in search of something or someone to smash, Dave snuck in the back door.

"Holy shit, he's pissed," Dave whispered.

"Ya think!" Julian said.

"What do I do? He's gonna kill me!" Dave whisper-yelled.

Just then, Smoothbore kicked in the door. "What the *fuck*, motherfucker?!" he roared.

Julian jumped between the two emotionally charged men and explained how it was all his fault and he was sorry and if Smoothbore wanted to punch somebody, but to punch him instead. Smoothbore backed down, and Dave headed off to go change his shorts. He swore never to throw another bucket again. And to my knowledge, he never did.

At Station 1, I was on the sled with Shane McKinley, son of Captain Peter McKinley. We'd just returned from an early morning call and Shane was sitting at the breakfast table, with his back to the apparatus floor, typing a run report on our laptop. I was in the kitchen making some toast for breakfast when I saw Engineer Slackwood sneak up on Shane and fire off the air horn from the high-rise bag, right next to Shane's head.

Shane winced in pain, and most certainly suffered temporary hearing loss. I threw my toast on a plate and went to check on him.

"You OK?" I asked.

"Huh?" he said back, his ears apparently still ringing.

"Be right back," I said, tossing my plate on the table and heading out the kitchen door. "What the fuck, asshole!" I shouted after Slackwood. He and I had come up together in rank, and he had a year or two on me. You don't fuck with my partner, though.

Let's review the rules of engagement when it comes to playing pranks in the firehouse. Don't mess with people's PPE, don't mess with their personal rides, don't throw water in the winter (AKA winter rules), and don't do anything that causes personal injury. It's easy: always operate your pranking within the rules of engagement, and you're good. Slackwood violated unwritten rule number four. As a member of the players club, I was duty-bound to confront him.

"What?" Slackwood said, turning around.

"Don't blow that air horn in my partner's ear," I said stepping into his personal space.

He looked back at Shane. "You mean that new kid?" he asked.

"That *new kid* is my partner today, and I need him at 100 percent so we can save people's lives together and go home to our families in the morning. What happens when he can't hear out of his right ear when I tell him we've got traffic at an intersection, and he doesn't hear me, or see it, and T-bones an old lady? All because you thought it'd be funny to blow his eardrums out."

"All right, calm down, man," Slackwood replied.

"Don't fuck with my partner. Nothing personal. I'd do the same if it was you," I explained and walked back to the kitchen.

Shane thanked me for standing up for him, and Slackwood didn't fuck with him anymore.

Ted Nester was the black shift captain at eights when I was stationed there. His engineer was Brett Davis. Nester couldn't stand Brett and went so far as to take the fire station copy of the dictionary, and next to every word that was synonymous with *idiot*, taped a picture of Brett Davis next to it as the new definition.

Moron—had a picture of Brett Davis. *Imbecile*—a picture of Brett Davis. *Boob, dummy, fool, stupid, dunce, nitwit, buffoon, sucker, clown, stooge, jerk, chump, patsy, dupe, oaf, blockhead, goon, nincompoop, klutz, slacker, deadbeat, slouch, bum, derelict, lazybones, jackass, dumb,* and *naïve*—all had pictures of Brett Davis taped to their definitions.

Fire department pranksters were absolutely relentless in their pursuit of hilarity and humiliation. Sometimes pranking feuds carried on for months, and the officers would have to order a cessation of hostilities. For the most part, though, pranks were considered harmless enough, and the players were usually good sports. I developed a sincere love of the game, and of witnessing a well-executed prank, even if I was the intended target. It certainly broke up the monotony of near constant death and destruction.

Chapter 11

Lucky Sevens

In the short time I was stationed at Sevens, we only made thirty runs. That's thirty calls in six months! Eleven of them were first-in fires, with the rest full alarms, medicals, and MVAs. To be clear, the word *slow* doesn't adequately describe the run volume and pace at The Cottage. I had plenty of time to reflect upon my life choices and their consequences.

It wasn't all that bad, though. I got high as balls in the basement boiler room with Koz and Young Dawg several times a day—if not all shift long—while they were there filling in as acting captains after Carl left. Usually, after just one pull from the bomber, Young Dawg would look over and say, "Just enough to put a smile on your face," then pass it back to me and walk off to work on a project or something.

Sevens was an old station, with hatches in the ceiling near the fire pole for storing hay from back in the days of the horse drawn fire pumpers. The lounge area, front desk, kitchen, and dining room were literally right next to the fire truck in the garage. When we had a call, diesel exhaust flooded the whole living quarters and drifted up the pole hole into the open dormitory.

I did make some notable fires from here. If we rolled out on a call, we could be certain it was on something legitimate. It was nice to have a reprieve from the bullshit EMS runs when I wasn't staffing the bone box, and Sevens provided me with plenty of downtime and some much-needed rest and recuperation. When a full alarm fire came in one afternoon, we headed out and arrived first. The home's chimney was puffing white smoke from its top and the eaves of the roof on both sides were belching a heavier, darker gray.

Marv Holcomb gave the report: "Engine 7 on scene, smoke showing, stretching pre-connect, next engine in grab a hydrant, Sevens has command," and we were off. I stretched the hose line out, the engineer charged it, and Holcomb met me at the front door after a walk around and a quick chat with the homeowner who assured him everyone was out of the structure.

We entered through the front door and the stairs to the second floor of the Cape Cod home were straight ahead of us. Visibility was good. I advanced up to the top landing and was immediately forced down to the floor by the intense heat.

Marv, several steps below, asked why I'd stopped.

I yelled through my mask, "It's too hot!"

I'm no sissy, OK; so when I say it was too hot, I mean it was melt-my-fucking-helmet hot; like ears dripping off my skull hot *while* wearing my fire-proof Nomex hood.

Marv figured I was just being soft, and pushed up the stairs around me, onto the landing.

"Oh my God!" he said, falling back down a couple of stairs.

"See?" I yelled.

The second-in engine crew from Ones was right on our asses coming up the stairs and there was nowhere to go.

"What's the holdup?" they hollered.

"Too hot!" Marv yelled back.

"Bullshit," came the reply from the perpetually gung-ho Ones crew as they pushed us to the walls of the stairway and moved up to the second-floor landing.

Seconds later, they were bailing headfirst down the stairs past us to escape the heat, their turnouts smoldering and singed. They didn't even stop at the bottom of the stairs. Just kept right on going out the front door to cool down. We radioed for a vent job from the truck crew and heard the chainsaw fire up. Then came the heavy clunk of the roof ladder being laid down over the shingles and hooked to the peak.

Someone outside smashed the second story windows on the gable ends with a pike pole, and the room lit up like the surface of the sun from a flashover. We kissed the floor. Thankful for the steps just below the top landing, giving us a few feet lower to wait for the vent job. As the hole was punched through the roof and ceiling, interior conditions improved dramatically. We advanced our hose line up to the landing and extinguished the room's contents.

It was still hot as hell in there and the exterior crews advised the flow of smoke chugging from the eaves was intensifying. With no more interior fire left to put out, Marv advised the fire was in the walls, and we began to punch holes in the three-foot-high knee walls along the sides of the long room. Sure enough, the fire was free burning, still roaring through the knee wall's void spaces. I stuck the nozzle through the holes in the drywall and with a fog pattern, swung it around in a circular motion until it was out. Then we did the same on the other side of the room.

Building construction for homes and businesses in the nineteenth and early twentieth centuries had lots of void spaces. There were often chases that extended from the basement to the roof, allowing fire to travel extensively throughout the walls, sometimes jumping multiple stories in an instant. It became very important to recognize this so-called balloon construction type when we pulled up, as it would dictate our strategies for fire attack. This fire had started from creosote buildup in the first-floor fireplace chimney. Then it moved through cracks and missing mortar between the chimney bricks and into the knee walls.

Over the following months, Lee and I would meet up at different places. I'd swing by her law firm, or we'd have lunch at a park. One morning on duty, I stopped by her house on the ambulance unannounced. When she answered the door in a bath towel, I kissed her in front of the neighbors, who were curious as to why the medic unit was there and gawking at the public display of affection scene we were making on her front porch. We were living dangerously, and I didn't care who saw us.

Stationed at Sevens, I was right on Lee's way home from work. She'd stop in when I was on duty, and we'd sit on the porch and watch the sun sink low on the horizon together. We'd rendezvous occasionally in the upstairs bathroom, or my dorm room on the second floor. Sometimes she'd stay for dinner with the crew, and we'd philosophize on the finer points of life over cigarettes and firehouse cuisine. One time she stayed the entire night with me, and we slept tangled up in each other's arms in my dorm room. It was perfectly blissful.

Out of Sevens on a cold, wintry night, I performed one of my first rescues from a burning structure. The full alarm came in for a structure fire at 01:00 hours. Russ Jackson was the captain and Bruce Owens was the engineer. When we arrived on scene, there was a man yelling from a second story window. He was trapped, and thick black smoke poured out from around him.

"Ladder that window!" Jackson yelled, then he gave his first-in report over the radio.

Flames were showing from the other windows of the second story, as I pulled a 24' extension ladder from the engine's side-mount rack and set it up under the man's window. Jackson met me at the foot of the ladder as I raised it into position just under the windowsill. Russ footed the ladder in the snowy front yard as I climbed up, tucked a leg into the rungs, hooked my foot around the rail, and swung out to the side of the ladder so the trapped man could climb onto it and scurry down. To my surprise, a young girl about six or seven years old climbed out from the smoke first.

"I gotcha," I said, helping her onto the ladder and watching as she made her way down to the ground where Russ was waiting.

Then came a little boy, four or five years old, coughing hard, and grateful to be free of the poisonous smoke.

Finally, the man emerged from the window. He thanked me between heavy coughs as thick black snot drained from his nose. He climbed down the ladder and was reunited with his children out on the sidewalk. The medic crews sheltered them from the cold in their ambulance and checked them for injuries.

Other rigs arrived and were engaged in various fire suppression activities. They'd taken our hose lines during the rescue, so we grabbed hand tools and helped support the attack crews. During overhaul, we learned from the Fire Marshal, the fire had been deliberately set on the exterior of the only entrance to the upstairs apartment. Possibly by the ex-wife's lover, who'd wanted the baggage of her previous family out of the way. Security cameras proved the theory right and the new boyfriend-turned-arsonist was convicted and sentenced.

Off duty, I was out at Agent's house riding his dune buggy around the property when Lee called. She wanted to meet, and when she arrived I introduced her to Agent as my cousin. He called bullshit right away and said something about kissing cousins—maybe. As we cruised around in the dune buggy, drinking our beers, and having a fun time, a bee lodged itself in Lee's shorts and stung her repeatedly. Thinking she was just having a really good time I continued to put the hammer down on the dune buggy. When we finally stopped, she asked me to help pull the stinger out of her butt cheek. Naturally, of course, I obliged.

Back in Agent's barn, he was trying to locate something that used to belong to his stepfather. Some documents of his time in the Navy. Lee suggested he look in the dresser drawers in the old chest in the corner. When he did, and found them, he was curious how she could've known where they were. Lee explained how Agent's *dead* stepfather was standing right there next to her, telling her where they were.

Agent was blown away. How could she be doing this?

Lee explained his dead stepfather was also showing her how he'd suffered a heart attack on the property.

Agent confirmed that, yes, in fact, he did have a heart attack while two snowmobilers were tearing up his property one winter day. He'd run outside to chase them off and dropped dead in the snow. How could she have known that?

Next, the dead stepfather showed her a little blond boy in a hole in the ground, with something in his hand. Agent's eyes welled up with tears.

"Now there's no way you could know about that," he said. "That was me when I was about seven years old. I had an M-80 and hid in the well pump housing to light it off. I almost blew my hand off that day, and my stepfather beat the shit out of me for it. He was a mean drunk."

Lee explained he was attempting to make amends for the regretful things he'd done in his lifetime and was always helping around the property. Atoning for his wrongs.

This was the first time I'd experienced Lee's psychic abilities. Agent's first time as well.

Things back at home came to a head for me on 9/11 of 2002, when a notice of default arrived in the mail from the district court, stating my divorce decree had been entered into public record. Sonya and I had both forgotten all about the court proceedings we'd filed a year earlier, and this was the first notice we'd received that it was final. My father-in-law phoned and was justifiably upset that two of his daughters had been sleeping with me at the same time, and now I was divorcing one of them instead of cleaning up my mess and making it right.

He said I was just like my father, and that was my tipping point. I threw the phone through the drywall, then did the same with the glass in my other hand for good measure and walked out. I packed my guns and bows in the Jeep and told my wife I was leaving for good. She stood behind me blocking the driveway and called the police, telling them I was suicidal. I wasn't—just fed up with this relationship and all its baggage.

The police showed up, running up my driveway with their guns drawn on me, right in front of the neighbors. My friends on the police force, like Ryan Nellis, showed up and helped to ease the tense situation. Chase was in the middle of a concrete side job across town and came screeching up in his pickup and trailer. Sonya had called all my friends and told them I planned to kill myself. Which was completely false.

The sergeant explained that based on Sonya's information he had to take me over to CMH (Community Mental Health) for a psychiatric evaluation. Ryan offered to take me, and I complied. I told Sonya we were through as I walked past her down the driveway and climbed into the front seat of Ryan's police cruiser. The cops took my guns, an official statement from Sonya, and away we went.

At CMH, Ryan and I sat in the waiting room until the psychiatrist was ready to see us. Ryan followed me in and gave the doctor a brief report and then left, wishing me good luck. I thanked him for being there for me. When the door shut behind him, the mood changed. The doctor was an attractive lady, in her mid-forties. She let her hair down and shook it out as we talked about the events of the previous few hours.

After explaining the situation and telling her I was only leaving the relationship, not suicidal, she seemed understanding. She certified my sanity and said she had the feeling she was talking to the wrong party in this scenario. That Sonya should be the one seeking therapy. She took a business card, wrote her personal cell phone number on the back, and asked me to call her when things settled down. Suggesting maybe we could get to know each other better.

I dropped the card in the trash on my way out of the building and called Lee to tell her about my crazy day. I asked her what the notice of default on the divorce decree meant. She explained it meant my divorce was final, and I was officially single. Her heart sank, as she realized she'd have to make a decision on her own marriage if she wanted to be with me.

She began looking for an apartment while her husband went on a month-long hunting trip, telling him if he left, she wouldn't be there when he returned home. He left.

A few days later I moved Sonya and the girls into an apartment and put our family house up for sale.

I helped move Lee's things from her marital home into an apartment. Her mother advised me not to get too attached because Lee had a history of messing her relationships up. Lee took that as a dare and became determined to prove her mother wrong. I moved in with her a few days later and we became an instant family.

Lee had a son from a previous relationship who was ten years old at the time. I'd always wanted a son and set to work being the father neither of us had ever had. We hunted and fished together, I helped him with his homework, we went on vacations and trips, and I tried to be there for him when he needed me.

Station 7 was quaint little place and fun for a short time, but I was on the phone with Carl daily, telling him to get me the hell out of there. The next round of transfers finally rolled around, and he made good on his word, bringing me over to Station 8 with him. Eights was a double company firehouse on the northeast side of town, with an engine and a ladder truck. In January 2003, I packed my things and left The Cottage for good.

Chapter 12

Body Fluids

People would come into my "office" all the time and bleed, piss, shit, and vomit all over themselves and my ambulance. My ambulance is my office, and I don't like it when people defile it with their body fluids, because then I have to clean it—again. Pretty much every day we'd have a half dozen or so of these patients who couldn't help but leak their body fluids all over our workspace.

A good EMT saw it coming and prepared in advance for it. Chance favors the prepared mind. Trust me. You need to stash an emesis bag behind the head of the cot between the padding and frame. While you're at it, stick a disposable blanket back there, too. It only takes five seconds to whip one of those bad boys over your cot before that drunk guy who just pissed himself sits down on it. Oh, he's feeling nauseated? Bam! Your vomit bag is deployed in two seconds and you're holding it right under his chin for him. ER docs and nurses love it when you bring them full barf bags, because they can get a thorough understanding of the patient's last meal.

As a patient, if you are bleeding profusely, have pudding in your pants, stomach chunks on your shirt, or smell like you just took a bath in ammonia, then you are getting a disposable blanket on your cot and I'm wrapping your ass in it like a burrito to keep the smell down. Speaking of smell, as a rescuer, don't breathe through your nose, or you'll be the next one vomiting in the trash can. Close those nasal passages off with the mental discipline of a sage. It's important. Turn the exhaust fans on full bore and open the porthole-sized windows. Stick your face next to them to breathe if you have to, through your mouth of course.

Speaking of puke, if a patient starts ralphing, for god's sake don't watch. That shit is like a chain reaction. I've seen a patient projectile vomit from his seat on the cot, bounce that shit off the back doors, my partner on the bench seat toss his cookies all over the patient, the poor new kid in the jump seat grab the trash bin and heave into it, and the engineer spiking a line in the ambulance stairwell open the side door just in time to blow chunks out onto the street. It looked like the freakin' Barf-O-Rama in the movie *Stand By Me*, complete with the Shriners yelling, "Boom-baba-boom," as a fat kid walked by.

My only saving grace was I hadn't eaten anything in damn near twenty hours, so I had nothing to offer to the festivities. Sometimes, the guys who'd just gorged at the dinner table would catch a full alarm fire directly afterward, and it was always hilarious when they'd fill up their Scott mask with stomach contents mid-way through a cock knocker. You had to be quick if you were masked up. Get low to the ground so it doesn't splatter, and with one hand, lift the bottom of your mask and let it rip. Then get your ass back in the game and finish the job. Be sure to brush your teeth back at the station.

For those of you who get woozy when you see blood, BREATHE. It took me months to lose the heebie-jeebies of seeing a person's insides on their outsides. If you feel lightheaded when you see blood, take a long breath in and long breath out. Now do it again. Keep doing it until you feel better. Through your mouth of course, don't you dare breathe through your nose with that funky stench in the air or it's all over. Remember to breathe. It's the first thing you did when you got here, and it'll be the last thing you do when you leave this place. Just breathe.

Early on in my career, we still got called to hose down the pavement at emergency scenes from body fluids. If there was a shooting in the street, or a stabbing outside the party store, we'd get called by the cops to come bring an engine over and flush the blood down into the sewer drains. Later, with bloodborne pathogen training, we realized this was not the proper sanitary way to handle these biohazards, and professional teams were called in to handle the cleanup.

Back at the station, it was a different story. Sometimes there'd be so much blood and other assorted body fluids, we had to hook up a hose line and spray off the inside of the ambulance. We'd flush it right out the back doors and down the apparatus floor drains. Which is probably why they smelled so horrible. On bad days, we'd have to do this more than once during the course of our shift. On good days, our disposable blankets would catch the majority of the flotsam and jetsam, and we could just spray some disinfectant and spot clean the overflow.

Sometimes, on an unconscious person not breathing, the medic would accidentally intubate the patient's esophagus and not listen for positive lung sounds before cranking away on the BVM. All the air they were pumping down that tube would be going into the patient's stomach. Their belly would slowly begin to rise like a volcano towering above the landscape around it. This was called gastric distension, and by the time you noticed, it was already too late.

Obviously, the tube was incorrectly positioned and needed to be replaced properly so the patient could get oxygen. In order to do that, we had to remove it first, which was treacherous. Usually, it went something like this: New kid pulls the BVM off the ET tube, then all the air pressure in the stomach comes shooting out the top of the tube like the Old Faithful geyser at Yellowstone.

Only it's not water, it's stomach contents, which, similar to Old Faithful, have been significantly warmed and come out steaming and piping hot.

There's really no good way to contain the catastrophe other than by rolling the patient onto their side to avoid aspiration and having them shoot it into the trash can, with a towel nearby to catch the overspray. After the geyser erupted, we were now clear to carefully deflate the ET tube cuff and remove the tube. Be sure to suction any remaining chunks from their airway, because stomach acid and lung tissue do not play well together.

Using the laryngoscope blade, the medic would then reposition a new ET tube properly into the trachea and inflate the cuff, this time listening for positive lung sounds in the apexes and bases bilaterally and checking for the absence of those strange gurgling noises coming from the stomach with each breath, called gastric sounds. Do it right the first time. It's important.

As time went on and my ambulance shifts became more frequent, there appeared to be no end in sight. What began as an eight-year commitment, turned into ten, then twelve, then fourteen years on the bone box. A good EMT developed an intuition over time for when and how to prevent massive bio-hazard contaminations of their office space. An ounce of prevention was definitely worth a pound of cure when it came to keeping things tidy in the back of the sled. And we've all got better things to do than cleaning up other people's body fluids.

Chapter 13

A Technical Rescue

As mentioned earlier, Eights was a double company firehouse with an engine and a ladder truck. It was the Technical Rescue focus station for our department and there I learned the specialty rescue disciplines of high-angle and low-angle rope rescue, trench rescue, structure collapse, and confined space. The station was situated in a large city park and had a quad-court sand volleyball feature directly behind the station.

As a favor to the volleyball players, the guys would sometimes place a charged 1¾" hose with a nozzle, strapped to the top rung of a 6-foot folding ladder. A makeshift shower so the ladies could rinse off the sand that accumulated on their bodies while playing. I felt it was a kind gesture and occasionally volunteered to supervise the operation to make sure things were functioning properly. Most of our significant others surprisingly disapproved.

Station 8 was only seven blocks away from our new apartment and Lee would swing by the station every time the opportunity presented itself. She was part of the firefighter family now, and Captain Carl had grown fond of her, calling her his daughter since he and I were known as Dad and Lad. We'd wash our personal vehicles together in the evenings and watch the sun set behind the park.

It felt exhilarating to be out of Station 7 and the run volume at Eights was steady. The ladder truck rolled on every north end fire response and there were several working fires every day. The engine typically made a dozen calls per shift between fires and medical assists with the ambulances.

There was a four-story Tech Rescue training tower beside the fire station where we practiced rope rescues and high-angle pick offs, setting bomb-proof anchors, tending belay lines, rappelling, Stokes basket evolutions, ascending and descending, swapping ropes, and window picks. We spent countless hours dangling from dizzying heights and practicing our craft.

One evening after dinner, Lee showed up. She called from the parking lot and asked if I'd come outside. When I did, she was absolutely stunning. She was wearing thigh-high black leather boots and a black, skin-tight short dress with a black trench coat covering it all.

She asked if we could go to the tower. We walked hand in hand and climbed the ladder up to the second story. There was a chair conveniently placed there from the previous crew's training exercises. I slid it over in front of the railing, and she danced for me. It was breathtaking.

We made it a personal goal to meet up and bang at every fire station in town. At Ones it was in my personal vehicle in the underground parking ramp and the administrative bathroom upstairs. At Twos it was in my Jeep in the parking lot and the weight room in the basement. Threes was on the hose tower catwalk. At Fours we did it in the bedrooms, in the cab of the fire truck, the women's restroom, a utility closet, and our own personal vehicles in the parking lot. At Fives it was the hose tower, EMS supply room, and the kitchen counter. We were busted at both Fives *and* Sixes, while shagging in the cabs of the fire engines.

Sevens was the bathroom, showers, and my dorm room. At Eights, we banged in the Tech Rescue tower, the weight room on the weight bench, and I won the dining room table bet as the first person to get a piece of ass on the new handcrafted table. Jake Slackwood affectionately dubbed Lee "stripper shoes," after the time she stopped by wearing her three-inch clear acrylic platform pumps that day. At Nines, we did it in the hose tower on the catwalk, and almost got busted in the cab of the engine. We were very naughty.

I asked Lee's father for permission to marry his daughter and he approved. The following week I popped the question by placing an engagement ring inside of a rose bud and presenting it to her. As she smelled the rose, the ring sparkled, and she cried tears of joy when I knelt down on bended knee and proposed. She said yes.

We picked out a wedding band at a local pawn shop and on August 10, 2004, were married at city hall by a Justice of the Peace. Our reception was back at home with our children, and we had ramen noodles for dinner. There was no honeymoon—we were living it. We were poor, but we had each other and that was all that really mattered to us.

On Engine 8 one night, Captain Denny Milton and I made a full alarm house fire on New York Avenue. We were first-in, and I stretched a pre-connect across the front yard and made entry into the one-story home. Heavy fire was in the kitchen and rolling over the ceiling through the living and dining rooms as we pushed inside. I opened the bale of my straight stream nozzle and hit the beast with it. An explosion lit up the room signaling I'd hit the electrical service panel with the hose stream. Sparks flew everywhere as the fire darkened down and then disappeared.

The next in crews set up a smoke ejector fan in the doorway and we opened the windows to ventilate. We put out the hot spots, then transferred the scene to the Fire Marshal, packed up our hoses and returned to the station. I remember thinking how easily that fire had gone out. It was so impressive initially and with the right technique, it just went away. Without even a fight.

Tyrone Blake was an enormous hulk of a man. He stood 6'3" and weighed around 280 lbs. As I arrived at Station 8 one morning, he was sleeping off his black shift hangover in a brown chair, waiting for his relief person in the lounge. The incoming red shifters were enjoying coffee at the nearby dining room table. BJ decided it'd be funny to put Tyrone in a rear naked choke hold from behind his recliner. He snuck up and grabbed the sleeping bear.

When Tyrone told BJ to quit fucking with him—that he wasn't in the mood—BJ ignored him and kept squeezing. Tyrone reached back over his head and grabbed BJ by the torso. He flipped BJ over the back of the chair and threw him right through a wall ten feet away and above a couch!

As BJ climbed out of the drywall covered in dust, Tyrone stood up tall and said, "I told you I wasn't in the mood." Then he walked out leaving BJ standing there dusty, confused, and embarrassed in front of the crews.

There's an awkward dichotomy that occurs when big city departments are called by the out-county fire departments to assist them with fires. I imagine it's like in the military, when Special Forces come in and take over a situation that's become out of control. We threw a lot of personnel at structure fires in our city relatively quickly and could accomplish all the important benchmark tasks with efficiency and speed. This isn't the case in the outlying communities, where staffing numbers are minuscule and they're far less aggressive in their fireground tactics.

They were content going defensive on just about everything if there were no life safety issues. That was an affront to all that we stood for at our department, and we'd be *damned* if we were going to stand outside and eat rehab station doughnuts in a heated bus while a taxpayer's house burned to the ground. We'd walk up to their scenes, check in with their command, offer our advice if their BC didn't have a freakin' clue on how to handle the situation, and steal the best assignments. We'd take their nozzles, put their fires out, and go home—leaving them to do all the overhaul, clean up, and paperwork. It was rude and we didn't even care.

As we prepared to turn in for the night at Eights, an alarm came in for a church fire in the next town over to the east. Marshall Harris was the captain and Willy P was the driver on Truck 8 as we headed out into the middle of the night and arrived to find the Jehovah's Witness Kingdom Hall fully involved. A sprawling church cock knocker with flames through the roof in three separate areas. Marshall told us to set up the elevated master stream on the east side of the building per their BC's orders, then he left to go talk with command.

We secured a relay pumped water supply line from one of their engines and started flowing water into the fire from the tip of our aerial ladder, into the spots where it had broken through the roof. Through the turntable intercom, Willy P bet me $5 we wouldn't see Marshall again until we cleared the scene, and he was right. I stood on the ladder seventy-five feet in the air and worked the nozzle controls as Willy P camped out on the turntable below.

We stayed there all night until the sun rose over the horizon, then made entry and finally extinguished the fire. We were standing in the sanctuary in front of where the alter used to be when I closed the bale on the nozzle, tipped my helmet to the fire gods, and declared the beast officially slain. Then Marshall poked his head through a window to let us know we could clear, and we moved out. Back at the station I handed a smiling Willy P his $5. Unreal.

On August 14, 2003, as blackouts darkened the entire northeast region of the country, Mark Taylor and I were on Engine 3 for the shift. Over the following twelve hours straight, we made *sixteen* calls for elevator rescues in the downtown area. Multiply this call volume by nine other engine and ladder companies all doing the same thing and that's a small picture of the utter chaos that ensued that afternoon. When the electricity went out, the elevator systems lost power, and most of them weren't supplied with backup generators. We rolled from building to building, working with security teams and facility managers to free the trapped civilians.

My wife is deathly afraid of confined spaces. She gets claustrophobic just thinking about elevators. We were stuck in one on a Vegas trip for a short time and it was absolutely terrifying for her. So, for those who experience the same trepidation of being trapped in an elevator, I offer this complete explanation of the procedures that we, as first responders, go about mitigating that type of emergency. Hopefully, it serves to ease the troubled mind and grants a new perspective on the things one can do to help save their own ass, if necessary.

If anyone ever happens to find themselves in this situation, first and foremost, remain calm. There are instructions on the elevator panel to help. Try pressing a button for a floor above or below, as sometimes an elevator can become stuck between floors, and this could remedy it. Next, try pressing the open-door button and then the close-door button and see if that works. Usually there's an emergency phone or a call button that can connect to someone able to help. Press the alarm button to alert building staff to the situation.

If there's a cell phone signal, call 9-1-1. Give the dispatcher the address, and how many people are trapped. Sit tight. Remember that help is on the way. It's going to take a few minutes for the rescuers to respond, so be patient. When they arrive, they're going to rendezvous with the building maintenance or security staff and retrieve the master keys.

They'll try to recall the elevator to the lobby, and if that doesn't work, they'll have to kill... hah, no I mean cut... or, let's say, shut off the power in the EMR (elevator maintenance room). They'll locate the stopped car and contact the trapped passengers to advise on progress and plans to get everyone out safely. If it hasn't been done already, stop the audible alarm from inside the elevator so everyone can communicate clearly.

As a responder, I usually liked to bring along with me on these calls a bag of life safety rope, a folding stepladder, a set of irons, and the elevator keys from either our fire department key ring, or the building's Knox Box. We may need to obtain a set of elevator keys from the EMR. On the West Coast they typically use a Z Key. These elevator keys open the hoist way doors, granting access to the elevator shaft.

As rescuers we'll insert the key and twist or lift the end of it, depending on the type, then force the doors open. USE EXTREME CAUTION when working around open hoist way doors, to avoid falling into the open elevator shaft. We'll use a harness and tie off if needed, for safety's sake. Next, we'll locate the stalled car and determine the best point of access for rescue. If it's stuck between floors, is it easier to access the car's top or bottom? Choose the method that provides the greatest element of safety to the occupants and ease of access for the rescuers.

Be sure to chock and block the hoist way doors open. We don't want them closing in the middle of our operation if the power is restored. Locate the release arm on the exterior of the elevator car doors. We may need to use a pike pole from a floor above (called poling) to reach the door release if it's blocked by the space between floors. Once it's open, keep everyone calm; there's still work to be done before everyone can exit safely. I like to use a step ladder here to bridge the gap between the hoist way doors and the car. I'll enter the car next and place a spare harness with a belay line onto the victims if needed, helping them exit one at a time.

If we're unable to free the victims from the floor below, and a car top rescue is indicated, we'll need to ensure the power is off, then get at least two ladders and our high angle rope equipment for rescuer and victim safety. Place a ladder from the floor above, down to the stalled car's top, and secure it in place with rope rigging. Locate the car-top power shut-off and light switch. Activate the power shut-off and, if there's power, turn the light switch on. If not, illuminate the area with a battery powered carpenter or floodlight. Locate the car top elevator access panel door and open it.

Insert the folding ladder and send a rescuer into the car to help calm and organize the occupants. Attach a harness and tag line to the victims and have them exit in an orderly fashion once the safety equipment is properly donned. Another rescuer should be stationed on the car top to assist the victims up the ladder and out of the shaft, where a belay line tender can assist them onto the floor level.

Give the newly freed occupants plenty of space to kiss the ground and offer supplications to their gods for having made it out alive. Some of the victims like to hug, so if you're not a hugger, you may just have to take one for the team here. Be sure to leave the power off and caution tape or close all hoist way doors when we're done, until an elevator technician has verified that everything's back in proper working order.

During my two years at Station 8, I was fortunate to learn the craft from some great firemen. They taught me all the latest Tech Rescue methods and protocols. Confined space was always my favorite. It was just me, in a tiny claustrophobic place: a man alone with his thoughts. The bigger guys had to stay outside and staff the air hoses and carts, while the skinnier firefighters made entry into the area. We had to be comfortable in there, remaining calm, not freaking out or we'd be screwed.

Trench Rescue was crazy. We don't ever really stop and think about the fact that if we're buried in dirt or sand, it compresses around our torso with every breath we take until it's packed in so tight, we can't expand our lungs to breathe anymore. We'd use giant "strong backs"—basically four by eight-foot sheets of 1 inch plywood with two by twelves screwed lengthwise into them for support, to build a box and then excavate around the patient. Those motherfuckers were heavy as hell to carry. The tools alone in that Tech Rescue trailer were a carpenter's dream!

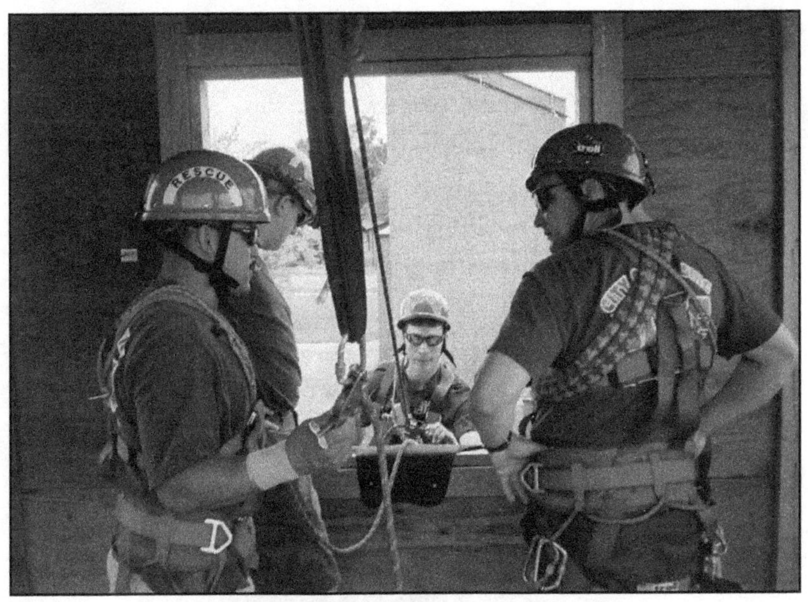

From left to right; Dan Martinez, Agent Mulder, Jason Hundt, and Dan Cooper

Structure Collapse was fascinating. We built bracing for shoring up destroyed buildings, learned techniques for searching them, and for locating where survivors were most likely to be. This was helpful when tornadoes or earthquakes ravaged a region. We had guys on staff who were actual builders and carpenters on their days off, so it worked out well on our shift.

I attended certification courses in high and low angle rope rescue. I learned a ton of knots and what seemed like a second language of vocabulary and terminology. There were things like; bombproof anchor points, strops, carabiners, belay lines, kernmantle ropes, Rollgliss pulley systems, double loop figure eights on bights, Munter hitches, double looped prusiks, ascenders, descenders, water knots, bowlines, load sharing anchors, delta maillons, bar racks, short snakes, long snakes, radium hitches, handcuff knots (also known as the Texas love knot), rope dogs, and alpine butterflies. It was the language of mountaineering.

We'd dangle off the practice tower out back, rappel from the tallest skyscrapers in the downtown area, and make rescue picks of people trapped on radio towers, roof tops, window washing platforms, and wind turbines. We'd do crazy things in terribly dangerous situations, and I loved every second of it. There's a great picture of me rappelling off the roof of city hall and giving the universal symbol for eating pussy, right outside the mayor's office.

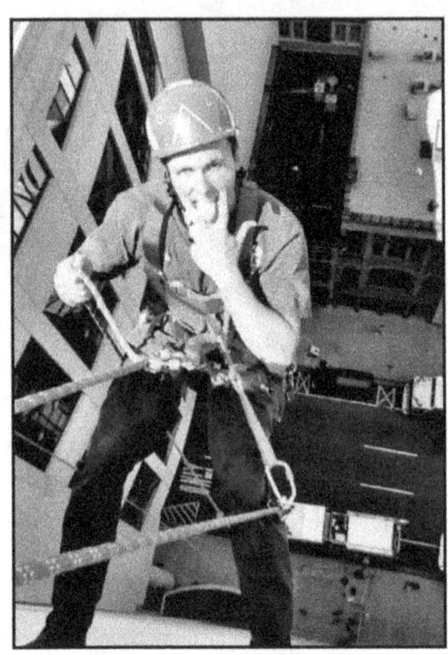

The author doing the high angle dangle

My biggest piece of advice if one ever finds themselves going over the edge of a building or a cliff and rappelling, is to lean *way* back. Lean farther back than you think you have to, then lean back even *farther*. Trust that equipment and lean back. Your back should be almost parallel to the ground, then bend your knees slightly, sit down into it, and adjust your angle for comfort. Picture yourself walking on the surface your feet are on. It's that far back.

The only real drawback to Eights was there was only one firefighter there. I was doing all the lowest seniority jobs for a double company station by myself. Nobody raced me to the phone—it was just my job. I cooked every day, swept and mopped the whole damn station, put the flag up and down, did the laundry, made the beds, and never got a break. The three engineers didn't help. They were too busy with the Tech Rescue trailer and training events.

The firefighter spot on the ladder truck was staffed by a third engineer in case someone had to drive the Tech Rescue trailer. It was an extremely long semi-truck. Think tiller truck length—the old ladder trucks that were so long they needed two steering wheels, one in the front and another in the back.

If a Tech Rescue call came in for anything in our region of the state, we were going. The back-end engineer on the ladder truck would drive the trailer, while we followed in the engine and ladder trucks. It was an impressive caravan of emergency vehicles to see rolling down the road.

Dave Bailey was a cigar guy. He always had a stubby cigar between his fingers or poking out from his mouth. Bailey was my engineer at Station 8. He always drove the ladder truck and I found out later he had more seniority than all the captains there. He never talked about why he'd frozen his rank at engineer, and it was only during a drunken deer camp poker game that I learned the truth.

It turned out that he'd stumbled into Station 7 one night, off duty and highly intoxicated. Thinking he was in the dormitory bathroom, he faced the urinal and began relieving himself. Only, he wasn't in the bathroom. He was standing over the bed of a sleeping female firefighter named Roberta Franklin, who awoke to a piping-hot golden shower courtesy of Dave Bailey. His brother Joe Bailey was a battalion chief at the time and lobbied Human Resources against the immediate firing of his younger brother.

The good ol' boy nepotism of the fire department and city government prevailed yet again over common sense and justice, and the issue was downplayed and simply swept under the rug. In the end all parties agreed to settling on a demotion to engineer for eternity without the possibility of promotion.

Dave was now a humble man, with a wealth of information, who knew his job inside and out, knew the streets and his rig like the back of his hand, and seldom drank to the point of blackout anymore. A great guy who taught me a lot about the value of a frozen senior engineer on your team. Although I'm certain Bobby Franklin would beg to differ with me on that one.

I discussed more frequently with Captain Carl about freezing my own rank at firefighter. He recommended against it and explained I had a lot to offer the higher ranks and would make a good officer someday. I brought it up around the department breakfast tables and asked the opinions of my colleagues. Everyone discouraged me from doing it.

Sure, it flew in the face of everything the rest of the department thought was good and right with seniority based promotional systems. But I was beginning to think it wasn't for me. I knew what I loved. The task-level stuff. It wasn't about the money anymore; it was about the mission. I wouldn't want to freeze at Eights, though. Only at a true double company station where I could ride the ladder truck every day, not make EMS calls, and have another firefighter doing the menial station work along with me.

I requested to leave Station 8 and was transferred to Fours in January 2005. The Dad and Lad era had come to an end. Carl made the battalion chief rank at the same time and left Eights for Station 1, and I just couldn't follow him down that road. It was a bittersweet goodbye, and I watched my once playful and jovial friend become an angry totalitarian ruler afterward. He disciplined everyone for the slightest infractions. Things he'd been guilty of doing dozens of times in his younger days and lower ranks. It was difficult to watch, and I knew right then, that would not be my legacy at the fire department.

Chapter 14

Making Rank

Let's talk briefly about rank structure. We hired on as a firefighter. We rotated shifts between a fire truck and an ambulance until we were promoted to engineer and got a small bump in pay to do so. However, at that time we also lost our ambulance incentive, which had given firefighters close to a lieutenant's wage if we were a paramedic.

So, now as an engineer, we made less than we did as a firefighter, only with the added responsibility of operating heavy equipment. We could choose to stay on the ambulance rotation after making engineer and keep our incentive, but not very many chose to do that, with all the added drama and sleepless nights it brought into our lives. Most firefighters had families by then and valued peace of mind over checking peckers (pecker checker = ambulance jockey).

Next was the officer's rank of lieutenant. Every new lieutenant did a six-month stint in Operations. After that was completed, the staffing rules had them working at the double companies, which comprised six of our nine stations. The captain's rank was next, and we received our own station with that. The junior captains were given the single company stations, and the senior captains were running the double companies.

After that came battalion chief and there were two of them on every day. Multiply all that by a 3 kelly, 2 shift scheduling system and we had a Fire Suppression division of 200 members strong. The support divisions of Maintenance, Prevention, Administration, and Training were all staffed with captains and chiefs ranks only, and we topped out at around 250 union-strong career firefighters when I hired on.

It wasn't uncommon to find the department seniority list, along with recent Fire Engineering magazines and updated AOGs (administrative operating guidelines) and SOGs (standard operating guidelines), strewn across the firehouse breakfast tables around the city. New kids would study the seniority list, trying to figure out how much longer they had in the ambulance rotation. Engineers wondered when they'd make the officer rank. Lieutenants wondered which station they might get someday. And the salty-dog captain old-timers would look to see how long until they could make the BCs rank and begin padding their pensions.

Everybody was jockeying for position, and they were all too happy to scratch out the name of a guy on the seniority list who'd dutied out, or quit, or transferred to a day division. They were moving up baby! One less person in the way of their promotional pay raise. The old-timers would ask the new kids how much time they had on and say things like, "Jesus Christ, I'd *hang* myself in the hose tower if I had that long to go," or "Holy shit, I've got underwear with more time in the stations than you."

As I got to know my colleagues by spending more time with them than their own loved ones did, I began to notice subtle changes that happened when they made rank. The engineers all put on weight; the "engineer twenty" they called it, while patting the sides of their bellies, and the ladies were no exception. Maybe it was a metabolic change associated with turning thirty. Or maybe it was a lack of required movement associated with the rank. Maybe they just ate more and exercised less. Whatever it was, they packed the pounds on. I won't even sugar coat it.

Lieutenants and captains seemed to struggle with letting go of their old, youthful habits and having to discipline their peers. It was a role reversal. Instead of rebelling against the establishment, now they were tasked with maintaining order in the organization and enforcing the very rules they'd earlier decried as oppressive to their basic human rights.

Some officers completely lost their mind on their troops. Upsetting certain ones would find us stripping and waxing the floors for punishment, all day long, until ten at night, on Christmas Eve. No shit—just ask Dan Martinez and Big Daddy about the time Fuckface ruined their holiday. Or enduring six-hour rope schools on fire service knots that were obsolete since the 1960s. Or any number of menial, bullshit tasks they could make us do for punishment.

BJ once had us change in and out of our dress uniforms four times, before noon, "just to fuck with the engineer," Wendy Simpson. Whom, incidentally, claimed harassment and discrimination against him and requested a battalion chief and union steward. The whole crew united against him, and BJ was sent home, transferred to the opposite shift, and busted down to engineer for life after that debacle.

Later, he'd sneak into the captain's quarters at Nines, off duty, drunk, and try to rape the female captain there. He was fired for that one, but somehow his attorneys convinced the city to give him his job back. They claimed the two had a previous sexual relationship. Teflon Don he was called, because like a nonstick cooking pan, no charges of wrongdoing would stick to him.

By far, the biggest personality change was at the battalion chief's rank. Guys' hair went completely gray or disappeared altogether within a month of making it. Once happy men no longer smiled. They were administrators now, calling a game of chess on the firegrounds, and we were the pawns. Some of them had heart attacks. Some had strokes. I think the best way I can describe it is that their joy was gone. Whatever image they saw themselves as, it was not what they'd wanted it to be. They did it for the money. And it wasn't worth it. Not even remotely.

When I hired on, the difference between a full paid firefighter and a battalion chief was around $13,500 per year. That's about $1,125 a month. I figured I could make that up on my twenty days off per month easily. Why would I want to make rank? Glory? Command? Please. I worked with a bunch of wackadoos. If I was their boss, I'd be the head wackadoo. No thanks.

I'd be writing them up daily for dumbass shit or get caught in a scandal or something. Ideas were brewing. I wondered if it was possible to freeze my rank at firefighter and get off the ambulance. All of the action with none of the bullshit. The union contract held the answers I sought. It was possible, with permission from the chief of the department.

There's another sinister change that happens toward the end of firefighters' careers: *Short-Timer's Syndrome*. It causes a pusillanimous reaction in their risk-taking abilities, and they turn into cowards. The ones who have three months or less until retirement, seem to stop trying so hard to get to their rigs fast. They drag their feet in hopes they'll get beat into their own area and won't have to go inside on structure fires. They're fine with being second-in and just grabbing a hydrant. Water supply was an important fireground task they'd say to justify it.

They'd stop asking for the good fireground jobs, too. Instead, opting for exposure control or staging officer. It broke my heart to be able to make a significant impact on the outcome of scenes and have my boss decline the opportunity to be heroes. These guys would literally disappear on us at the scene. They feared action, and it was disgusting to watch them turn tail and run for cover when shit was going down.

Doug Gordon or "Gordo" as we called him, hit his retirement eligibility as a captain because the BC ranks were full of old-timers getting their full two years in at that rank. After his classmates had all retired, he took the promotion to the BC spot. He stayed another two years past retirement eligibility and held up promotions at every rank, just to pad his wallet with an extra hundred and fifty bucks a month for life.

Personally, I spent an extra *two years* on the medic because of it. Those waiting on him to leave began ruthless campaigns to make his station life hell, hoping to force him to retire. They felt like he was taking money out of their pockets. Elderly walkers with tennis balls on their legs, adult diapers, and geriatric equipment were stuffed into his locker and BC car daily, for two years straight, every day he came in to work. Just to let him know he was old, and it was time for him to retire. It was brutal on both sides.

I mentioned earlier I was the first in my class to break-in on all the department's fire apparatus. A necessary step to becoming a second driver. I acted engineer for the first time when I had three and a half years on. At Station 8 that day, we made a small house fire, first-in. I stood outside at the curb and pulled the pump levers, while my brothers were inside. I was alone, outside of a burning house, while we waited for more rigs to respond. Everything went fine and we packed up our gear and headed back to the station. But I didn't really *enjoy* it.

That night, I woke to the medical alarm and rolled out of bed. When the dispatcher said the address, I drew a blank. I didn't know that street. It took me a moment to find the street in my map book. Hell, it took me a moment to realize where I was at in the city. The boys were already in the rig waiting for me and as I cruised through the streets, I'd made up my mind.

I knew then I was freezing my rank at firefighter. Fuck writing reports and pulling levers. I was going to be a nozzleman and a truckie. Every goddamn day. To be the guy working the tool, saving the day, directly impacting the situation's outcome. I would lead from the bottom rank and give my officers someone they could rely on. A partner with just as much experience as they had. Someone who knew the ropes inside and out, like Engineer Bailey did.

The senior members of every rank enjoyed certain benefits. Roving was based on seniority, so I could be at one station every day I worked. They got first pick of the vacation and personal leave days, so I could get holidays off and spend them with my family. They were able to choose their station assignments, too. This decision was starting to look better all the time.

When the chief of the department granted me the ability to leave the ambulance rotation, in writing (when the person behind me in rank made engineer and passed me), I submitted my request to freeze at the firefighter rank. I was instantly the senior-most firefighter in the department and would stay there for the next thirteen years. Everybody was always jockeying for rank, and I didn't give two shits about it. *Fuck* academia. They say those who can, do. And those who can't, teach. I didn't need any letters after my name to be a hero. Real-world experience is far more valuable than what's taught in a classroom or in a textbook.

Some said I was crazy.

Granted.

Some said I was a fool.

Hardly.

Some said I was a genius, and they too followed suit. Soon, there were frozen firefighters at the top of the rank structure on every shift. We ruled the roost. Money was not a factor in our decisions. We did it for peace of mind, and we did it for a deep and abiding love of the game.

I worked with the best captains, in the best stations. Our engineers were frozen too, so they were the best and most experienced. We ruled firegrounds. We rode ladder trucks every day, and we didn't do any bullshit. We rolled on every fire and every rescue. No more EMS calls, no more report writing. Everything had a purpose and was carefully calculated, and it was one of the best times of my life.

Chapter 15

All Kinds of Awkward (Character Shorts)

All right, I'll go ahead and start this one off. If there's a chapter here that pokes fun at the stupidity and lack of fire service intelligence of others, I'll willingly sacrifice myself and jump on that grenade as the first burnt offering to the fire gods. Martyrdom being a hallmark of the best heroes and all.

On the day we drew for seniority in rank at the training academy, the department mentor of trainees gave a speech before the entire recruit class of nineteen probationary firefighters. Tim Sanchez began his tutelage of how to act and perform our duties in the fire station with those famous words: "There are no stupid questions." Followed by: "If you don't know, ask."

My friends, that is absolutely *not* true. He went on to say how fighting fire is much more than just "putting the wet on the red." My mind spun. Having no previous fire training to fall back on, I'd never heard this saying before. So, like an idiot, I raised my hand.

"Yes, in the back there," Tim said.

"Yes, sir. What's 'put the wet on the red' mean?" I asked.

Immediately, I began to sweat as every person in the crowded room turned around slowly to see who it was that had just asked the dumbest question in the history of the US Fire Service. With all eyes on me, and most staring in disbelief at what they'd just heard, some shaking their heads that we'd hired yet another jackass off the street who knew nothing about the job and all of its intricacies, Tim explained, very slowly, so the idiot in the room could understand, how putting the wet on the red was a *firefighting* term describing the act of putting *water*, which was wet, onto a *fire*, which was red.

"Oh, thank you, sir," I said, my face turning as red as a fire truck. The captains, engineers, chiefs, recruit firefighters, and union officials continued to stare at the moron in the room while Tim went on about the difference between Signal 1s and 2s, making sure there was always a fresh pot of coffee on, giving station tours, and night watch. Remember the saying that goes, it's better to keep your mouth shut and be thought a fool, than to open it and remove all doubt? They wrote that one about me, right there. I spent my next twenty years internally attempting to live down that first impression from the fire academy.

The great thing about our department was if we did something stupid, we just had to wait about two weeks, and someone else would top our act of foolishness and everybody ridiculed them instead. There were plenty of morons at the fire department so I could blend right in and disappear. You don't have to be smart to be a firefighter. In fact, it helps if you're not.

The fire department had some crazy characters staffing its many stations and rigs. Some of the most interesting people I've ever met were coworkers of mine. Not all of them are worthy of mention here, but a few of them hold dubious distinctions of hilarity and insanity. These are a few of the more noteworthy, short descriptions of them, and their greatest faux pas.

There was a black shift captain at old Station 4 who had narcolepsy. Max Costanza was legendary when I hired on; for one thing. One day, while sitting in the engine, waiting for his crew to finish grocery shopping, he'd fallen asleep. When dispatch tried repeatedly to raise them to respond on a call, but couldn't, the battalion chief was sent over to investigate.

Upon finding Max sleeping in the fire truck, the BC was understandably upset and banged on the window, startling Max, and waking him from his narcoleptic slumber. "What the fuck, Max? Dispatch has been calling you for an alarm."

Max smacked his lips, rubbed his eyes, and said to the BC, "You can't make 'em all."

The BC lost it on Max, and before writing him up for being an idiot, he explained that yes, in fact, we are expected to make them all; that's the reason they pay us.

At Station 1, in the dead of winter, a young firefighter named Marky Mark read on the daily duty list, the words "Windows Up." For many generations, this had been the phrase to inform the firefighters to clean—with glass cleaner—the upstairs windows. Mark understood it differently and took it to mean that he was supposed to put all of the windows in the fire station up, and open.

When the battalion chief came out of his office and into the freezing cold station, he was curious to know why someone had opened all the windows. Mark explained how he was just doing the daily chores, putting the windows up, like the duty list says, and thereby cemented his place of distinction in the annals of our fire department's history.

Then there was Josh Porter, who, as a new kid, called in sick one day because he cut his penis while showering and had to get stitches. You'd better believe Ops spread his new name "Stitch" all over town in minutes. Questions like, how, and why, with their associated theories and conjectures floated around the dinner tables that day, and poor Stitch had some splainin' to do when he returned to work the next week.

Our very own union president, we'll call him Felonious, was a convicted felon. How he kept his job, I have no clue. Felonious was off duty at a bar up north when a local resident began making advances on his wife. He and the guy got into a scuffle, and it spilled out into the parking lot. Ol' Felonious pulled out a gun and fired it into the air to ward off the attacker. The police arrived as he discharged the weapon, took him into custody, and hauled him off to jail.

It's always awkward when one had to call the station and tell them they wouldn't be coming to work that day because they're in the slammer. Felonious spent three weeks in jail and was sentenced for his crimes to something like six months in the county lockup. Through trade time and backdoor deals he made it out and kept his job. That's union-strong, bitches.

Bruce Allen went bat shit crazy one day. He decided he was going to break into Station 1 and steal the half bill and contingent money to pay off his spiraling debt. Ever since the murder of one of our on-duty firefighters, which Bruce had witnessed right in front of him after surviving the attempt on his own life, he'd been barely holding it together. His family had been crying out to everyone, including the fire department for help, but no one listened.

After midnight one evening, Bruce falsely called 9-1-1 and reported a shooting, then watched as Station 1 emptied out into the night. He made his move when the alarm lights went out, sneaking into the firehouse and lifting the lock boxes from their cabinets. Chase Powers was the on-duty battalion chief and had just returned from the false alarm, opening the garage doors, and flipping on the apparatus floor lights as Bruce was walking across it with his treasure chests full of booty.

When Chase asked what was going on, Bruce confessed, and Chase called the police. Bruce was arrested for larceny and reporting a false alarm and sentenced to probation and mandatory rehab. The department shipped him out to Maryland to the IAFF (International Association of Fire Fighters) rehab program on a prison bus that was heading that way. Bruce ditched the program, fled the facility, and returned home by hitchhiking from truck stop to truck stop. He was fired, then claimed a PTSD duty disability from the murder incident. After some legal wrangling, he was granted his job back with the condition he complete the rehab. Which he did… eventually.

Wendell Turner was a captain at Nines and a rather short and portly man. He would tell his crews he was going upstairs to work out each afternoon after lunch. When they passed by the workout room later, Wendell would most often be lying on the weight bench fast asleep in his workout clothes, and the Wendell Workout became synonymous with taking an afternoon nap.

Darren Komm was a black shift firefighter at Station 8 who was about five feet eight tall and weighed in at close to three hundred pounds. When it was his turn to cook the night meal for the crews, he would routinely say he was calling Domino's because he was "fuggin' tarred" (fucking tired). His black shift brethren began calling it "Komm"-ino's because Darren ordered it so often for them.

Mandy Thorn hired on just before me. Her first and second husbands both passed away on her and she'd taken up bodybuilding to deal with the grief. As she cut weight and lowered her body fat by refusing to eat, she developed deep, dark eye sockets and gaunt cheekbones. The joke was that her body resembled She-Ra with Skeletor's face, in reference to the *Masters of the Universe* characters.

At the dinner table at Fours in the evenings, Mandy would be off the mess, but would come sit with us and longingly watch us all eat. She'd take one large spoonful of peanut butter and lick it repeatedly until the spoon shined clean. One day during this activity, I noticed everyone at the table had stopped eating and was staring at Mandy, licking her spoon like a lollipop. The next morning, Joe Collins had written her name on all the jars of peanut butter in the cupboard.

Mike Rhodes and Tim Warner were two of the tiniest men I'd ever met. Small in stature, they were both big on ego and would argue their points to no end. Both officers at the time, the two had pushed each other to the limit one day, and a fight broke out at Station 6 on the black shift. It was worse than a cat fight with the two of them slapping and clawing at each other until Mike latched onto Tim's pinky finger and twisted it. Tim cried out in pain and holding onto his mangled digit, declared the fight over. They both had to go visit Human Resources over that one and the broken pinky finger fight became a black shift legend.

Jason Hundt had been at the fire department for a few years when I hired on, and some of the guys I was working with told me his name was Mike. So, for the first six months I worked there, that's what I called him. Until one day he calmly explained to me that his name was really Jason—not Mike. Not Mike Hundt. He went on to inform me that I'd been duped into saying "my cunt." I was so naïve, it's scary. Poor Mike… I mean Jason.

Dan Milton was a firefighter and the son of Denny Milton, an active-duty captain on our department. One Saturday, while helping the crew clean the apparatus bay, Dan found himself on a slippery cement floor covered in water and soap. His portly stature and lack of ice-skating prowess led to an unfortunate slip and fall. His feet went completely out from under him, and he landed flat on his back in the puddle. As he struggled to move and regain his breath, one of the crew suggested he resembled a fish out of water and "Flounder" became his new nickname.

Flounder, unfortunately, was not the only nickname young Dan Milton had. At Station 1, he was assigned to the engine, when a fire alarm came in. He hustled to the rig, donned his gear, and climbed aboard as they rolled out of the station. The rig made a hard left onto the street and continued its left turn onto the adjacent street.

With the acceleration of the pegged throttle, and the resulting G forces of the sharp turn, Dan fell over from the momentum and landed against the door. His weight pushed down on the latch, causing the door to fly open as they rounded the corner. Dan fell from the truck and went rolling across the intersection, earning him the dubious nickname of "Tumbleweed" as well.

For physical therapy at Station 6 one day, the crew decided to head over to the local track and run laps for a nice cardio workout. Ken Nelson was a socially awkward, yet friendly new firefighter. He was excited for the field trip and arrived ready to workout. He had a red, white, and blue headband around his freshly shaved bald head, short shorts, and white knee-high tube socks with the red and blue stripes to match his headband.

As the crew stretched out and readied on the line for their one-mile jog, Ken took off and, doing a high-knee 360 to look back at everyone, yelled, "C'mon guys, let's go!" and he sprinted off. The veteran crew calmly paced themselves, and as they returned to the starting line after one lap, there was Kevin, beet red and lying on his back, out of breath. The official report describes him as "turtled up" and unable to continue his shift due to exhaustion. He had unfortunately become incapacitated after just one lap. So goes the legend of "Nelson's ¼ mile marathon."

Marky Mark again, of the previous "Windows Up" legend, was on duty at Station 6 one day and wanted to go play in an intramural soccer game at the local indoor arena. His fire department team was playing that night, so he asked the station captain for permission to take the ambulance over there. Scott Sherman was the officer and begrudgingly agreed to allow it, stating bluntly, "If your dumbass gets hurt, I didn't know about it."

Mark agreed, and when the time came to join his teammates, he changed out of his uniform and took the field. Midway through the match he was checked into the boards and received an awful compound fracture to his radius and ulna. His ambulance partner drove him to the ER, where the battalion chief met them; since they were obviously not in service anymore, and with a little interrogation, Mark explained he'd received permission to play from Scott. Throwing his captain under the bus to save himself. Everyone got written up with formal discipline for their roles in the "Soccer Debacle."

Incidentally, that same night a fight broke out between the two teams at Soccer Zone when one of the opponents decided to send the ball into low-earth orbit by bouncing it off Ginger McEntire's face. She was about five feet away in front of the guy when he let it rip from mid-field, and her face absolutely exploded. I've never seen an impact like that, full frontal, head snapped back, took her right off her feet. The benches cleared, and a brawl ensued.

Speaking of full frontal, Scott Sherman (from our previous story) has a blunder of legendary status himself. The "Sherman Face Plant" occurred when he was a younger lad, on the ambulance for the day. He was standing over his naked male patient, straddling the cot while the sled was en route to the hospital, attempting to start an IV in the patient's far arm. This, we are taught, is a dangerous and compromising position to be in, as Steve was soon to find out.

While transporting a patient to the ER, the driver must deftly maneuver through the city streets. Dodging potholes and traffic and carefully negotiating turns so the crews in the back can administer patient care effectively. Smooth is the name of the game. Easy on the stops and goes. When the ambulance driver had to slam on the brakes to avoid T-boning a car in an intersection, poor Scott wasn't holding on to the grab bar and took a header directly into the fully exposed patient genitalia. Straight cock to lips—no word of a lie.

We were at the hospital finishing our report one day when Medic 1 rolled into the ambulance bay with a woman in labor. I opened the back doors to help unload the cot and Brad Perry gave me a horrified look as he jumped out to help make sure the cot legs locked properly into place, as I pulled it from the rig.

"Get me the hell out of here," he said under his breath.

They wheeled the expectant mother off to labor and delivery, and after Brad made it back to the ambulance report writing room, I asked him what happened.

While his oblivious partner was outside cleaning the medic unit after the call, Brad explained how he'd asked his EMT, Julio Torres, to check for crowning on the pregnant woman. Julio, not fully understanding how to do this, reached his hand between her legs and inserted it into her vagina, replying to Brad matter-of-factly, "She's dilated to four fingers."

Brad, assuming his brief career was in jeopardy because of Julio's abhorrent actions, asked his partner to please get out and drive, while he spent the next three minutes en route attempting to soothe her pain and be as nice as he could to dissuade the young lady from suing them for negligent malpractice. Fortunately for Brad and Julio, their patient was not aware of the abuse, or in too much distress to care, and nothing came of the incident except an ass chewing for Julio, courtesy of his partner that day.

Later in his career, when Julio was appointed to the Q/A (quality assurance) committee—the group that reviews customer complaints and hands out penalties for procedural violations—there was a collective uproar given his own checkered past. Cries of "How does ol' four fingers get to be on the committee?" and "Mister Fister probably isn't the most qualified to sit on the board," were levied against him. They weren't wrong.

There was *another* narcoleptic man on our department who suffered from a skin condition as well, earning him the nickname "Alligator Hands." Marshall Harris could often be found standing in the back of classrooms to avoid falling asleep during the presentation. The scary thing was, if a person ever went to shake his hand, they would unknowingly close their hand around the freakiest palms humankind had ever known.

They were scaly, like the back of an alligator, and usually soaked in gobs of moisturizing lotion. So, it was sweaty, sticky, and scaly. The faces people would make while shaking hands and trying to say, "Nice to meet you, Marshall," were hilarious. Some would jerk their hands away and scream. Some would twitch and crack horribly twisted smiles. But invariably, once you shook his hand, you would never ever make that mistake again.

There was a black shift fire at a nine-story brick, turn-of-the-century residential death trap. Firefighter Kyle Locke was told to take a coiled manila rope to the seventh-floor stairwell window and drop it down so the engineers could begin tying tools to it. Then Kyle could haul them up the exterior of the building, as opposed to climbing the stairs with hundreds of pounds of equipment in his hands.

Kyle, as a new kid, didn't quite grasp the concept, and as he leaned out the window, dropped the rope down to the ground. All of it. Still in the neatly tied bundle he'd just carried up. Which, obvious to everyone but Kyle, left him without an end to pull the tools up with.

This method of bringing tools to the fire floor was archaic, outdated, and lazy in my opinion. I never used it and just viewed the extra weight and stair climbing as a good workout. Residents fleeing down the stairwells would cheer us on as we climbed, looking like pack mules and Sherpas scaling the peaks of Everest. That's how the real pros did it.

Walter Spidel hired on with me in 1998 and was assigned to the black shift at old Station 6. On his very first day of work, he came into the dining room and introduced himself at the head of the breakfast table saying to everyone in a cheerful tone, "Hi everyone! I'm Walter Spidel, but my friends call me Spidey."

After an awkward silence, one of the red shifters spoke up and said, "How 'bout we call you asshole." Walter's smile disappeared from his face, and he left the room dejected amidst the raucous laughter of his new station mates.

Big Daddy hired on with me. When we were both new kids, he left me alone on the scene of a highway PI accident when he decided to ride into the hospital with a critical patient on a different medic unit than the one we were assigned to. I asked one of the engineers from the engine company that responded, to drive our sled to the hospital to retrieve him, while I provided treatment for the basic patient in the back. He apparently didn't realize at the time that it took at least two people to operate an ambulance successfully.

Prior to that one, he almost got himself fired by calling in sick after attending the red shift Christmas party the night before. Operations tended to frown upon new kids boozing it up and then reporting to work drunk. It was even worse as a new kid, to party with the same guys he proceeded to call the next morning and request to be placed on sick leave, because he was still drunk from the night before. Especially since he'd only accrued twenty-four hours of sick leave during his short, one-month tenure there as an employee.

September 1, 2004, was a beautiful sunny afternoon. I was washing my car in the driveway at home when Operations called. I sent them to voicemail because I didn't really feel like working callback that day. My neighbor Norma came out of her house and asked if I'd seen the news, that there was a big fire downtown, and she pointed off to the north. I looked up to see a huge plume of heavy black smoke chugging upward into the sky.

It was a massive oil distribution company fire that burned all day and into the night. Brent Gillette tells a hilarious story of the initial crews and their struggle to contain the fire. He says it was like the old Keystone Cops—only with firemen.

"With the fire load, there was no way anyone was putting that fire out," Brent recalls. "The only way it was going out was after it had exhausted its fuel supply. Protecting exposures was the only option."

As they crested the bridge over the river, Brent and Todd Heyward on 6 Engine, had a bird's eye view of the scene. Fifty-five-gallon drums of oil were exploding and being launched into the air like mortars. The plume of smoke from the scene was the size of an entire city block and extended into the air as far as they could see. They were the third-due engine company, and when they arrived, people were running everywhere.

Brent says Engine 8 with Engineer Tyrone Blake was parked ten feet away from the oil storage building. His crew had made entry, and Tyrone was at the pump panel, on air, wearing a Scott pack because the smoke was so heavy next to the rig. Brent asked why he was parked so close, and Tyrone replied that's where Captain Ron Finkle had wanted him.

Engineer Rob Osborn had backed Truck 8's turntable up to the scene and Captain Leon Walker was dragging a five-inch hose he'd just uncoupled from an engine bed, over toward the ladder truck. As he hooked it into the rear of the truck, the ladder was still in the bed and pointed directly at the cab of Engine 1.

The windows on Engine 1 were rolled down because it was a nice summer day outside. Its crew had received an assignment and were deployed elsewhere on the scene. When Captain Walker radioed Patricio Mendoza at the hydrant and said to charge it, Brent recalls a strange hissing sound coming from the nozzle at the tip of Truck 8's ladder. Everyone turned to try to comprehend the noise. It was the pressurized air from inside the five-inch hose escaping through the nozzle, being pushed by thousands of gallons of water. Seconds later, water came shooting out the end of the still-bedded aerial master stream and flowed directly into the cab of Engine 1.

At 1,000 gallons per minute, it didn't take long for the stream, which was cascading off of the interior of the windshield, to completely fill the cab up and start spilling out over the doors. Rob Osborn ran to his turntable and tried to raise the ladder from the bed. As he did, he rotated it away from Engine 1, saving it from the deluge. However, as he rotated it to his right, the water stream sliced right through the recently established rehab and staging areas the medic crews had just set up.

People were completely soaked and dove for cover from the non-elevated master stream that carved its way through the troops. Rob finally navigated his ladder through the crowds and underneath the power lines—which were now on fire above him—and positioned his water stream at the fire, helping to cool it. As the water lazily drifted onto the flames, some noticed that the stream didn't have the correct pressure it normally should have.

Herein lies the lesson, my friends. With a hydraulic pump, there are ports for intake, and ports for output. If we don't connect our water supply line to the correct port, our equipment doesn't function properly. Usually, the intakes are down lower, and the outputs are up higher, and they should always be labeled. When Captain Walker hooked the hydrant supply into the rear panel of the ladder truck, he connected it to the wrong intake. The pipe he hooked into was separate from the pump and had no gates to control the pressure or flow of water. It was straight hydrant pressure, and the only way to turn it off was to shut down the fire hydrant.

As is often the case at these cock knockers, Brent relieved himself the following morning because he'd agreed to trade time with another engineer. So all the oil-covered hose that he'd packed up from the scene in the middle of the night was sitting in a twelve-foot-high by twenty-foot-wide pile at Station 8 when he arrived there. He spent the whole next day, until 22:00 hours that night, cleaning it off with a pressure washer and degreaser. Good times.

Rocky Faust was a black shift engineer who would always one-up our stories. If we told a tale of a rough night on the sled, he'd reply how that was nothing, and then go into his own story on the matter. His name became synonymous with the verb for having just had a story one-upped. We'd just been Fausted.

He'd also frequently say the words *god dammit*. However, Rocky spoke with a nasal inflection to his voice, and it often came out sounding like "nyod nyammit." If someone remarked how they'd just been Fausted, it was customary to reply with a nasally sounding "nyod nyammit."

Like I said earlier, if one screwed up and made a fool of themselves, they only had to wait a week or two and someone else would be the talk of the town. Guys were worse than a bunch of little old ladies gossiping at the breakfast tables in the fire houses. Seriously.

Chapter 16

Stuck

All of us have, at one point, found ourselves in a position in life where we acknowledge we've become stuck and need to ask for assistance. The fire department is imminently qualified to help with all manner of "stuck," given its plethora of forcible entry tools and extensive body of rescue knowledge. From being pinned inside a wrecked car, to finding oneself trapped within a burning structure, to any other conceivable situation one could possibly need rescuing from, the fire department has a knack for saving people from their predicaments.

For me personally, vehicle extrications are the most exciting of these. I've always enjoyed being on the tools and cutting cars. Most of my career was spent at extrication focus stations and the runs and memories are extensive. Some stand out above the rest.

With a year or two under my belt, I roved up to Station 2 on the north end of town. That afternoon around 15:00 hours, we were dispatched to a head on collision. It was about ten blocks away from the station, so we arrived quickly. Two Pontiac Grand

Ams had struck each other head-on, and the damage was catastrophic. The speed limit was 45 miles per hour, and the eastbound driver had fallen asleep and crossed the center line.

As the officer and I walked to different cars to check on the patients, we found both drivers were pinned inside their vehicles, and both were in critical condition. As my officer relayed the information to dispatch and requested a second sled, the engineer and I prepared the extrication tools and positioned the hydraulic pump between the cars so we could work on both simultaneously.

I started on the green one. The man was unconscious in the driver's seat and his legs were pinned beneath the dash. My officer began on the blue one. The woman was still conscious in the driver's seat, and also pinned by the dashboard. As I began to pop the door with the spreaders, 5 Engine radioed that they were delayed by a train and needed to find an alternative route. That's when shit went downhill fast.

After the door pop, I could see the man's leg was fractured midshaft at his femur and nearly severed. He had an arterial bleed, and it was spurting bright red blood into a puddle in the foot well. I applied a tourniquet and twisted it tight, as my engineer switched the hydraulic tools. When he was done, I picked up the cutters to snip the A pillar for a dash roll. I twisted the handle, and nothing moved. When I looked down, hydraulic fluid was squirting out from the handle in a steady stream. The tools wouldn't work, and a man was dying right in front of me. With no operational extrication tools, I prayed for 5 Engine to hurry the fuck up.

I glanced over and saw my lieutenant pop the driver's door on his Grand Am.

The first medic unit rolled up, and I waved them over and reported my priority patient's condition. "Thirty-five-year-old male, unconscious, airbag deployment, dashboard impingement on his legs, compound femur fracture with an arterial bleed."

They went to work packaging the patient for transport, while our engineer tried to figure out why the cutters weren't working.

I could hear 5 Engine screaming toward us in the distance.

The *hoses*.

I remembered from our in-service training, if the hydraulic hoses weren't seated properly in their couplings, hydraulic fluid would flow in, but it couldn't flow back out the return line. That was it. I checked the connections, and the return line was barely seated. Covered in hydraulic oil, my gloves slipped as I tried to twist and pull back the coupling. Finally, it clicked together properly.

I swung into action with the functioning cutters—shearing through the A pillar, B pillar, then C Pillar of the driver's side.

5 Engine rolled up with pre-connected extrication tools and their firefighter jumped on the other side of the car with his cutters while I prepared the dash roll. I set the rocker panel brace and disconnected our cutters, replacing them with the hydraulic ram.

Setting one end on the brace, I twisted the handle, extending the ram until it bit into the A pillar at the curve of the dashboard. The roof was off, and the medics pounced on the patient like vultures on a carcass, starting multiple IVs and placing the C-collar. I twisted the handle on the hydraulic ram and the dash rolled up and off the man's legs.

My god, I thought. The rising dash revealed both legs were nearly severed clean through. Two jagged femurs were sticking through ripped blue jeans and as the medics rotated his torso to lay on the backboard; his legs below the fractures were barely hanging on by thin pieces of skin. If it wasn't for the blue jean denim, they probably would've fallen right off. I was impressed the tourniquet I'd placed earlier had stopped the arterial bleed. Either that or he'd simply run out of fluid. When we grabbed his lower legs from the pool of blood in the foot well, they were soaked in it and dripping. I helped load the patient into the sled and then went to check on the other car.

They'd just finished the roof removal and were preparing for the dash roll. Their patient was in significantly better condition than mine was—conscious, though still critical. I positioned the rocker panel brace and the ram. As I twisted the handle on the ram, the dash raised up and released its victim. The medics removed her from the vehicle and transported her to the hospital.

There's usually a moment of pause after the patients leave the scene in the medics. Time to breathe. I explained to the engineer what happened—why the tools weren't working. We piled the car doors and roofs back into their original cars and swept the street clear of glass and plastic trim pieces. We dumped HyDry onto the asphalt to soak up the oil and coolant. The wreckers came and hauled away the vehicles and we went home. Both patients survived.

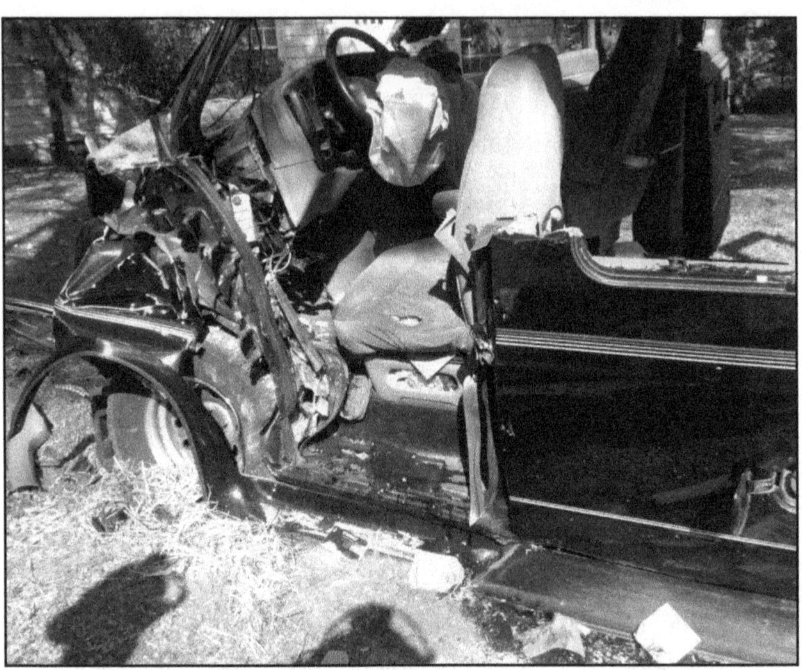

A typical extrication scene after the patient has been transported

At Station 5 one overcast afternoon, "Cowboy" Dan Henry and I were on the medic unit, when a call came in for a three-year-old with an airway obstruction. Children in trouble always brought out the best in us, and we raced to the scene with reckless abandon. Cowboy parked the sled out on the road, which was a long way from the house in an upper-class neighborhood. We ran our equipment up to the door and an elderly lady—still on the phone with dispatch—let us in.

Just inside, a little girl was lying face down in the thick plush carpet. I rolled her over and she was purple, still conscious, unable to breathe, and staring at me with the biggest blue eyes about to pop out of her head. Cowboy scooped her up in his arms and like a fullback running down the football field, took off for the ambulance across the yard. I heard the fast-paced thud of back blows on the child as he carried her over his left arm and beat on her back with his right.

Her grandmother explained the girl was running and eating popcorn and began to choke. She didn't know what to do, so she just left her there on the floor, and called 9-1-1. Doing the math in my head that meant this child hadn't taken a breath in over three minutes. I got her name and told the grandmother to meet us at the hospital, then sprinted to the ambulance with our gear.

Dan was working feverishly to get air into the child with hard chest thrusts and back blows, followed by two vents with a BVM (bag valve mask). The girl was still conscious and looking up at me with those big blue eyes that begged: *Please don't let me die*. Another round of chest thrusts and back blows, another two breaths. They went in this time. The kid started making a squeaky, whistling noise every time she took a breath, but she was breathing.

The popcorn kernel stuck in her throat had been pushed down farther into her right main bronchi, allowing the left lung to get air flowing again. She sounded like a squeaky toy, but her eyes held the look of relief. Her skin color returned almost immediately, and I drove like the wind to the ER. She survived and made a full recovery. I had a hard time understanding how a person could just leave their grandchild face down in the carpet, not breathing. We'll file that one in the fucked-up shit folder. At least she lived.

Linda Gross, one of the town drunks, had a sister named Betty Gross, who stepped on a railroad tie one afternoon and had a twelve-inch spike pierce clean through the middle of her foot. Engine 9 was toned out after Krishna and Showtime on Medic 6, made the decision to cut the railroad tie and leave the impaled object in situ. This was in line with what we'd been taught; however, it turned into quite an ordeal.

I was riding Engine 9 that day and prepared to cut her loose. Showtime was explaining the procedure to Betty, while Krishna started an IV and snowed her with morphine for pain. The spike was stabilized with gauze and cravats, and I began to cut through the railroad tie with a Sawzall. Just for future reference, most railroad ties have an S-shaped metal band running through the length of them. If we don't have a blade that can cut through this metal, there's going to be a lot of vibration and torquing on the tie. There was a lot anyway.

This of course caused Betty a tremendous amount of pain, which she verbalized to the entire neighborhood, which had gathered around and stood watching in nervous anticipation. I pretended not to hear and gritted my teeth, finishing the cut. Let me tell you, a one-foot-long chunk of eight-inch by eight-inch railroad tie hanging from your foot by a twelve-inch-long spike is quite unwieldy and much heavier than it appears. It's also very difficult to find the illusive "position of comfort" driving down the pothole-strewn roads of inner-city paradise.

Betty was transferred to the hospital staff with the chunk of railroad tie still impaled in her foot, and the removal operation was a smashing success. The lead emergency department doctor seemed frustrated with Krishna's overly literal translation of the protocol on impaled objects, and while looking him in the eye, proceeded to yank the chunk of railroad tie from Betty's foot and toss it across the trauma room floor, much to Betty's disapproval. Apparently distal appendages didn't qualify on the list of impaled body parts that required an object to be stabilized and left in place, only to be removed by the hospital staff.

On Engine 4 we responded to Fred Street for a young boy with his head stuck between the balcony bars on the deck of his apartment. Pat Duncan and I tried to pull the spindle bars apart like two supermen, but it wasn't quite enough. Fergie got some dish soap and dumped it along the sides of the kid's head, but he remained stuck. Pro tip: If you ever find yourself stuck between two objects, try using dish soap to lubricate the surfaces.

We were an extrication station and had the Jaws of Life, but that was a little too much brute force for this delicate situation. The decision was made to utilize the air bags that we had for lifting and stabilizing heavy vehicles. It would be less traumatic for the child and less destructive on the property. Duncan and Fergie gathered the equipment while I comforted the little boy.

An SCBA bottle was hooked to hoses and a regulator, then to an airbag placed just above the boy's head. The lines were charged, and the bag slowly inflated until the bars spread enough for the child to slip his head out. The neighbors cheered, the mom hugged her boy, then slapped him, and all was right with the world. We packed our gear and headed home.

The local minor league baseball team's stadium was located right across the river from Station 1. One evening, during a hot dog eating contest at home plate, the team owner's son, who'd just shoved an entire dog down his gullet, began to choke. The call came in for Engine 1 and Medic 11 to respond to the stadium at home plate. As the crews arrived and were ushered down to the field, event staff were doing chest compressions on a young man whose skin had turned a deep shade of purple due to lack of oxygen.

Taking control of the scene, Jughead opened the man's airway. With a laryngoscope blade and forceps, he reached into his trachea and removed a completely intact hot dog from his throat. The man immediately began to cough and breathe on his own, to the cheers of thousands of fans. The umpire, who'd been looking on from the backstop, ran up as the man started to walk off the field and yelled "Safe!"

Hank Brooks had a few years on me and was always a friendly face to see on the scenes or in the fire house. He was another stoner firefighter who was always high when I'd see him, although we never got high together, which was strange. He was injured in a fire truck accident where he'd herniated several disks in his back and had unwittingly opted for surgery from the city's doctors as a fix. Thinking optimistically, they could actually help him.

It ended up doing more harm than good and he could barely walk after they cut on him. The doctors installed a cage around his spine to give it support, but it ended up puncturing his liver and spleen and Hank almost died from internal bleeding and infection. He received a line-of-duty injury disability at twenty-seven years old and can barely stand up and walk today.

One of the low-rent hookers and a frequent flier on the medic unit in the downtown area was Candy Gagnon. One evening we were called to her favorite Motel 6 hangout for a woman requesting transport. We arrived to find Candy in her hotel room, complaining her "butthole had been stretched out" and asking if we could "tuck it back in for her." She removed her towel to reveal a prolapsed intestine hanging from her rectum. My partner and I simultaneously cringed.

She explained the John she was with earlier was violent with her, but she didn't want the cops to be informed, given her profession. I poured sterile water onto a large trauma dressing and wrapped it around her insides, which were now on the outside.

We covered her up in a blanket and transported her to the local hospital on her side—we call it lateral recumbent—in a position of relative comfort. It's always an adventure on a medic unit in the big city.

Rings were sometimes converted from finger decorations into painful torture devices that refused to release their wearers. Every ambulance carried a ring cutter in its jump kit. It had a protective metal piece that went between the finger and ring, and a grinding wheel that was hand cranked, until the soft metal ring had been sawed through.

Pro tip: if a ring cutter isn't available, or dish soap has failed to work as a lubricant, try wrapping a long strand of dental floss or sewing thread tightly around the skin at the distal end of the ring. The wrapped thread compresses the swelled tissue to the bone and makes room for the ring to slip off easier. We handled hundreds of calls from citizens who'd tried on a ring that once fit, but the years since had determined otherwise, and the ring had become stuck.

Such was *not* the case one fateful evening when a call came in for a citizen assist with a ring stuck on a finger. We responded on Medic 6 to a gentleman who explained he'd been masturbating, almost three days ago now, and was unable to remove the metal cock ring he'd used to enhance his experience. He wanted our ambulance crew to use the ring cutter to help him escape his entrapment and flatly refused transport to the local hospital. Ginger McEntire declined to touch the man's member, while Cain Long felt pity for the poor guy and offered to take a look and see what he could do.

The man dropped his shorts and revealed a purplish-black penis that appeared like it could fall off at any moment. The shiny metal ring had been restricting blood flow like a tourniquet for the past three days. Both paramedics immediately suggested transport to the hospital, citing infection and possible amputation as legitimate reasons. But the man adamantly refused and was too embarrassed to let others know about his predicament. He begged them to attempt cutting the ring off.

Long swung into action with the ring cutter, but after several awkward minutes of turning the hand crank, the cock ring had barely a scratch on its surface. All three faced the reality they'd have to transport to the ER to free the man from his trap. At the hospital, it was determined the ring was made of titanium. A grinding wheel with a diamond blade was secured, and the man was released with only minor lacerations to his member.

On the way back to the station, Long made Ginger swear to secrecy about the details of the call. Neither could keep the secret, though, and soon the entire department had heard about the "cock ring" run. At the training tower the following shift, Ginger was spilling the beans to a dozen or so firefighters. While describing Long's intense concentration and focus in extreme detail, Cain walked up to the group and stood behind Ginger as she revealed the rest of the juicy story. When asked why he did it, Cain responded, "Hey, I guess I just felt bad for the poor guy."

There was a park where a stairway of nearly 150 steps led down the ravine to a fishing dock on the river. On Medic 6 one day, Brad Perry and I were called for a girl with a fishhook stuck in her eye. We headed out and drove the sled through the park to the stairs.

With the blue bag in hand, we set off to find the patient. One hundred fifty steps later, we met up with a three-hundred-pound young lady whose friend had cast their line and hooked her right in the white meat of the eyeball. We cut the line and stabilized the hook with a gauze dressing. "Can you walk?" Brad and I said simultaneously in stereo. She didn't think she could make it.

"Ohhh, sure ya can," Brad suggested, attempting to use his Jedi mind tricks.

What he really meant to say was, "Bitch there is no way we are carrying your fat ass up 150 stairs while you just sit there. Your legs ain't broke!"

"C'mon, let's try," I said, thinking there was no way we were carrying this she-whale up those steps. The girl winced in pain as she took the first step.

"Good job, keep going," Brad encouraged her.

It wasn't working. She quit walking, and Brad and I stepped away from her for a sidebar.

"Dude, this is gonna take all day," Brad said.

"Oh yeah, what do you suggest? A helicopter? A crane maybe?" I asked.

"Let's just go get the cot and bring it down here," Brad suggested.

"You're crazy, bro. We are *not* carrying her," I replied.

"Yes, we are. End of discussion," Brad said, and he headed up the stairs.

I explained to the patient and her friend that we were going to get our stretcher and we'd be right back.

"This is stupid, dude," I whisper-yelled as I chased after Brad. "I bet if you told her we had tacos up there, she'd walk. She'd prolly float right up these fuckin' stairs."

We climbed back up the steps and then back down them carrying a cot. Then we carried her giant-ass back up fifteen stories of stairs!

"I got my workout in for the whole week," I said when we hit the top landing. We transported her to the hospital, and I slugged Brad hard in the arm for being an idiot.

"Scary" Sherry lived in an apartment near Fours and was a frequent flier on the citizen assist airline. She was scary because she weighed 450 pounds. One day, Duncan, Fergie, Natalia, and I were on 4 Engine and were called for a citizen's assist. Sherry had slipped to the floor from her bed in the living room and needed help moving back to the bed. Her boyfriend was 150 pounds of skin and bones and refused to help. Even when Natalia tried to shame him for not helping his own girlfriend, he replied, "That's not my job, it's yours."

Sherry and Natalia both evil eyed him as we prepared to lift.

Natalia and I each got under an armpit—yes, I know, I get grossed out just thinking about it—and Pat and Fergie each grabbed a thigh, which was probably worse, I don't know. On the count of three, we lifted. When we did, a cat howled and ran out from underneath her, and a TV remote fell out from under one of her breasts.

"Hey, I was looking for that!" her boyfriend said.

We tucked her in bed and promptly left to gouge our eyes out and shower. We felt dirty all over. Morbidly obese patients often have a white creamy substance between their layers of folded skin that doesn't get washed as much as it should. The medical term for this smelly cheese like substance is *smegma*. We called it "Fomunda Cheese." Because it came fom unda their rolls.

Jonesy was a rather eccentric red shift captain at Station 2. He often had an unlit stogie in his mouth and left a trail of peanut shells on the floor everywhere he went. His side gig was a scrap metal and trash hauling business, so folks called him Junkin' Jonesy.

Twos was an extrication station, and one day after a training session at a local junkyard, Jonesy found three unopened tins of old popcorn in the trunk of an abandoned car. He decided it would be a kind gesture to give them to the three red shift battalion chiefs as a Christmas gift. The grateful BCs devoured them and then the secret of the popcorn's origin came out—only after they'd been fully consumed. The BCs tried to discipline Jonesy for poisoning them, but they could never prove anything.

On an MVA scene one day, Jonesy came up to me while I was sweeping glass from the road and said, "If you ever come up to Twos, you'd better cover those fucking tattoos up."

I told him, "Don't worry. If I ever get sent to Twos, I'll just call in sick," and went back to work sweeping the road.

When I did finally rove up to Twos, he never said a word about them. Dispatch called the station directly that day and advised a civilian had called for a cat stuck in a tree. She added that she told them we didn't do that sort of thing anymore but wanted to give us the lady's address and phone number just in case.

Jonesy decided it would be a great public relations opportunity and ordered us to roll out. We arrived at a house with dozens of tall pine trees on a sleepy street. Jonesy made contact with the resident, and then explained to us, "Ahhh yeah, so the old broad says the cat's been up there four days and won't come down."

"Want me to grab a ladder, boss?" I asked.

"Nope. The cat's up too high for that. Wilson, you put the rig in pump. New kid, pull the booster line and stretch it up the driveway." Jonesy explained his plan was to shoot the cat off the limb it was on, about forty feet in the air, and knock it onto the roof of the one-story house with the hose stream.

What a crazy motherfucker, I thought as I pulled the hose up the drive and into position. The sun shone brightly through the pines and highlighted the cat's silhouette as I bled the air from the line and readied my nozzle.

The resident looked on in horror as she realized this was not going to be the storybook rescue she'd imagined.

"Now!" Jonesy yelled. As the cat turned curiously to look at him, I opened the bale and struck it broadside, sending the ball of soaked fur writhing through the air. Water droplets gleamed in the sunlight as the cat fell nearly thirty feet, in what seemed like slow motion, and landed on his paws, unscathed, on the roof of the house.

The owner screamed obscenities at Jonesy as he told her to just relax, put some food and milk out, and her cat would be back in her loving arms in a few minutes. I shook my head and laughed as Wilson and I reeled up the booster line and prepared to leave.

"That's how you do that shit!" Jonesy yelled as he walked down the driveway and set his helmet on the engine bumper. He reached into his turnout coat pocket and produced a shelled peanut. He smiled as he cracked the shell and tossed it on the street, and then explained how that lady would never again call us for that. The irony that he carried around a sack of peanuts everywhere he went is not lost on me. Jonesy was the living embodiment of a giant nut sack. That was my one and only cat-in-a-tree rescue.

We had a call that resembled the scene in *Gilbert Grape* where the firefighters had to remove the mother from the house by cutting the wall out. Ours was a 725-pound woman right across the street from the hospital, having chest pain in her second-story bedroom. She was too big to fit down the stairs, and hadn't been out of her bedroom in months, so they decided to remove the exterior wall and take here out by hoist and crane.

The Technical Rescue team was activated and promptly cut her wall open from floor to ceiling with a chainsaw. Then the Rollgliss was placed onto the tip of the ladder truck and raised into position outside of the bedroom. The patient was placed on a cargo tarp, dragged over to the edge of the wall opening by a team of eight firefighters, and hoisted up into the night sky. Then she was lowered by pulley system into the waiting ambulance below.

The cot had to be removed and the patient was laid directly on the floor of the meat wagon. During the entire operation, she was receiving excellent patient care for her cardiac-related medical condition. She was transported directly across the street, where she spent the next few months in the hospital's cardiac rehab to lose the weight.

There was a drunken man trippin' balls outside his house one night. We were called for a stabbing and arrived to find a man wielding a Katana in the front yard. The cops seemed to know him well and pleaded with him to drop the weapon.

"Martin, put the sword down or I'm gonna taze your dumbass," the officer said.

Martin simply ignored the orders and waved the sword around like he was Bruce Lee readying for battle.

"Martin, you've got to the count of three to drop the sword," the cop advised, resorting to toddler bargaining tactics. "One..."

The police officer fired the electrodes right into Martin's bare chest and he dropped the sword, shaking and twitching on the ground as voltage pumped through his body.

"What the hell happened to 'two' and 'three'?" I asked.

"I decided: fuck it." The officer shrugged.

While Martin got stuck with the tazer, we went inside and took care of the patient who'd been sliced with the katana. She attempted to grab the sword away from her drunk friend and received a nasty slice on her hand for her efforts. We hauled her to the hospital for few dozen stitches and a tetanus shot. The cops hauled Martin off to city hall to spend the night in jail.

Out of Fours, I was on the Engine when a call came in for a man in a creek stuck under a lawn mower. It's crazy some of the things we respond on. The man was mowing just down the road from the fire station when he drove his mower off the retaining wall above a drainage creek. The wall was around ten feet high and when he fell, the tractor pinned him in the frigid October water.

When we arrived, the man was suffering from hypothermia and a broken leg. We pulled the mower off and hauled him out of the creek and onto the embankment. We splinted the leg and wrapped him in blankets, then carried him on the cot across the field and over to the sled waiting at the road. Thanks to the quick work of Station 4's crew, the man still mows to this day.

Spike Young was a lieutenant when I began working at the department. He and Matthew Hawk were the quintessential badass prototypical firefighters. They could make anything go their way, were calm in the face of overwhelming odds, knew all the tricks of the trade, and partied like rock stars.

I loved the days when Spike and I worked together. He was a god to me. He taught me a hell of a lot about firefighting and life in general. He was like a fucking father figure for my puberty years in the fire service, he was that important to me. When I was stuck at Sevens after Carl ditched me for Eights, Spike was the junior captain there with me every other shift. When we're not making emergency runs, there's not much to do at The Cottage but get high, tell stories, work out, cook, eat, and sleep. He kept me sane and engaged. I met Lee then, and we'd all sit around the firehouse and shoot the shit together.

After I left Sevens, Spike hurt his back on a call. The city doctor prescribed Oxycontin and some time off for recovery. The Oxy led to a dependency and when the refills ran out, and the docs cut him off, he turned to street dealers to feed his addiction. The dealers introduced him to heroin, and it was all over. A couple of shady deals near the fire station from a house under surveillance by the narcotics unit, and he was busted. The brass in upper management had a hard on for Spike for his less than stellar attendance record as of late, and he was immediately fired.

Spike hired an attorney who claimed his duty injury was to blame, and a lengthy court battle ensued. Having sympathy for Spike and his plight, I'd hang out with him occasionally on my days off. Lee reviewed his case file and with her legal background, identified a few loopholes and angles to exploit. It worked out for Spike, and he was granted a line-of-duty disability. Not ideal in his eyes, but at least he was somewhat vindicated.

At one of the red shift golf outings, Firefighter Steve Bishop was running the fifty/fifty raffle and cruised around in his golf cart, selling tickets and prescription meds to all the foursomes. When Doctor Bishop approached me and asked if I wanted some Oxy, I politely declined and asked if this was his new side hustle. He explained it was the only way to fly and he had the Oxy connection for the entire department if I ever needed any. Spike Young was in the cart beside Steve, and it wasn't very hard to put two and two together.

Steve was my FTI a few years earlier when I was being broke in on the ambulance. He'd recently hurt his back on a medic run and was currently on duty injury. He'd been prescribed Oxycontin by the city doctor just like Spike Young and had yet to turn to street drugs as his supply of prescription meds had evidently continued unabated.

A while later, Smoothbore, who was in the foursome ahead of us and, as rumor has it, had taken some of the meds from Steve, promptly took a face plant into the floor as he passed out cold, double fisted, while returning from the clubhouse bar. A little too high on the wave was the diagnosis from Doctor Bishop, and he had a wipeout.

I ran into Steve at the movie theater a few months later. His skin was gray and pale, and he walked like ninety-year-old man. He'd had back surgery and they'd fucked it up worse.

"Jesus, Steve, you look like hell," I said.

"Thanks. Feel like it, too," he replied, adding that his line-of-duty disability had just kicked in and he was pursuing a career in real estate. I wished him luck and we parted ways.

Sometimes vehicles left our roadways and ended up in the river. This was the case one night when a car jumped the curb, flew over a guardrail, flipped over midair, and landed on its roof in the middle of the river. We scrambled our water rescue boats and picked the driver off the underside of his car where he'd climbed to escape the cold water. A wrecker cable winch was run out to the vehicle and secured. The car was hauled back ashore and towed away. The driver was drunk and barely had a scratch on him—as is often the case with drunk drivers—and he was transported to the hospital for observation.

Another time on a road that followed the river, the same thing happened when a car left the roadway and broke through a guardrail, ending up submerged. The drunk driver swam to shore uninjured. He spoke only broken English and was unclear about whether there were more people in the car with him at the time of the accident.

We scrambled the boats and were having trouble locating the car in the murky water because the river was nearly two hundred feet wide. Damyon handed me the TIC (thermal imaging camera), which Ginger McEntire, Paul Shaheen, and I—as the coxswain of our boat—used to locate a temperature variance from the still-warm motor of the car, under fifteen feet of water, at night. The wheels were still faintly visible as well on the camera. We dropped a buoy to mark the location. Then the search was called off when the man finally acknowledged he'd been alone in the car. We had to be innovative and adjust our strategies to fit the situations that we found ourselves in. Creative, out-of-the-box thinking was essential for survival in the field.

We were called on Medic 1 to an industrial plant one day for a fork truck that pierced through a man's boot and foot. The lift had been removed prior to our arrival and the sole of the man's foot was separated from the bones, like a flap, only attached near the toes. The yellow fat beneath the skin was visible, oozing from the flap on all sides, and it smelled absolutely horrible. I wrapped the foot with a trauma pad and a cravat, and we transported the man to the hospital. After surgery to reattach the sole of his foot, he made a full recovery and soon returned to work.

Regardless of how or why a person was stuck, if the fire department couldn't get them out of the jam, it probably wasn't possible. We rescued everything and everyone we could. We laid it all on the line for our communities and their residents. We were our city's heroes, and we gave our all every time we put on the uniform and raced out on a call.

Chapter 17

The Big Top

Station 4 was the newest firehouse at our department. It had a giant red domed roof over a triple company drive thru apparatus bay. There were single story dorm rooms on the west side and living quarters on the east. The large domed roof earned it the nickname the "Big Top" as it resembled a giant red circus tent from back in the old days—before animal rights activists and creepy circus clowns destroyed the industry.

In January 2005, I requested and was granted a transfer to Station 4. I'd stay there as the senior-most firefighter on the department for the next thirteen years. It was my home away from home. I served through twenty-three engineers, seventeen captains, and eight BCs, before they eliminated the battalion chief there due to budget cuts.

Station 4 had brand new beds in the private dorm rooms, a ladder truck, an engine, a medic unit, a battalion chief, and most importantly for me, a set of extrication tools. There was plenty of mess money to make great meals and it was in the first due area of my family's home, so it only took about three minutes to get to work in the morning. Bud Adams was my station captain and Chase Powers was an engineer. Everything was looking up. Absolutely everything. I've learned now I should prepare for a disaster when that feeling arises.

Sam Sullivan was an amazing, down-to-earth guy. A portly, jolly old soul. He was an FTI, paramedic, and engineer who still rode in the ambulance rotation. At Station 6 he could be counted on to do his job well and was a stabilizing force on the fireground in chaotic situations. We noticed he was losing weight and complimented him on looking well, right before he developed a persistent cough and went to see the doctor. Stage 4 lung cancer was the diagnosis, and within a month he was reduced to skin and bones from chemotherapy.

Then he was gone. Just like that. On February 8, 2005, the frailty of our lives had been exposed and one of the best at our craft had succumbed, unexpectedly. He'd suspected the cancer was caused by a Hazmat fire he made as a new kid, when no one used their Scott Paks. But there was no way to prove that was the case now. He was granted a posthumous line-of-duty death so his widow could receive his full pension and the funeral was planned.

It took place in his hometown, just south of the big city, and the department sent over two ladder trucks, two pumpers, and the Honor Guard in a battalion chief's car for the funeral procession. A huge American flag was suspended from between the two aerial ladders above the funeral home's parking lot entrance and the services began.

I was at Fours on the medic with Cain Long and around one o'clock that afternoon, a car plowed into a bank of apartment gas meters in Sullivan's old Station 6 first due. The initial engine arrived on scene at the gas leak and began evacuating the twelve-unit apartment building. The initial medic transported the car's driver, who'd apparently suffered a seizure and mashed the accelerator as he ripped the meters off the building. As the last resident exited the structure and the engine crew returned to the parking lot, the apartment building exploded.

Captain Ginger McEntire was launched through the air by the blast and landed in the middle of the parking lot. Engine 6 was riddled with flying debris and looked like it'd been through a war zone on the driver's side. Ginger got on the radio and yelled for dispatch to send a full alarm. This being my partner's not-so-undercover lover, we were already on the rig and rolling out of the station when the alarms lit up for us to respond.

As we turned down Miller Road, we could see the plume of smoke from the other end, miles away. Racing toward it with lights and sirens, we couldn't help but think of Steve. His spirit having one last hurrah and going out with a gigantic cock knocker of a fire. We heard the rigs from the funeral clear and go en route to the fireground.

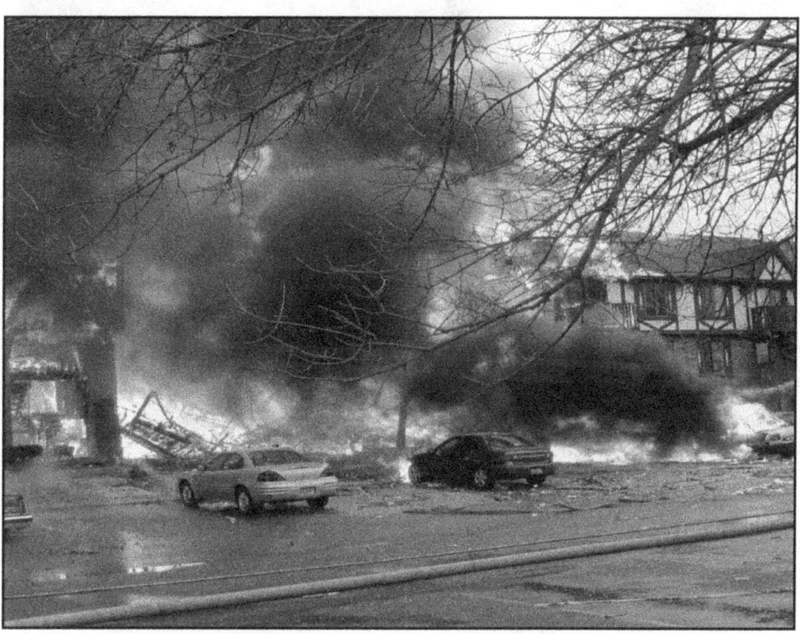

Gas main explosion during Sullivan's funeral

We arrived and immediately took medical control as there were multiple patients with burns and internal injuries from the explosion. A gas-fed fireball had turned the front of the three-story building into a volcano and was acting like a gigantic blow torch on the front six forward facing apartments. The fire raged on as incoming rigs screamed through the complex, hooked up water supplies, and stretched their hose lines.

We triaged patients and rehabbed the firefighters as they came through, changing air bottles and handing out cold water and dry towels. The beast still roared through the building as the media rolled their cameras and a crowd of hundreds of onlookers swelled around to watch. The crew from Eights with the Tech Rescue trailer arrived to shore up the collapsed structure and I was pulled from my medic duties to join them because of my structure collapse team training.

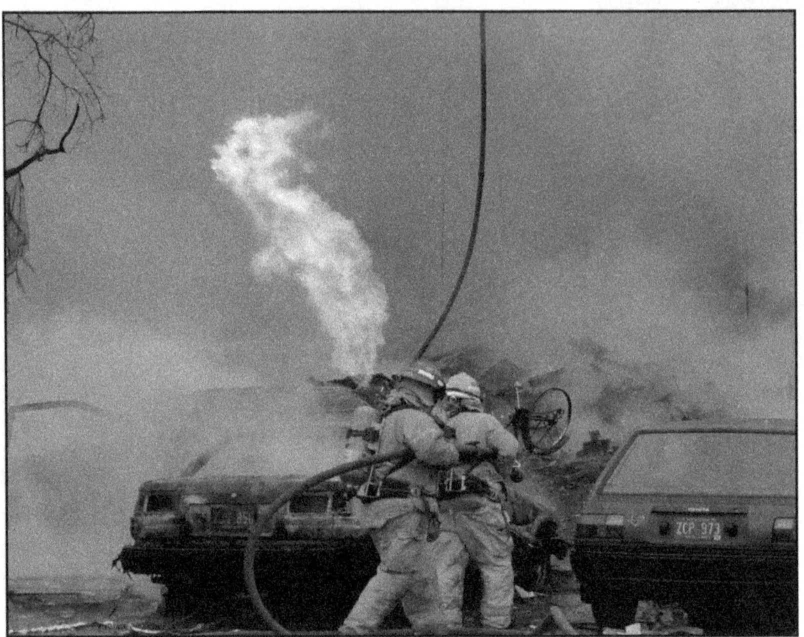

Fire demon about to be slain by The Bravest

I joined Captain Carl and we surveyed the collapse zone as the gas company finally shut the fuel source down at the road. It was like a bomb had gone off and the interior of the front apartments had been demolished all the way back to the dining room and kitchen areas. The floors were gone and so were the stairs leading up to them. We commandeered a ladder truck with a bucket and raised ourselves up to the carnage, putting out hot spots with a 1 ½" booster line that was pre-plumbed into the bucket. Half the structure was a giant crater now.

It was pure destruction, and everyone knew it just had to be Steve. It was how he would've wanted to go out. Not with friends crying at his funeral service, but with everyone battling the beast in a well-coordinated attack. As a team—one unit—with a common goal.

All the bullshit seemed to go away when we were on the fireground. Petty squabbles, rich or poor, black or white, male or female: nothing else mattered except mission success.

Remember when I mentioned one could murder someone at the fire department and not get fired? Here's why. Mid-way through my career, the black shift was called out of Station 1 for a full alarm structure fire. The ladder crew was using an old straight-stick Seagrave reserve truck because their frontline rig was out of service at the garage being repaired. Pat Hopkins was the engineer, Jeff Oliver was the captain, and Erica Hanson was the firefighter.

As they pulled out onto the apron and turned left onto the road, they had to make a quick right turn onto the cross street to head to the address. Those old Seagrave trucks had power steering systems that borrowed from the throttle, and if we let off the accelerator, we lost damn near all our steering assist power. As Pat slowed down to make the turn, he realized he wasn't going to make it and tried to whip the wheel back around, continuing down the initial street.

Unfortunately, he was too deep into the turn by then and didn't have enough throttle to crank the steering wheel far enough. There was an elderly lady standing across from the station on the sidewalk, waiting to cross the street. The ladder truck went up over the sidewalk and ran her over—her head struck square in the middle of the rig, leaving a dent in the sheet metal.

Oliver screamed at Pat from the boss's seat. Later he said when he looked over, Pat's eyes were closed, and that he'd probably passed out from the shock and horror of it all. As the ladder truck rolled over the elderly woman's body and slowly crept farther down the street, Erica and Jeff jumped out of the still moving truck and rushed over to help.

The woman sustained massive traumatic injuries and died in their arms while they waited for the ambulance to arrive. Our ladder trucks weren't licensed as medical responders and carried no EMS equipment at the time. There was nothing they could do besides start CPR and pray. Pray that God had a miracle for them, or that the medic unit would hurry the fuck up, or that it was all just a nightmare they could wake up from. Oliver retired a month later and Hanson quit the department soon after.

The woman's family promptly hired an attorney and settled out of court for a healthy sum. Engineer Hopkins went on to not only continue his firefighting career, making captain and battalion chief, but then applied for and was awarded the Chief of Fire Administration, the top job on the Department. How you ask?

Our union contended, and successfully proved through litigation, that faulty ladder truck mechanics were to blame, not the negligence of Engineer Hopkins, and that the city themselves were responsible and should shoulder the burden of this woman's death because of their refusal to purchase updated equipment to replace its antiquated fleet. Yes, my fire chief murdered a little old lady trying to cross the street. Ran her right the fuck over, then was rewarded by being put in charge of the whole fire department. That's union-strong baby.

Over the course of my career, I've participated in two hundred seventy-four CPRs (with only *seven* saves), eleven successful childbirths (with three more stillborn), and witnessed hundreds of dead human bodies or DOAs (dead on arrival).

One morning out of Station 1, Jason Hundt and I responded on Medic 1 to a police officer who—when called for a welfare check on a civilian—reported a deceased man lying on the porch of a shack on the north side of town.

As we approached, the officer was standing over the body and kicked the corpse in the shoulder while he explained how he was "pretty sure this guy's a goner."

Jason canceled the responding engine as I hooked up the three-lead for an EKG. We had to verify they were pulseless and apneic, or not breathing. Based on the body's condition and length of down time, a decision was then made to either "work" the patient (perform CPR) or call the ER for a time of death. Viability was the key factor in making this determination.

Just as Jason leaned down to look at the monitor, the man took a goddamn breath.

"Holy shit!" the cop said, startled. As if a zombie had just risen from its grave.

We went to work on the man, initiating CPR, and told the engine company to turn back around and meet us again. That was always fun to explain to the engine crew when they showed up on scene. The man ended up making a full recovery after we transported him to the hospital.

The same damn thing happened when Pants and I were riding Medic 5. We responded to what we called a granny stacker, or high-rise apartment building where the aged and low-income folks lived. Dispatch requested a welfare check on an elderly woman last seen a week ago. When we hit the address floor and stepped off the elevator, it immediately smelled like decomposition, and we'd both smelled that before. Many times.

The manager unlocked the door, and we filled our nostrils with the rotting flesh and body fluids scent of human decomp. Switching to mouth-breather mode, we pressed on. The living room and kitchen were empty, and the bedroom door was closed. As I tried to open it, the door hit a body. I could see through the crack in the door frame, there was an elderly woman lying on the floor, blocking the door. Pants and I both put our shoulders into the door and forced it open, sliding the body across the tile floor in a smear of urine and feces.

She was on her back facing up, her eyes were opened wide, glazed over with the haze of death. As I checked for a carotid pulse with my gloved hand, a cockroach ran out of her rigored open mouth and back into her nostril. Another one ran out of her ear and scurried off across the floor. Then—with my hand still at her throat—she took a fucking breath.

Pants and I both jumped a mile, then got to work packaging her in a disposable blanket and hauling balls out to the cot in the hallway. The back of her satin night gown had completely disintegrated from lying in her body fluids for days—maybe even a week.

We dropped an oral airway and breathed for her with a BVM as we rushed down the hallway and into the elevator. We were only a few blocks away from the hospital and Pants called them on his cell phone from the elevator to let them know what we had and that we'd be there in thirty seconds. We found out later that shift she'd suffered a stroke about five days earlier. She'd lain there on the floor, dying, for five fucking days.

Out of Fours one night, we responded for a motorcycle versus pedestrian. Upon arrival we discovered there were actually *two* pedestrians that had been hit. A motorcyclist was traveling close to 100 mph when a couple—a larger woman and a smaller man—began to cross the street together, returning from a trip to the party store and heading back to their apartment.

They walked hand in hand as the crotch rocket hit them both perfectly in line and obliterated most of their bodies. There was a debris trail of blood and body parts for nearly one hundred feet. From the intersection to where the bike had come to rest on the shoulder of the road. There sat a drunk man on the curb, completely uninjured, as is often the case, wondering how he was going to live with himself. Two counts of vehicular manslaughter were the cost of his joyride.

One sunny, summer afternoon out of Nines, Big Daddy and I were on the medic. We were kicked back in the brown chairs after lunch when we heard a motorcycle peel out of the gas station next door and speed away.

Big Daddy joked, "There goes our next patient."

He was right.

The alarm came in a few seconds later for a car versus motorcycle PI (personal injury) accident.

We arrived to find a debris field of motorcycle parts extending from the intersection to a car sitting a hundred feet away, sideways across the road in the southbound lanes. The rider had crotched the car's front tire between his legs and was lying on his back motionless. As I took C-spine control, the bones in the man's neck crunched terribly and his torso was oddly twisted. He wasn't breathing and had no pulse.

As Big Daddy arrived with the backboarding supplies, I said to him, "I think this one's a K." As in the military acronym *KIA*, or killed in action. He always reminds me of that. Apparently, it was the first time anyone had ever referred to a patient like that around him. Guess I'd just seen too many old war movies in the brown chairs. The bystanders said the rider had been going around 70 mph when he laid his Hayabusa bike down to avoid hitting the car that had pulled out in front of him.

He slid across the pavement ahead of the bike, crotching the front tire of the car, right before the heavy motorcycle slammed into the top of his head, crushing his entire spine between it and the car tire. We called it a fatal accident right there and didn't work the patient. There was no survivability, and everyone knew it. The police closed the road for hours while they investigated the crash.

I have another grisly motorcycle story—not that I'm against bikes of course. I moved out of my parents' house at age eighteen after I bought a 1978 Suzuki GS 750. They gave me the ultimatum of either sell the bike or move out, and I chose the bike. This story just happens to be about another fatality involving a motorcycle. Which is fairly common, unfortunately.

Our local bus agency had an old-time trolley they'd converted into a bus for nostalgic public relations events. It was returning home to the bus garage after a summertime event in the evening. A motorcyclist had taken off from a stop light about a quarter mile away and was using the straightaway as a drag strip, redlining the tachometer, as it approached speeds topping 100 mph. The trolley driver began his left turn, not seeing the speeding bullet heading directly for him, and was positioned sideways across three of the five lanes of traffic when the motorcycle slammed into the side of the trolley.

The bus didn't move very much, but the bike and its passenger exploded into a hundred pieces. They'd struck the fuel tank on the side of the trolley, and diesel was pouring over the intersection. One of the biker's boots had landed in the convenience store parking lot, kitty-corner from the accident, with the rider's detached foot still inside of it.

I was riding Engine 6 that day and we were called to bring the Hazmat truck, with its extra supply of HyDry absorbent to help control the fuel spill. Let me just say, when the human meat in the middle gets sandwiched between two pieces of machinery, there isn't much left for the rescuers to work with. It was extremely gory to say the very least.

Nothing wakes one up in the middle of the night, quite like stomping the bushes alongside a highway after a rollover accident, looking for ejected passengers. That's a stroll through the woods I'd just as soon pass on, if left up to me. Probably because I've *actually* come across several mangled human bodies that way.

Some of them were wrapped around trees, some impaled on branches, some eviscerated by fences and smaller brush. It's amazing the crazy things one can find walking the medians and drainage ditches along our highways at night. It's always creepy, like in a horror flick, when my flashlight came upon a body in the brush.

Other times, people just became roadkill themselves. Out of Fours one night, I was riding the engine when an alarm came in for a PI accident on the highway. We headed out, hit the emergency turn around, then rolled down the shoulder to the accident scene. We arrived to find two carloads of teenagers talking with police at the roadside. A badly mangled body lay in the middle of the road, and a stream of bloody human debris stretched along the center line for about fifty feet.

I grabbed the blue bag and stepped over various body parts in the road as we made our way to the victim. It was a young girl, covered in abrasions from road rash, pulseless and motionless, obviously dead. I covered her with a disposable blanket. On our way to check the teens, Fergie alerted me to a human tongue sitting in the road, so that I wouldn't step on it.

The hysterical kids explained their deceased friend had been trying to cross between two cars as they traveled down the highway. They'd been drinking and had seen this stunt in a movie, so they figured they'd give it a try. When one of the drivers veered a little too far away from the other car, the passenger in the opposite car lost their grip on the girl and she fell to her death onto the highway pavement, to everyone's shock and horror. Her severed tongue lying in the road.

In early 2005, a group of firefighters on our department registered and began training for the Scott Firefighter Combat Challenge. This was a nationally televised firefighting obstacle course that pitted individuals and teams against each other in a timed competition. In October of that year, we headed off to Janesville, Wisconsin to test our mettle.

Kyle Locke rode with my wife and me, and on the way, the Phil Collins song "In the Air Tonight" came on. Kyle said from the backseat how much he liked this song, and could we turn it up. Surprised that our aspiring rapper and former Kappa step-team member even knew a Phil Collins song, Lee turned it up and we vibed down the highway for the next few minutes. I glanced in the rearview mirror and saw Kyle looking exactly like Mike Tyson in *The Hangover* movie, grooving to the song, singing, and even playing the air drums at the breakdown.

Our relay team of Dwight Hopewell, Matt Baker, Roger Colavincenzo, Don Harrington, and me qualified for the event finals. We faced off against the defending world champs from Windsor FD. They smoked us, of course. But the healthy competition helped us push hard and we became the Relay State Champs from our home state, with a time of 1:39.53.

I gave it my best in the individual rounds, but having just smoked a joint in the parking lot and finished it off with a ciggy, I was completely out of breath at the dummy drag. I wasted a good thirty seconds standing over top of the dummy just struggling to move air in and out of my leather lungs. The course proctor came over and asked me if I needed the medical staff, and, out of breath with my hands on my knees, I held up one finger, asking him for just a moment. A few seconds later, I dragged the dummy across the finish line for a time of 2:44.13. Not my best time, but hey, at least I did it. Which is more than most of our nation's firefighters can say.

Bud Adams and Tommy Rush both retired from Station 4 a short time later, and things just weren't the same without them there. Tommy was the black shift Yin to Bud Adams's red shift Yang and the two of them—both old salty fire department dogs—had kept the new Fours humming along quite nicely.

The next group of captains seemed to come and go every six months or so. They were all a little quirky and odd for the next couple of years. There was John Dryer, Marv Holcomb, Frank Ford, Tim Sanchez, and Jimmy Knight—until he became a raging, dysfunctional alcoholic and dutied out from PTSD.

A few months after retiring, Tommy Rush was diagnosed with ALS. He'd just begun his second career as a fire instructor at the local community college and was teaching new recruits the tricks of the trade. One day he was with us, the next he retired, then he was gone. Another funeral, for another dead firefighter.

In December 2005, Lee and I had our son, Banks. I helped with the delivery at the hospital, and we welcomed our little boy into the family. The following night as we slept at home in our bed, she woke up crying. When I asked what was wrong, she said she'd seen how our future together was going to play out. She explained I was going to cheat on her, we were going to come close to divorce, and I'd attempt suicide. I told her she was crazy, to relax, and to go back to sleep.

Life was difficult living on one quarter of my income now from paying child support, but it was good to have each other, and we made the best of our circumstances. Lee left her position at the law firm and opted to stay home and raise our family while I was away at the firehouse. Our blended family was melding well, and she did an amazing job of coordinating the various school activities and visitation drop offs and pick-ups that were required of divorced, blended families with four children.

Captain Carl was always a fun-loving guy coming up through the ranks. When he made BC his demeanor changed, and he was always angry about something or other. There were two red shift BCs then; one was John Dryer whom we called the Velvet Glove, and the other was Carl whom we called the Iron Fist. Carl would go into firehouses and staff meetings and rile everybody up, then storm out. John would stick around afterward and calm everybody down. Carl incidentally survived a massive heart attack within a month after he'd retired.

John Dryer was an engineer when I'd first met him. Kind and inspiring, he'd served as my captain for a short time at Fours before making the battalion chief rank. John passed away a month before his retirement from a brain aneurism. He'd lived in the same neighborhood as I did and while bending over to pick something up from his yard, ruptured a blood vessel in his head. It started with a terrible headache and by the time his wife rushed him to the hospital minutes later, he was projectile vomiting. Through slurred words he told her he loved her, and then he was gone. Another dead firefighter, another funeral. The battalion chief rank was truly brutal.

Next up at Fours was Captain Tim Sanchez. He was the mentor I'd asked, what "put the wet on the red" meant back in the academy. Tim was a volleyball aficionado and his sister had moved to L.A., became a radio personality, and ended up marrying the rapper Coolio.

After a few years together, their *Gangsta's Paradise* turned into more of a bad decision and their *Fantastic Voyage* ended in Splitsville. I always asked Tim what the holidays were like with a famous rapper at the Thanksgiving dinner table. And what does one get their celebrity rapper brother-in-law for Christmas anyway? Tim would just laugh and say how he was just Artis, a regular guy when not performing in character. I learned Coolio was an actual firefighter too at one point. Go figure.

Out of Fours one afternoon, the ladder truck caught a full alarm at the opposite corner of the city. Bubbles was our engineer and we headed off in the general direction of the scene. About two-thirds of the way there, she turned off onto a side street and proceeded through several neighborhoods until she turned down a road that had a "Dead-End" sign posted at its entry. Several hundred feet later, Bubbles coasted to a stop at the end of the road.

Looking over at Captain Sanchez she said, "I have no idea where I am."

Tim turned off the lights and siren and just shook his head in disbelief. He asked me to get out and back us down the dead-end road, because it was too narrow to turn the ladder truck around on. By the time we reached the cross street, the fire had already been extinguished, and rigs were clearing. We just turned around and headed back to the station, having never made it to the address. I don't know how Bubbles could even live with herself; she was so oblivious it was scary.

Tim Sanchez made the battalion chief rank in mid-2007 and transferred back to the black shift. Marv Holcomb and Frank Ford each spent about six months as captains at Fours before making the BCs rank themselves. Captain was more of a stepping-stone for them, and they cared more about advancing their careers, than the crews they oversaw. They spent most of their time studying for making rank and we rarely saw them, outside of emergency runs and dinners.

Next up on the seniority list for captain of Station 4 was Jimmy Knight. A man's man. Tall and brooding, he had a commanding presence wherever he went. He'd hit home runs repeatedly on the softball diamonds and was a former quarterback in college before deciding to be a firefighter. He was kindhearted, fun to party with, and wise to the politics of the fire department. He'd married a nurse, had a nice family, with two kids and a vacation property on a lake northwest of town. Life was good for Jimmy Knight.

That all changed when he made captain at Fours. His vices of alcohol, drugs and porn began to catch up with him and he fell hard into the bottle. His wife found out about Vegas and filed for divorce, taking everything with her including the kids. Having lost all he valued in life; Jimmy embraced the only thing that had never left his side—booze.

He'd go on benders for days at a time. Neither sleeping nor eating, reeking of alcohol, and then passing out cold in a fire station bed somewhere. The medic units began picking him up around town and running into him passed out in the ER hallway beds, like one of our frequent flier vagrants. It was tough to watch. At work he'd scream at his troops over seemingly minor infractions, sleep all day, curse the BCs to their faces, and cry full blown crocodile tears to new kid firefighters as they tried to console him in his misery.

Jimmy ended up claiming a PTSD disability and walked away from the profession an addict and an alcoholic. When he'd stop by the firehouse to see his old pals, there'd be patches of hair he'd missed while shaving, or open sores on his face and head, always smelling like he'd just bathed in a liquor cabinet.

In July and August 2007, our city was home to a serial killer. Someone would break into single women's homes, beat them unconscious, then sexually assault and murder them. The killer unknowingly targeted the seventy-six-year-old mother of a city councilwoman for his initial victim. So, the pressure was on the police department to find a suspect.

Over the next month, the body of a thirty-six-year-old woman, naked from the waist down, was found in the same park I'd found my first murder victim, ten years earlier. A 46-year-old former prostitute turned house cleaner was found two days later. The cops didn't have many clues and had arrested and charged a mentally challenged homeless man while two more of the murders were committed.

A 64-year-old woman was found dead in her home two weeks later. The next day a 41-year-old prostitute was found in a vacant home that was for sale, when potential buyers came by to inspect the place. It wasn't until the seventh victim, a fifty-six-year-old woman, was discovered barely alive that police finally had a description of the suspect and enough evidence to identify him.

The elderly lady fought hard to survive after being hit repeatedly in the head with a toilet tank lid. The woman's dog managed to scare the attacker off and he fled. Left for dead, and critically injured, she crawled to the phone, leaving a massive blood trail, and called for help. Police and paramedics responded and saved the woman's life. It was Krishna, as a matter of fact.

Shortly afterward, the murderer, a twenty-seven-year-old former convicted sex offender, was captured, tried, and sentenced to two consecutive life terms of imprisonment without parole, ending a spree of terror that had gripped our community with fear. He also confessed to the 2004 murder of a sixty-year-old community college professor, a case in which the police had wrongfully convicted another man.

The innocent man was subsequently released from prison after having served a year and a half behind bars. After reopening the case, video surveillance footage, DNA, and fingerprint evidence all linked the real murderer to the crime. Though police had this information in their possession during the initial trial, they failed to produce it in court and knowingly prosecuted the wrong person. After being exonerated and set free, the innocent man and his attorneys settled out of court for $2 million in damages for the wrongful conviction.

In January 2008, continuing its downward trajectory of liquid assets, the city made one of the dumbest financial moves I've ever seen. They offered a buyout for any battalion chief that wanted to leave early, before retirement eligibility. So, for $50K each, Frank Ford and Lenny Smith left just two months early. The buyout was also erroneously figured into their FAC on their pension, and they both received six-figure annual salaries for their retirement income. A short time later, due to constant attrition of the workforce, and with fewer employees making payroll contributions, the city began complaining that the police and fire pension system was strained and had unfunded liability. I wonder why. Bureaucrats, man. I wish I could've made a backdoor deal like that.

After Jimmy Knight went Section 8 and dutied out, things got even worse when BJ showed up as the new boss of Fours. He seriously had no business being at that rank. He was a child in a man's body who made daily station life hell on his troops. One day he had us training for six hours on a 1960 IFSTA (International Fire Service Training Association) ladder manual. He told us to write essays on the Bangor ladder, a gigantic one with guide poles on the side of it, no longer in use.

Another day it was a four-hour school on ropes from the same 1960 series of IFSTA manuals. We had to demonstrate tying knots that were obsolete in the fire service. It was always some kind of baloney he tried to pull on us just to make himself look smarter or to put us down and make us do busy work while he flexed his officer muscles.

One night at Station 4, BJ was the boss, Chase was my driver, and I was on the back end of the engine ridin' dirty. Chase came out to the apparatus floor around 23:00 hours and made sure his rig was ready before turning in for the night. He noticed the captain's truck door was closed and decided to open it and hang the boss's coat up proper.

When he opened the door, several empty beer cans rolled out from underneath the officer's seat and clanged across the concrete floor. Chase cleaned up the mess, covering for BJ who was a raging alcoholic at the time. He knew BJ functioned better drunk and had a habit of sitting in the fire truck, late into the evenings and knocking back a few cold ones.

On a Spring day in the early morning hours, Captain BJ, Engineer Bruce Owens, and I were on Engine 4, when an alarm came in for a CPR in progress at an adult foster care home. As we arrived at the facility, the circle drive approach to the building was packed full of cars. It was about a football field's length away, from the road to the entrance, so BJ advised Bruce to just drive across the lawn.

About halfway up to the building, the engine slowed from its uphill crawl through the mud of the spring thaw and became stuck in the front lawn. The three of us piled out, grabbed our EMS equipment, then took off across the lawn to locate the patient inside. While BJ yelled at the administrators to clear the driveway for the incoming ambulance, Bruce and I took over the chest compressions and breathing on an elderly male who was pulseless and apneic.

The ambulance arrived and brought their equipment inside, the patient was loaded onto the cot, and moved to the sled. We helped them run through the protocols of starting an advanced airway, getting an IV established, and pushing the first round of cardiac arrest meds into the patient. The medic crew had a third rider that day, so when they were ready for transport, we hopped out and they went en route to the hospital.

As we surveyed the situation with our engine, Bruce thought he could just back it down the hill the same way that he'd come in and most likely free it from the mud. BJ and I took up positions in the rear and watched as Bruce rocked the rig back and forth.

"That dumbass ni&&er," Captain BJ said. "What a fuckin' idiot."

Offended by his racist remarks about my friend, I replied, "He just did what you told him to do. Don't call him that."

"Shut the fuck up! What are you gonna do about it?" he said, turning his ignorance to me.

Bruce freed the rig from the lawn and backed it down to the street. BJ told us to grab shovels and pitchforks from the truck and get to work trying to lift the ruts we'd made in the yard. As Bruce and I dug in the lawn, BJ just sat in the officer's seat of the engine, watching us work. I told Bruce what BJ said to me and asked if he wanted to take it up the chain of command, adding that I'd testify against that asshole any day.

Bruce said, "Nah, that's just BJ. He's an ignorant bastard, but that's not my style. Karma's a mother… and he'll get his."

We kept on digging until Bruce felt we'd done enough to repair the ruts from the engine. Later, he'd make the assistant chief position after BJ was busted down to engineer for harassment, and it seemed like poetic justice had been served. Bruce was a great man, who did his job better than most and always treated me well. It pained me to see him treated that way over the color of his skin.

On Truck 4 one day, we were called to Target (department store) for a worker on the roof who was having a cardiac event. The man was an employee of the contractors that were repairing the roof. He was incapacitated with chest pain and unable to climb down the ladders and make it to the ambulance. We sent the medics up to the roof and set up our aerial ladder for a roof pick-off with the Rollgliss pulley system and the Stokes basket.

As the medics started an IV and placed the man on the heart monitor, we attached the basket and guided it up to the rooftop. The engine crew on the roof secured the man in the basket and we raised him up, then over the side of the building, guiding him with ropes attached to the ends of the basket, lowering him to the ground beside the ambulance. The medics transported him to the hospital, and he received excellent life-saving care, surviving his heart attack.

BJ ordered us in and out of our dress uniforms three times by 11:30 hours one shift. As I was cooking lunch on the grill outside, he walked over and told me we were going to do it again "just to fuck with Wendy (Simpson)," the engineer that day. Then he keyed the mic on the station PA and gave the order.

When Chase came out to the grill to see if I needed any help, I told him what had just happened. He was upset and went to tell

Wendy what I'd said. They both met me by the grill and Wendy asked if I'd tell the battalion chief what BJ had said to me. I agreed. Bubbles was the lieutenant and promptly called up the chain of command to inform them of the harassment going on at Fours that day.

The battalion chief, Denny Milton, showed up a few minutes later and asked to speak to BJ in the ACR (the ass chewing room, formerly the south-end BC's office). BJ flipped a dining room table chair across the lounge as he walked away with Denny. A few minutes later, they came out of the office and Denny explained to Wendy she'd have to go home for the day—without pay—for insubordination.

Wendy was livid. "I called you here to investigate harassment against me, and you're sending me home?"

Chase stood up from the table and said if they were sending her home, then they needed to send him home, too. I did the same, and when Denny turned to look at Firefighter Dwight Hopewell at the end of the dinner table, he said, "I suppose you want to go home too, right?"

Dwight said he didn't want to be the only one left at the station with "angry BJ" and agreed to stand united with us. We were all so sick of BJ's bullshit. Bubbles just quivered over in a corner and did absolutely nothing out of fear for her life.

Denny went back into the ACR with BJ and called the chief of the department. A few minutes later, BJ was smashing furniture and screaming at the top of his lungs at all of us. They sent *him* home without pay instead, and we all had to go down to Fire Administration for investigative interviews with Human Resources.

BJ was busted down to engineer without the possibility for promotion and earned himself a transfer over to the black shift. He'd still occasionally catch engineer overtime on the red shift, and we'd all have to work with him again, which was awkward. But at least he wasn't the officer in charge of our daily lives anymore.

Bubbles and Wendy feared reprisals for their testimony to HR of the heinous things they endured under his leadership, or lack thereof. They would both call in sick if the running chart ever listed them together with BJ, and Ops had to juggle some creative staffing protocols to keep them from crossing paths at shift change.

Dan Cooper stepped in to replace BJ and instantly brought an abundance of street cred and leadership ability. He was calm, cool, and collected under pressure and excellent officer to work with. At least he wasn't a maniacal racist.

When a full alarm fire came in for a cold storage warehouse, the entire north end of town cleared their stations and rushed to the scene. The three-story brick building had very few windows and was a heavy timber construction that belched thick brown smoke from every opening upon arrival. We made it on the second alarm from Fours on the ladder truck and manned 2 ½" lines supplying ground monitors for several hours during the defensive operations.

After several hours, a team of trusted bad-ass firefighters were assembled to make entry and we prepared a plan of attack. Two engine crews with two ladder companies backing them up readied at the loading dock doors with a pair of charged 2 ½" hose lines. We'd advance with thermal cameras and search for the seat of the fire.

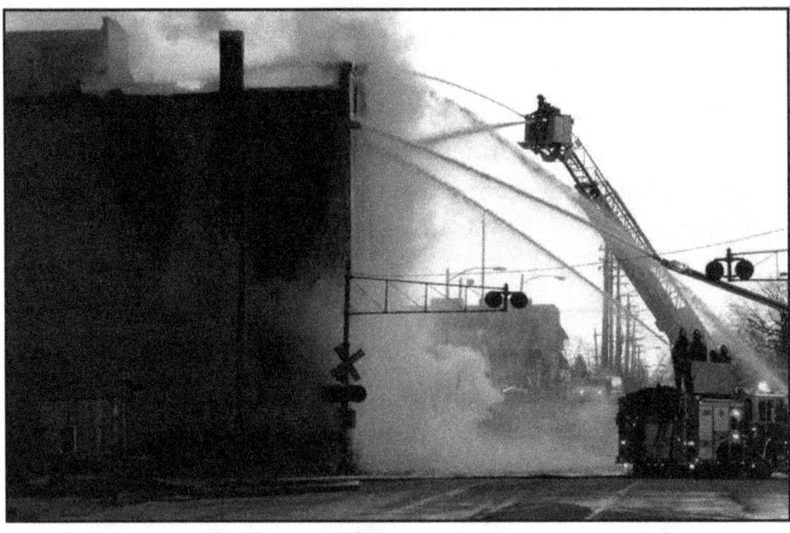

We entered the building and were met with high heat and zero visibility. The 2 ½" hose lines were difficult to maneuver through the cut-up maze of hallways and refrigerated storage rooms that lined the interior. Unable to make headway with the unwieldy hoses and dangerous conditions, we were forced to back out.

Outside, the decision was made to resume defensive tactics. We maintained exterior operations throughout the evening and into the night. Around midnight, an excavator arrived and began punching holes in the brick exterior with its bucket so our hose streams could penetrate the building. As the night wore on, we rotated crews to and from the scene, to give fire companies a well-deserved break.

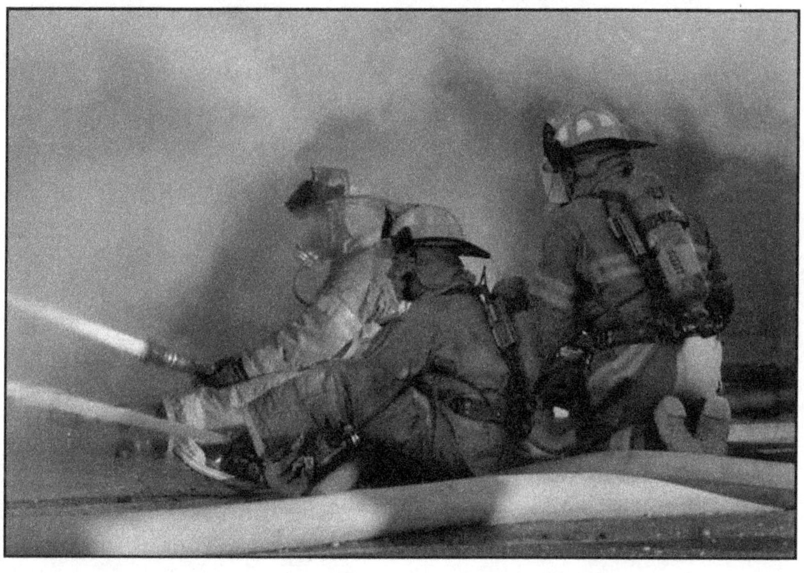

Firefighters sitting on 2 ½" hose lines during defensive operations

As the sun rose over the horizon, the building was reduced to rubble and the elevated master streams soaked down piles of debris made by the excavator. It was a total loss. The destroyed building sat there for three years while the owners and insurance companies squabbled over the cause of origin and payout amounts. The owners had recently placed the building up for sale, and it sat on the market for a few months with no interest, until the fire broke out. Arson was suspected, but there was no way to prove it, and the property sat as a testament to the city's blight and financial ruin.

Dan Cooper, Spoons, Kyle Locke, and I were called out to the highway for a semi-truck versus a pedestrian. The line on this was 1,000 to 1 in favor of the truck, so the odds weren't even remotely in favor of the person, who, strangely, had been on foot walking down the highway. We arrived to find a perfect human being indentation in the front grill of the semi, with about three feet of impingement into the motor area, dead center on the front of the truck.

The driver, visibly shaken, stood at the roadside talking with police and being examined by the medics. Apparently, the woman had just jumped out in front of him. When he slammed on the brakes, she flew off the front of the truck and fell beneath the eighteen-wheeler. At least nine of them ground her body into the freeway asphalt as the truck skidded to a stop.

Later that same night, within hours of the previous suicide, we responded on a man who'd hung himself from the rafters of his basement. Dan cut him down as I bear hugged the man's dead body and lifted him up. Once free, he fell over my shoulders. I laid him down on the concrete basement floor, and we began CPR. The ambulance arrived minutes later and transported him to the hospital. It was too late for him, though.

Thirty minutes later we rolled out to Vincent Drive. A father had hung himself in the garage after his old lady broke the news that she was having an affair with his brother and leaving him. We cut him down and pumped away on his chest while his kids watched. The meat wagon pulled up and we continued CPR en route to the hospital.

What are the odds of three back-to-back suicides in our first due in the same night? I think when I die and get to the other side, I'd like to visit the statistical odds department there. Maybe check in on the crazy, never in a million years, types of things I've witnessed in my lifetime. Or view the otherwise meaningless statistics, like how many hours of my life I'd spent mating socks during laundry activities, or picking my nose, or cleaning up dog poop in the backyard, or some other bric-a-brac shit like that. You know, the worthless things that fill the seconds and minutiae of our days here.

Dan Cooper made battalion chief a short time later and in 2008 Hector Garcia became the captain of Fours. The next group of officers were from our stoner group, and we partied our asses off day and night, with very little in the way of the traditional hard-nosed captain disciplinarian type of leadership. It was more along the lines of, "Everybody feel free to do your own thing and then when the tones go off, switch into ass-kicking motherfucker mode."

CHAPTER 18

Town Drunks and Frequent Fliers

Every city has them. Patients and locations we respond to nearly every single day on duty. We call them frequent fliers and we could bet our paychecks we'd be picking up several of these folks and transporting them to the hospitals every shift. They never paid their medical bills, but we were obligated by law to provide care for them anyway. Their stories are infamous in the police and fire station break rooms around the country. These were my regular customers.

Willy Mills was probably *the* most frequent flier we had for our ambulance service when I joined the department. On a good day, we'd pick him up once or twice. On the bad ones, it was four or five times. He be passed out drunk, somewhere downtown, and most likely have a stream of piss running downhill away from his body. We'd wake him up and he'd mumble at us like Mush-Mouth from "Fat Albert"—always unintelligible until he said the words, "Suck my dick!" Like clockwork, every time. Those were the only words we could ever understand from him. Clear as day.

"Ol' Hibbity Bibbity" they'd call him because of the slurred words. Sometimes we'd drop him off at the hospital and he'd walk right out the door before we could finish our report. Dispatch would call for us to go pick him up again down the street a few minutes later. The smart medic crews would transport him to the south end of town and drop him at the other hospital so it would take him a few hours to walk or hitchhike his way back north again.

Betty and Linda Gross were sisters, and both were drunk and disorderly almost daily. Linda more so than Betty in their later years. One time Linda had a sixteen-year-old boy convinced that he was her true love. She was herself, near fifty, had no teeth, talked with a lisp and this poor kid was infatuated with her. She'd cut her foot while walking barefoot, hand-in-hand with the boy, down the middle of the road and we were called in to assist.

The two lovebirds appeared inseparable and when the boy turned his head to talk to my partner, Linda whispered for me to please get her the hell out of there now.

"He thinks he's in love," she said in the ambulance, "I just wanted a young piece of ass and now he won't leave me alone." She confessed. Drunk and bleeding from her foot wound, we transported her to the hospital and advised the young man to get checked for STDs.

Another time I picked Linda up outside of a party store. She was incapacitated on the sidewalk and incontinent. As we helped her onto the cot, she asked if we wanted to fuck. I politely declined but advised my partner, Shane McKinley, was recently single and looking to get back in the game. He passed on the offer as well, and we loaded her into the sled.

On the way to the hospital, we stopped at a red light and Linda stood up and dropped her pants, touching her toes and hollering for me to look, while I was on the phone with the hospital. As my eyes burned out of my skull, my partner hit the gas and Linda, with her pants down around her ankles, took a header face first into the back doors. The whole ambulance smelled like a crab shack, and we had to leave all the doors open for the next hour to ventilate.

Every night on the ambulance downtown, we were pretty much guaranteed a run to the VOA. The Volunteers of America was a homeless shelter just across the river from Station 1. It was a four-story building with administrative offices, patron lounges, a kitchen and a cafeteria on the first floor, and hundreds of bunks in large dormitories on the floors above. If the patrons were drunk, they wouldn't let them in, or they'd eventually get kicked out. That's where we came in.

We could also bet our firstborn son on a run to the city jail. There was an incident right before I'd hired on in 1998 in which an inmate was killed by the guards when he was handcuffed and restrained in a kick-stop restraint device that ties the hands and feet behind the suspect's back and then to a waist belt. After that he was left to lie there on his stomach. A method specifically warned against by the device's manufacturer because it can potentially cause suffocation. Tragically, it led to the 260-pound man's death.

He was denied repeated requests for medical assistance after a severe beating by multiple officers, right on the heels of the Rodney King debacle. A large police officer stood on the inmate as he was restrained in the device by the other officers, and the medical examiner concluded that this maneuver had caused the death of the inmate from postural asphyxia.

As he was dying, the man urinated himself and the officers cut his pants off with a pocketknife. Then they left him face down in a puddle of his own piss. At this time, the guards cinched the kick-stop restraint so tight the straps broke. The officers rigged it back together with chains and handcuffs, then they left, as the man remained motionless on the ground.

It would be ten minutes later before the guards checked in on him and moved the unconscious man over to another cell, re-manacled him there, then left his lifeless body in *that* cell for another four minutes before calling an ambulance. Steve Bishop, my FTI a few months later, responded as the lead paramedic, and his crew performed CPR. They transported the patient to the hospital, where he was pronounced dead a short time later.

After a twenty-seven-day trial and two days of deliberations, a jury awarded nearly ten million dollars to be paid to the victim's family. The order came down the administrative pipeline that all inmates were now allowed to be transported to the hospital upon request. And really, who'd rather sit in jail than a hospital?

Not many, we found out, and so we began making EMS runs all day and night to the city's police lockup facility. It was a regular chest pain factory, and those two magic words got the inmates a get out of jail reprieve for the next few hours. A hefty medical bill came along with it, but most everyone in jail had no intentions of paying for those types of things anyway.

Bobby Buxom was a young, mentally challenged woman who suffered from, and frequently faked, seizures. Most of my faker detection techniques were developed and finely honed on her, while trying to determine if it was an attention-seeking moment or an actual postictal situation after grand mal seizure activity. She lived in an adult foster care home, and we'd run on her several times a week.

She became quite fond of me and after a while would recognize me on arrival. If she'd been faking it, she'd snap right out of it when I tried to wake her. Probably out of fear of having her eyeball poked with a gloved finger or her hand dropped from above her face. If we held the patient's hand directly above their face and then let go, it would strike the patient in the face if they were legitimately unconscious. If they were faking, their hand would veer away and miss their face, to avoid injury to themselves. Hey, everybody has their methods. Don't judge.

Bob Boone was a regular drunk for about twenty or so years when I hired on. I'd made dozens of calls to pick him up, usually lying drunk in puddle of his own urine. But after a while he just sobered up and stopped drinking. We'd see him around town, always on foot and looking disheveled, and he'd swing over and tell us how many days he'd been sober.

"Two hunderd n' sixty fiiiiive," he'd rattle off the number of days that he'd been sober in his southern drunk stoner voice. He'd stop into the fire stations sometimes and greet us with a "Three years, a hunderd n' twenty onnnne," brandishing the AA coin in his pocket.

We'd all congratulate Bob on his sobriety and the guys that remembered him would tell their best Bob stories.

"There was this one time Bob was passed out cold and another bum dropped a steaming deuce right on his forehead!" or,

"One time I picked him up passed out drunk on the sidewalk and it was so cold out, his pissed soaked pants had frozen solid as a board!" or,

"Another time in the tent city, the other bums had ol' drunk Bob tied up, bent over a 55-gallon drum, and he was passed out with his pants around his ankles and Vaseline caked all over his ass cheeks."

Bob would just smile and say, "Yep. Yep. I don't remember those par-tic-ular ee-vents, but I sure am glad they don't happen anymore."

I wasn't really sold on his act though. He still looked awfully sketchy, stumbling down the sidewalk and drawing out the vowels in every last syllable as he spoke. He was probably lifting his flask full of swill right now as he turned the corner. But I was thankful at least we weren't running on him anymore.

One of my old babysitters as a kid in elementary was named Ruby. She lived right across the street from my best friend and would feed us PB&Js with lemonade and let us watch cartoons at her place after school until our parents got home from work.

Fast-forward twenty years and she was a widow now, in her late seventies, who liked to get into the sauce a couple of nights a week, dress up in her nightgown, or nothing at all, call for the ambulance, and try to seduce the strapping young lads who responded. I get it. She was lonely. Is that a crime? Apparently so.

A couple of crews complained to the red shift battalion chief, Marv Holcomb, and he went over to have a chat with Ruby one afternoon while she was sober. He explained that if she kept going down the road she was on, he'd have her committed to an adult foster care home. She acknowledged her wrongdoings and swore not to let it happen again.

But come on; who can let a good thing like that just go away, and with the help of a little dementia, she was soon back at her old shenanigans.

"She's my babysitter, Marv. You can't commit her," I begged.

"I can and I will," he said matter-of-factly.

Once a douche—always a douche, I was resigned to admit. He committed my former babysitter and had her removed from her own home for trying to get her dementia freak on.

There was one drunk who'd walk through the supermarkets and drink all the vanilla off the shelves. Not the imitation stuff, but the real extract. I was surprised to find out it had real alcohol in it and if one drank enough of it, they got buzzed. Our local guy was named Richard, but we called him Vanilla Dick. He single-handedly caused the lockup of all the local stores' supplies of vanilla extract. Yep, first the razor blades and now the vanilla. Now we needed a store clerk to come unlock our vanilla for those yummy no-bake cookies we were making later.

There was a lady who lived right down the street from me, named Cheryl Barbaro. She was about six feet tall, had enormous boobs, and a thicker mustache than I could grow if I wanted to. She'd tell us, when we responded for her almost daily chest pain, how she used to be a stripper and the years of cocaine use had caused her heart condition. We'd shudder to think of her in her glory days and then rush her off to the ER, happy to conclude that call and move on to the next.

There was a frequent flier named Dory, who called for us for chest pain nearly every day at 4 p.m. like clockwork. She was a former rock n' roll groupie of various bands, including Bob Segar, Ted Nugent, and Eddie Money and admitted doing "mountains" of cocaine in the '80s and '90s. Now, as expected, her heart was not what it used to be, and she suffered chest pains because of it. We assumed she just wanted a certain type of medicine that was only offered in the ER. Morphine maybe—who knew—but every day we transported her.

Bernice was an old bird. She'd call at two or three o'clock in the morning, always drunk off her ass and say she'd hurt her toe or something. I figured it was just to have some hunky firefighters carry her out to the sled. She talked liked Droopy Dog and always wanted us to put her shoes on for her or put her coat on for her or help her do some menial bullshit task before we all headed out the door.

One night, we got toned out to her place for the usual. She met us at the door and said her husband had cut his toe. I found it interesting that we weren't there for her bullshit this time, it was for her husband. We followed her to the back bedroom where her old man was sitting on the bed holding a towel over his foot.

"All right, let's take a look, big guy," I said.

As he pulled the washcloth away, a stream of crimson shot across the room about five feet, stopped and then did it again a second time before I could say, "Oh my god, cover it back up and hold pressure on it!"

We dug into the blue bag and grabbed the bandages, replacing the washcloth with a 5 x 9 gauze pad and cling, for the man's arterial bleed. He said he'd been trimming his toenails, which, judging by the others he had yet to trim, looked like an eagle's talons. He'd cut deep into the flesh somehow, and we transported him to the hospital for treatment and a blood transfusion.

In our town, there were many high-rise buildings that served our city's population as low-income, subsidized-housing apartments. These "granny stackers," as they came to be known, included Friendship Circle, Mount Hope Manor, Edgewood Acres, Holmes Village, Shady Pines, Jolly Farms, Burneway Place, Ottawa Towers, Porter Apartments, Edgewood Villas, and the list goes on. We'd made fatal fires in at least four of them, and we could bet our firstborn son that we'd be running to at least two or three of these addresses every shift. Sure as shit.

On EMS calls to these places, it never failed—the patient's apartment was at the end of the hall, almost always the one farthest away from the elevator. We'd better take all the equipment we could possibly need, based on the dispatch chief complaint, or the run gods would see to it that we'd have to go all the way back down to the ambulance to get it, while our partner stayed up there, with a patient dying in their arms. Chance favors the prepared mind, my friends, and this was definitely one of those times it paid to be prepared.

If we took it all, most likely we wouldn't need any of it. If we didn't, it was a sure thing we'd be up shit creek without a paddle. We'd load the blue bag, drug box, and heart monitor onto the cot for everything, even a cut finger. If we didn't, the odds were the person who'd cut their finger would've hit an artery, and bled out, then gone into V-fib, leaving us needing to start an IV for a fluid challenge and deliver a shock in between rounds of CPR. Remember to bring that backboard along, too, for a nice hard surface to back up those chest compressions.

Granny stackers were also high probability zones for food on the stove fires. Low-income housing crammed people of all walks of life into their cramped corridors. The one thing they almost all had in common was making poor life choices. Putting food on to cook, for example, then running off to the laundry room or to the party store. One of those frequent bad choices, and we'd be called to extinguish their smoldering pan of whatever-it-used-to-be and ventilate the building of smoke. We'd make bets as we walked up to the doors on what type of food the person had burned this time, based on its pungent odor at the street.

The Provencial House was a sprawling single story adult rehabilitation center. We were always going there for people who'd coded or were simply rotting away in the filthy living conditions. I must have personally made at least a hundred runs to that place alone. There were elderly folks just dying off in droves in that place. We'd tell each other, as ambulance partners, to swear to just put a bullet in our skull if we were ever sentenced to stay in that facility.

The Armstrong Center was another three-story adult rehabilitation care center that we ran to almost every day. I'd watched my own grandfather wither away and die in there, and, like The Provencial House, the standard of care was atrocious. I'd made hundreds of calls there, too. The living conditions were filthy, and we tried not to set our EMS equipment down on the floor for fear of MRSA (methicillin-resistant *Staphylococcus aureus*) contamination, bedbugs, or cockroaches crawling inside of it. We'd also respond frequently on engine companies to calls for fire alarms, CPRs, code reds, code browns, code blues, and I *always* felt dirty after leaving there.

The trailer parks in our town were absolute shitholes. Literally, two entire parks of them were condemned by the city because the sewage systems had backed up, and there were infestations of bedbugs, head lice, cockroaches, and rats the size of cats. Bunnel's trailer park was the first to go, and then Life O' Riley was next on the list. The residents were given thirty-day eviction notices and told to vacate the premises. "Public health hazard" was the official condemnation reason given by the code enforcement officers.

The other ones around town were significantly better than these, but the living conditions were still pretty bad. We were constantly running over to Windmill Village in the south end, and to the Riverview Estates in midtown. They must've thought by calling it Riverview Estates, it somehow made the fact the homes still had taillights on them more appealing to the residents. Kensington Meadows was in the southwest corner of town, and I'd never seen a single meadow over there. Just a bunch of people with gunshot wounds, overdoses, and domestic violence calls. Lots of blood and drugs. No meadows, though.

Patty Buttons was a drunk lady we ran all the time. She lived on Torrent Court, and we were guaranteed at least one call to her place a night for EtOH, the chemical compound for ethyl alcohol, and the code word or hospital-speak for being drunk. One day she complained of chest pain, and Krishna, always the thorough paramedic, decided to take her at her word.

I rolled my eyes as he put her on the heart monitor, and we were surprised to see a rhythm called bigeminy. She actually *was* having a dysrhythmia with her heart. It was prematurely beating and not firing properly. We call these extra beats PVCs (premature ventricular contractions). She won herself an IV with a dose of lidocaine for her condition and we rolled up to the hospital. Krishna's paramedic skills had helped save the day.

Jennifer Florida was a young woman who fell deep into the bottle and never climbed out. We'd find her all over town in precarious situations, usually barely able to walk or talk, and generally incapacitated and having been taken advantage of. One night, Krishna and I found her at the recently shuttered Deluxe Inn, which was now a vagrant heaven with real former hotel rooms to sleep in, instead of on the street or under a bridge overpass.

She was unconscious on the floor, and we loaded her on the cot and into the sled. As I prepared to take patient care, Krishna decided he was going to take her in tonight. He checked her respiratory rate and tried to wake her. At some point he decided to intubate her just to see if she'd tolerate the airway. She sure did. He dropped an 8.0 ET tube right between her vocal cords and she took it like a champ. He assisted her ventilations all the way to the hospital, and we transferred patient care to the ER staff. An hour later, she stumbled out of the hospital past us and into the parking lot as we were wheeling our next patient in. Good ol' Jennifer Florida!

There was an old hotel that had fallen on hard times in the south end of town. The Magnussen—an eight-story former Days Inn, former Holiday Inn—had trouble filling its rooms during the recession of 2008 and partnered with some of the local homeless shelters who were at full capacity to house some of their overflow residents. It was in our first due, and this development caused an immediate uptick in runs to this address.

Two of the frequently drunk and disorderly new tenants looked exactly like Santa Claus, with his long white hair and beard, and the Wicked Witch, complete with long dark hair and facial warts. One day Santa Claus overdosed on heroin and died in his bed. It's true, I saw him purple and rigored. I even ran an EKG strip on the monitor to confirm. Then we had to take his girlfriend, the Wicked Witch, who was high on either meth or crack—I'm not exactly sure which one—to the hospital for tachycardia and anxiety related chest pain. It was tragic.

The rats in that building were huge, like small dogs (think

ROUSs from the *Princess Bride* movie) and would scurry across the rooms and hallways as we made our way past piles of garbage and old broken hotel furniture haphazardly strewn about. The elevators were in a perpetual state of disrepair, and we were lucky if we happened to find one in working order.

The whole place was one big code violation and even the hotel restaurant had major termite damage as well. With the tiny bugs' mud shelter tubes running along the outside of the walls, around the peeling paint, and right in plain view of the staff, who couldn't have cared less. The restaurant also served as a storage area for hundreds of old hotel mattresses stacked on end and no longer in use. The fire load was atrocious, and we all knew that someday, she'd burn.

Chapter 19

A Generality of Fires— The Basics

There were numerous types of fires we could be called upon to suppress as firefighters. It was important to know which techniques worked well on the various kinds we were dealing with. The following is just a sample of the basic firefighting runs we'd respond to on a regular basis, along with a few pro tips to help mitigate them quickly and effectively.

Car fires were always interesting. The length of involvement and how fast we responded usually determined how much of the vehicle was salvageable after the fire was out. Most of the time it was an engine fire caused by motor oil leaking onto the manifold. After a while of driving, the oil would reach its ignition temperature and begin to smolder, then burst into flames. Hopefully, the firewall at the rear of the engine would stand as a barrier long enough for us to arrive and extinguish the flames before they advanced into the passenger compartment.

Sometimes the fire burned through the hood release cable, and we'd have to find another way to access the engine compartment. Halligan tools were great for this endeavor, and a real crowd pleaser, too. We'd raise the bar high above our heads and drive the spiked adze deep into the corner of the hood, near the hinges, by the windshield. Then we'd pry the corner of the hood up enough to cut the hood's hinges, or jam a fog nozzle into the opening, then spray and pray.

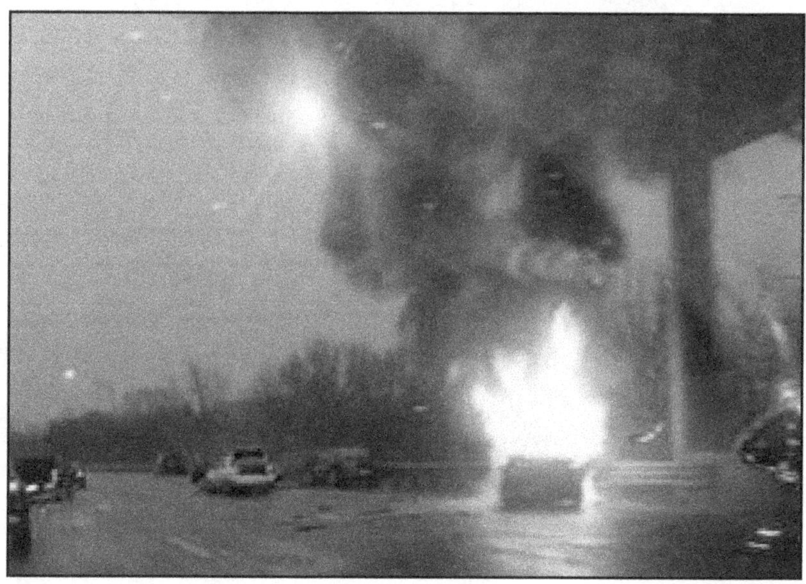

Never stand right beside the tires during a car fire, either. They can explode and send flaming rubber in all directions. Listen for a slight whistle as a precursor to the loud *boom* of the tire explosion. That always scared the crap out of the new kids.

If the fire burned through the firewall or melted the glass of the windshield, as was often the case, then the interior would quickly ignite and the whole car soon became fully involved with fire. At this point, we smashed glass and twisted steel with reckless abandon to gain access to the involved areas.

Our hose line of choice for car fires was the trusty booster line. Smaller in diameter than the pre-connect, yet still pre-plumbed into the pump, the booster line was mounted on top of the engine with the deck gun and conveniently stored on a hose reel. The reel made cleanup and repacking hose much easier than pulling a cross lay.

Specialty car fires were unique and posed interesting challenges to the responders. High-end and commercial vehicles used engine parts made from magnesium, which reacted violently when exposed to water. I recall Dave Owens shitting his pants when the Comcast van that was free-burning next door to Station 4 exploded as he opened the nozzle on its engine. Not gonna lie, I wasn't expecting it either, and everyone was startled when it burst into a shower of sparks and flame.

As I was winding up my career, EVs (electric vehicles) were becoming more prevalent on the road, and we attended training events at the local dealerships to familiarize ourselves with the intricacies of handling these fires. If an EV was involved in an accident or fire, there were certain areas we'd need to check, depending on the model, to find the electrical shutoff switch. Once the power was off, we could safely extricate a patient or extinguish the fire without risk of electrocution to the victims or rescuers. We trained constantly on the latest techniques for vehicles in this new and emerging type of response.

There was a gasoline tanker that jack-knifed and rolled over on the highway, dumping its payload all over the interstate. Police and firefighters closed the highway and evacuated the driver, just before the whole thing exploded into a huge fireball and mushroom cloud of napalm. The news photos of it are insane, and the guys still talk about the heat that melted their helmet visors and anything else that was nearby.

If anyone ever sees a semi-truck involved in an accident, be sure to look for the diamond-shaped placards on the sides of it that can reveal what it's hauling. There's a paperback guide put out each year by the DOT (Department of Transportation) that lists all the placard numbers and what chemicals and products they stand for. 1203 is gasoline, and the only way we're going to put that fire out is with AFFF foam, and lots of it. If it's leaking from the truck's container, get far away and call for help. Unless you *are* the help, in which case, start damming and diking with absorbent materials to protect the environment, and get a pumper with lots of foam coming; you're going to need it.

Dumpster fires are smelly—but easy. It's basically a giant metal container with a fireball in it. So, if we have no exposure concerns to worry about, like flammable objects nearby, we can just surround and drown it. The rookies would stretch pre-connects to flow water into the bins.

After a while, guys got sick of folding that two hundred feet of hose back into the bed and started pulling booster lines on hose reels so they could be reeled back in with the push of a button. That button, incidentally, was almost always broken, and we'd have to climb up to the top of our rig and rotate the hose reel by hand to rewind the booster line.

The real pros—engineers who'd frozen their rank or senior captains—would pull up alongside the container and, from a safe distance of course, open the *deck gun* right into the dumpster. The deck gun is piped directly into the pump and sits midship, atop the fire engine. It's like a mounted .50 caliber machine gun on top of a military truck.

Capable of flowing hundreds of gallons of water per minute, we'd pull up, dump our water tank in the dumpster, catch a hydrant on the way out of the complex, and be back in service in five minutes tops. It was the perfect technique. No trash container could burn once we'd filled it with water and saturated everything within, and there was no need to stir it up and flip the smoldering trash over with a pike pole to make sure it was out. That fire was done.

No fire was more hated—at least by me anyway—than the dreaded food on the stove. We could usually tell when we pulled up out front if that was the case. The stench permeated everything and wafted its pungent odor downwind thru the hallways and out to the road. The aroma of burnt ox-tail soup or briquettes of crispy chicken tits in a skillet stuck to our turnout gear for days and reeked of culinary disaster.

We never used water on a kitchen grease fire because it just flared up and pushed the fire around. Dry chem or, better yet, a CO_2 extinguisher worked great for these. Most of the time, the first-in firefighter could just grab the pan of smoldering charcoal and move it to an exterior patio to cool. Then we'd open the windows and place a smoke ejector in the doorway to ventilate the structure. The smell always stuck around, though, as a lingering testament to the terrible cook who'd inadvertently neglected their cuisine.

High-rise fires in my department were classified as anything 4-stories tall or higher. They hold a special place in my heart because they're *way* more physically demanding than an average structure fire. I've made hundreds of them, most as a Truckee, and they're by far one of my favorites. High-rise operations are different too; the first due engine company secures the elevators and master keys for the incoming ladder truck crew, and the truck crew advances to the fire floor first. While the first-in engine outside hooks to the stand-pipe system, the second-due engine grabs a water supply at the nearest hydrant.

The first-in ladder crews grab their high-rise bag and forcible entry hand tools, secure the master keys, and head to the fire floor to locate the seat of the fire and begin search and rescue operations. The second-in engine crew brings up the high-rise hose bundles and hooks to the stairwell standpipes one floor below the fire. Every crew after them brings up multiple SCBA bottles, high-rise hose, and hand tools to the stairwell staging area one floor below the fire.

We never wanted to be performing operations directly above the fire because it could burn through the floor, and if we fell through, we'd end up in the fire and most likely be toast. So, we always staged the crews on the floor below just to be safe. At least, as safe as we could be running into a burning building. The first ladder crew would radio the incident commander regarding conditions on the fire floor, and a plan of attack would be put into motion.

The closest stairwell to the fire was usually designated for ventilation and had its roof hatches opened, creating a chimney of sorts. Resident evacuation occurred in the other stairwells, to account for proper smoke direction away from the civilians. It was a beautifully orchestrated symphony of perfection when performed as intended. If the crews deviated from the protocols, it could lead to disaster.

As medical marijuana was legalized in our state and dispensaries began popping up throughout the city, old rental homes were converted into grow houses. With little to no inspection processes, the home grower was relatively unchecked in their electrical and plumbing rigging. We began seeing an increase in grow house fires and upon making entry, would often find ourselves in veritable jungles and greenhouses full of marijuana.

Inevitably, we'd come out for bottle changes with stalks of weed, top colas and popcorn buds stuck in various places on our gear. The stickies for the ickies, the *Chapelle Show* stoners would say. We were constantly finding buds in our boot treads, or hiding beneath our collars, or stuck in our helmet visors. Any pinch point that could rip them from their stems.

At a warehouse on Sunset Boulevard, we found ourselves in a large open area with hundreds of plants. Ganja was everywhere and when we were done climbing through it, our Scott Paks resembled little Charlie Brown Christmas trees on our backs. Guys kept making entry and hanging out next to the warehouse doors just to breathe the smoke that was rolling out. Nobody wore their respirators on that one. The fire trucks and our apparatus floor locker rooms smelled like weed for weeks and we kept finding buds in the fire trucks for the next two or three rig days after that one.

We also made fires in houses that had been converted to meth labs. The chemical processes of manufacturing the drug created volatile gases that were easily ignited by a careless source. A cigarette or even turning on a light switch in a flammable atmosphere could cause a massive explosion, and we'd be called in to extinguish the flames.

Toward the end of my second ambulance tour, people started committing "chemical" suicides in hotel rooms and cars. They'd mix common household chemicals in coolers or buckets and the resulting chemical reaction would produce Hydrogen Sulfide. A toxic and deadly gas that binds to iron in the blood and prevents oxygen uptake.

Often there'd be an odor of rotten eggs or "swamp gas" and we'd find notes taped to windows warning the responders not to approach due to toxic vapors. We made several of these calls and they always turned into a Hazmat scene, with the victim perishing. At least they tried to protect others, including the responders, even as they ended their own lives.

Fire alarms are loud. Like *really* loud. When we're going door to door, checking every apartment to make sure the residents have all evacuated, or looking for the cause of the smoke in a church or a warehouse at midnight, it damn near shakes the brain it's so loud. Like the sound of the siren or air horn on the front bumper of the fire truck loud. Like we can hear it from a mile away level of loud. So, there's a certain level of hearing loss one has to deal with if they want to make it through a career in the fire service.

Waterflow alarms were always a treat. Sometimes at a fire, the sprinkler system would activate, causing a waterflow alarm to be called in by the alarm monitoring company. Usually, it was still smoky inside and water would be flowing out from under the doors as we arrived. Most of the time the fire was out. We just had to shut down the water that was saturating the home or business and protect the building from impending water damage.

It was the always the lowest seniority person's job to climb up a ladder to the activated sprinkler head with the sprinkler shutoff kit. Inside the bag were various wedges and cones made of wood and rubber that the new kid was expected to jam into the sprinkler head to stop the flow of water that was gushing out at high pressure. The officers would go try to shut down the fire suppression system, while the engineers would stand back at a distance and laugh their asses off at the new kids getting soaked to the bone.

This exact scenario played out as Ellen Voss and I, both new kids on Engine 1, responded to a waterflow alarm at a storefront on Washington Avenue. I climbed the ladder while Ellen steadied it from below. When I reached the ceiling level, I lowered my helmet visor to avoid being sprayed directly in the face by the water, as it careened off the sprinkler's deflector plate.

Every sprinkler head is different, so we had to choose a stopper that fit properly between the discharge hole and the deflector plate. I'd seen new kids in training try to jamb giant pieces of wood into the sprinkler head and break it right off at the pipe. So, to be successfully performed, it had to be a delicate and precise operation. After going through what seemed like the whole bag, I finally found a wedge that fit. It never stopped the flow of water completely, but I managed to find two that fit nicely, and inserted the wedges in opposite directions. Then I carefully tapped them with a rubber mallet until the streaming water slowed to a trickle.

With the head stopped up, we squeegeed the standing water out to the sidewalk. The officers finally managed to gain access to the sprinkler standpipe and shut the water supply off. Ellen and I could wring water from our turnouts and every other piece of clothing on our bodies. We dumped the water from our boots into the street before getting back on the trucks to leave. It was a crazy job, but somebody had to do it.

There was a water flow alarm at one of the local apartments where the college co-eds lived. The management there would shove a dozen or so kids into a four-bedroom unit with a shared lounge and kitchen area. When the fire alarms went off one day, and a sprinkler had activated in one of the kitchens for a culinary mishap, we were called in to investigate and handle the emergency.

College Towne Apartments was a wonder to behold. In Station 4's first due, there were parties there every night. If it wasn't someone smoking weed in the hallways, it was an idiot spraying the dry chem extinguishers and pulling the fire alarm box just for shits and giggles. When we arrived this time, it was a kitchen sprinkler going off in an all-female apartment. It was like a wet T-shirt contest at a sorority house.

There were young women running everywhere in their pjs and underwear, soaked to the bone, trying to figure out what to save and how to save it, carrying possessions, running into each other, slipping and falling on the wet floors, body parts exposed, and clinging to firefighters for safety. It was an absolutely glorious moment of mayhem.

The kitchen fire was out when we arrived, extinguished by the apartment's sprinkler system, but the alarms were still blaring, and the unit was filled with a light haze of smoke. I carried smoldering pans of whatever it used to be, chicken of some sort I think, to the open slider door and placed it on the ground outside to finish cooling off. When I turned and saw the chaotic scene from my vantage point it was reminiscent of a shower scene from the 1980s movie *Porky's*.

I opened the windows to ventilate the smoke, and the captain gained access to the water supply in the hallway closet and shut the water and alarms off. We grabbed squeegees from the ladder truck and began overhauling the apartment. We pushed the water from the kitchen and lounge, out the slider door in waves. The residents sheltered in their cars in the parking lot while management got to work finding them temporary shelter for the next few nights.

Later that same shift, we made three different CPR calls on Engine 4. It just goes to show the up and down roller coaster of emotions we go through daily, as a firefighter. One minute I'm in an apartment with a dozen half naked co-eds clinging to me and calling me their hero, and the next I'm touching three dead people, doing chest compressions, hauling their lifeless bodies to the ambulance and hospital, and consoling their grieving families.

This was a microcosm of the fire department as a whole. For every perceived good thing, there were three times as many bad ones, and when we stood back and looked at the whole enchilada, it was honestly all bad. Even the things that seemed fun at the time, were highly inappropriate and ethically questionable at best. The terms legal, moral, and ethical were all subjective terms where I worked. They were flexible concepts that could be manipulated to fit our particular circumstances at the time, swayed in our favor, and interpreted in various ways based upon our point of view and level of intelligence quotient.

Wildland fires or brush fires popped up occasionally in the city I worked in. There were areas of overgrown property, especially where the giant power lines ran their current through the city to smaller substations and then into the neighborhoods. Grass fires in the medians of highways, school fields, and boulevards were always favorite spots for discarded cigarettes to start fires in the dry summer months.

We had ATVs with small water pumps on them and would scramble the fleet to quench the burning bushes and grasses when one of these alarms would come in. If we ran out of water deep in the bush, there were stiff fiber brooms that we'd have to beat the burning brush with, much like fighting a structure fire with no water, then stomp out the smoldering ashes, until the ATV returned from a water resupply run.

On the wide-open fields, if the ground was hard and dry enough, we could catch a hydrant and set up the deck gun. Sitting atop my engine, I felt like a soldier on a mounted machine gun, directing the master stream over the enemy field of engagement. That was the way to beat a brush fire with an overwhelming display of blitzkrieg force. No ATV required.

In the big city, folks needed a burn permit to have campfires within the borders of town. It cost residents $50 annually and was valid from the beginning of spring until the end of fall. They could only burn natural wood and had to have their burn pit inspected and approved by a Fire Marshal. Occasionally, someone would violate the rules, or an angry neighbor would call Dispatch for an illegal burn.

We'd roll over in the fire engine and ask to see the resident's burn permit. If they didn't have one, the officer had the choice to issue a temporary twenty-four-hour permit—if the fire was acceptably compliant with the rules—or we could make them put it out, which always sucked. Being the dude that killed the party was not my *modus operandi* and we usually found a way to let people continue their festivities. Unless they were total assholes. If that was the case, we'd shut them down and make them extinguish their own fire with a garden hose, while we stood there and watched, until their conflagration was sufficiently snuffed out.

FYI, if I ever didn't want to pay for that $50 burn permit, I'd just go ahead and burn my natural wood safely in my fire pit, with a charged garden hose nearby in case things got out of hand. If the fire department showed up and asked for my permit, I'd just tell them I'm cooking food. Cooking fires are allowed nearly everywhere—without a permit—and we're good to go. Check the local rules to be certain of course, then enjoy those hot dogs and s'mores!

Odor or smoke investigations were when a civilian smelled something odd like smoke, or rotten eggs, or decomposition, or their CO (carbon monoxide) detector was alarming. Sometimes it really *was* a dead body, or an animal carcass in the attic, or a natural gas leak. Whatever the reason for the call, we always tried our best to eliminate the most dangerous potential causes and make sure the citizens involved had peace of mind before we left the scene.

Sometimes a passerby would call in a house fire when they'd see a laundry vent emitting steam from a home, or a back porch grill was smoking and they thought it was a house fire, or a car that was parked over a steam vent on the road as a possible car fire, or a campfire in a backyard.

We'd show up to check out the situation, often scolding the child who'd just burned his homework in a trash can. Or monitor the air for CO, only to find the civilian's detector was expired for five years now. Or locating a fluorescent light ballast that had recently shorted out and left a light haze of smoke in the business. We could pinpoint the problem rather quickly with our thermal cameras and a well-trained nose for trouble and soon we'd be on our way back to the station, having put the resident's mind at ease.

Chasing tiny issues around were more time consuming than productive and it was greatly preferred, among professional firefighters, to let the beast rear its ugly head and make itself known, rather than trying to hunt it down. The old saying "Where there's smoke, there's fire" is a fallacy and not true in many of these instances. Most of the time on these types of calls, the officer would end up advising Dispatch, upon clearing the scene, that there was no cause for alarm, and we'd head home.

If a structure fire was discovered in its incipient stage, we'd often find only one room burning at the time. This was referred to as a "room and contents" fire. I know, genius, right? If we arrived at the incipient stage of a serious situation, and upon discovery of an impending disaster, the officer would ask for a full alarm, or request additional resources like a truck company, and we'd snuff the fire out before it had the chance to grow into a bigger incident.

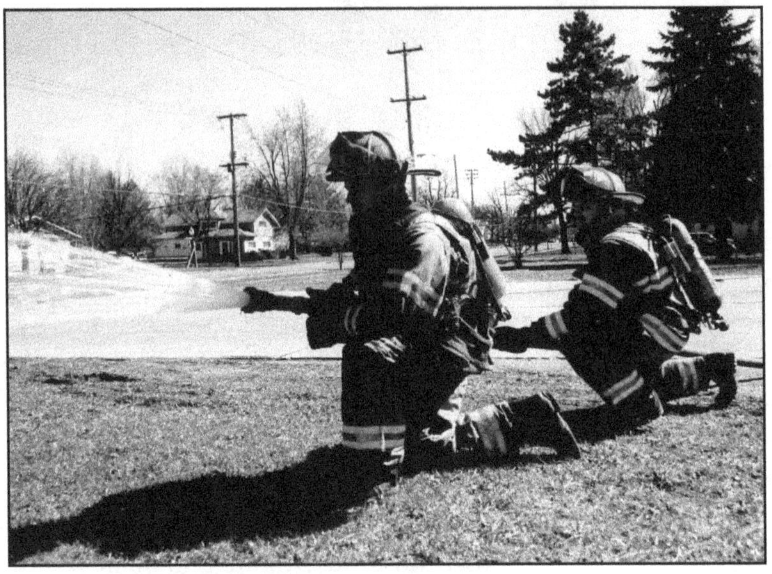

The author with Fergie backing him up on a 1 ¾" hose line

If the fire had more time to grow before discovery, as was often the case at night, then it could advance to include multiple rooms burning at the same time, or even the entire dwelling. The pros refer to this as being *fully involved* with fire.

Chapter 20

High Times

Hector Garcia stepped in as the next captain at Fours. I was excited to reunite with my former engineer from Fightin' Fives and looking forward to having an aggressive officer who could get us in a position to do the real hero jobs. Hector fit the bill and under his leadership station life was just like it was at Fives, minus Chase and Mumbles. We had a blast over the next year or so, raising hell and kicking ass on the fireground.

In the introduction, I mentioned smoke boxing a ladder truck while driving through the city. The truth is, it happened twice, while going down the road, driving through the city, each time with completely different crews: once on the black shift on our way to the garage to transfer rigs, then again on the red shift. The officers both times produced the spliff, sparked the bomb-bud, and proceeded to pass the joint around the cab like it was nothing at all. Smoking it down to the roach, then flicking it out the window onto the street.

At Fours one sunny summer morning, the engine had a training gig all day, and it was just Hector, JT, and me in the gigantic triple company station. It was lawn day, and after we'd returned from the grocery store, JT began push mowing the three-acre lot while I prepped the noon meal. Hector came into the kitchen a short time later and stopped me, saying Jerome wasn't feeling well. He was pale and sweaty. I'd never seen JT so ashen colored and when we checked his vitals, Hector decided to take him to the hospital, thinking he might be having a cardiac event.

He called the BC and received permission to take the ladder truck up to the ER and we headed out the door. As we pulled out, Hector torched a Marley and we passed it around the truck the entire way, from the south end of town to the north. When we reached the hospital, JT turned into the parking lot and crashed the aerial ladder right into an elevated sign. The impact knocked the speaker and a bracket from the aerial oxygen supply tank off the ladder truck.

Hector escorted JT into the hospital and told me to inspect the damage. When he returned, I'd gathered up all the broken pieces and was ordered not to breathe a word of it to anyone. We threw the pieces into the dumpster back at the station. No one even noticed until the following week on rig day. By then it was too late for anyone to pin the damage on us.

The captain of Station 9 at the time, Peter McKinley, busted me smoking weed one evening around bedtime while I was on the medic. After blazing in the parking lot, I passed him and Pants in the stairway and they smelled the ganja on me. The next morning, he called me into the office and closed the door.

"Listen, Shit Boy, don't ever do that to me again," he said.

I knew exactly what he was talking about and answered with a "Yes, sir."

"If you do, I'm going to report you. Don't ever put me in this situation again," he said calmly.

I promised him, and I never did. At least not when I was stationed with him.

Earlier I mentioned the two mothers who lit their children on fire. The first one did it on purpose in cold blooded murder and the second was more an act of pure stupidity, than anything else. Either way, the poor kids in both situations paid the price for their mother's crucial lack of mental acuity and poor decision-making skills.

The first was a Mexican immigrant mother who wanted so desperately to return home, she made up a story about drug lord mobsters threatening their family. When the local police disproved her theory, she waited until her husband left for work one day, locked the doors of the family home, doused her entire house in gasoline, then dumped it all over herself and her two young children, lit a match, and *BOOM!*

I was assigned to Truck 4, and we were the second-due ladder company when the call came in for a full alarm. A house explosion, the neighbors were calling it. Arriving on scene, we found the glass from the front picture windows in the street. The doors were barred and locked from the inside, so it took a moment for the crews to force entry through the side door. The neighbors said they'd just seen the family enter the home twenty minutes earlier and the mother's car was still in the driveway.

While the first-in engine crew extinguished the fire, we assisted Engine 6 with search and rescue in the still smoldering home. Downstairs in the walkout basement, we found the mother still clutching her two children. They were in a pile on the floor together, unconscious. Showtime grabbed hold of the mother's arms and lifted. I watched as the skin sloughed off her forearms and slipped over her hands like a pair of dish gloves, as Showtime struggled to hold her.

Cain Long stood holding the mother's feet, while Showtime continued to struggle with her arms, dropping her a second time. Captain Benny O'Brien, apparently tired of waiting for Showtime to quit fumble-fucking around, wrapped his arms around the mother's waist and suplexed her body up onto his shoulders.

I scooped up a kid and we headed for the walkout sliding door another firefighter had just opened nearby.

In a train of bodies, we traveled out the door, up the hill, and down the driveway to the front yard where the engineers were triaging victims. The first due ambulance was already full of responders working on the first child. Medics were frantically performing CPR and trying to save the little girl, but they were having trouble keeping the melted skin on her body.

People were running everywhere. My lieutenant, Bubbles, was performing CPR on the second kid on the front lawn with two engineers as they waited for more ambulances to arrive. I headed back into the house and met up with Koz on Engine 9. His company was first due, and they were finishing up with the hot spots. The smell of burning dreams inside the house seemed a welcome respite from the chaos of death and soul-reaping going on in the front yard. Through the recently-exploded front window we could see the poor husband arriving home in agony to find his hopes of a better life in America shattered.

The second mother-of-the-year award goes to a lady on Glendale for her DIY lice treatment on her two young children. Evidently, shampooing kids with gasoline *IS NOT* an effective treatment for a lice infestation. Especially when performed in the kitchen, and in proximity to the burners and pilot lights of a gas stovetop.

We were the fourth engine called for manpower on a house explosion and arrived in time to see the mother—with two bloody stumps where her hands used to be—walking to an ambulance with assistance from two firefighters. The skin from her face was dripping off her chin and there was no hair left on her head.

The kids had already been transported by the first two medic units on scene and our crew rushed mom to the burn unit hospital in the third. I drove like the wind and soon we arrived at our destination. I remember the whole ER smelled like gasoline, burnt hair, and singed flesh when we walked in, from the children who'd arrived ahead of us. Two kids lost their faces that day because their mother was a moron. The whole family survived... pretty sure the lice weren't so lucky.

On a cold, snowy day in January, Bubbles was standing inside the apparatus bay at Fours, just as Connie Wagner pulled in driving the Maintenance division's snowplow truck. As she began clearing the parking lot, Bubbles yelled out to Connie through the glass, "Yeah! Girl power!" Seconds later, while Connie waved back at her, she backed the plow truck right into Bubbles's pickup truck. "That Bitch!" Bubbles screamed as she marched outside to check the damage. Bubbles was clueless and rode the emotional roller coaster of her life with hands in the air and reckless abandon. Trouble in paradise was always brewing when she was around.

At a softball outing one year, around the bonfire, after we'd won the championship, Bubbles leaned in and kissed me on the cheek from behind my chair, telling me how cute I was right in front of my wife. A catfight ensued, with Lee telling her to "back the fuck off my man," and Bubbles saying she was my lieutenant and could do whatever she damn well pleased.

"Bitch, you're damn near fifty! I'll whoop your ass and throw you in that fire!" was the witty retort from my wife, as other firemen began to restrain the inebriated Bubbles.

Chad Roberts stepped in and soothed her wounded ego as only he could, and the two walked off into the darkness together.

Big Daddy stumbled over next, slurring something about how he could smell the "devil's lettuce" and was anyone doing anything inappropriate over here.

Lynn Palmer arrived back from the head a few minutes later and told everyone he'd just witnessed Bubbles deep throating a grinning Chad Roberts while he'd been in there. Such were the typical softball tournament afterparties.

Around midnight, on a sultry summer evening out of Fours, I was on the truck with Hector and Bubbles when a full alarm came in directly across the street from the station. It was an apartment fire with a second-floor unit that was fully involved when we pulled up. Hector and I went to work going door to door, waking and evacuating the residents, while Natalia had trouble getting her engine to go into pump. The fire spread quickly out of the apartment, into the eaves, and along the roof line. Soon, all the eaves were puffing with smoke.

I rescued a cardboard box full of tiny puppies from one apartment that a fleeing tenant had left inside. He was so thankful when I returned them safely to him outside. Hector met me in the parking lot and advised everyone was out. We turned our attention next to ventilating the roof. It was a three-story building, so we decide to use our aerial ladder to access the roof. As we turned to help Bubbles set up the truck, she already had it done. It was fully extended a hundred feet in the air, and nearly straight up into the night sky.

As we came around the back of the ladder truck to grab our tools and head to the roof, she was hooking the five-inch hydrant supply line into the main pipe that was plumbed into the aerial ladder. The problem with that was there were no gates or controls for it. When the boys at the hydrant got the green light to charge it, she still had the ladder damn near straight up in the air and no one was on the ladder or turntable to aim the elevated master stream nozzle.

"Isn't that the—" Hector started to say, but it was too late.

He tried to stop her, but the hydrant was charged, and water came spraying out from the elevated master stream into the Earth's upper atmosphere. It was on a full fog pattern and shooting straight up into the sky over the fireground. There was no way to control the water pressure or turn it off except for at the fire hydrant. She'd hooked straight into the ladder pipe and not into the pump intake. We had two engineers there, and both had fucked up their only goddamn job. This is exactly what I mean about the first-in crews doing their jobs right and setting the tone for the entire incident.

As hydrant water rained down over the scene, we radioed for the engine crew who'd charged it to return and shut it down. The hose continued to flow water downhill into the truck for a few minutes, while the fire raged unchecked through the roof of the apartment building. After a while, enough water had drained from the hose that we could disconnect the supply line from the rear of the truck. It was still loaded with water and heavy as hell to drag over to the pump intake. Finally, the hydrant was charged again. The BC made the call to go defensive at that point and I reluctantly climbed the ladder and manned the nozzle controls for the next hour.

We lost the roof on that one. Six apartments suffered a roof collapse on top of all their possessions, and the ones on the lower floors got a swimming pool full of water on theirs. It was a disaster. We were there all night, and as the sun rose, I sat on a remaining peak of the burned-out roof with a hose line, soaking down the last of the hot spots.

This is exactly why you need to have renter's insurance if you live in an apartment. You never know when some dumbass is going to burn the whole place down. Even if you're careful, there are plenty of other idiots around you making terrible decisions.

Hector transferred up to Station 2 soon afterward, because it was the closest station to his home on the north side. When he didn't show up for work one day, we found out through the grapevine he'd been caught growing weed on the public land surrounding his property. He was arrested and charged with possessing and cultivating marijuana. The county narcotics squad had noticed it while doing aerial reconnaissance in a helicopter. Over 110 plants were surveilled and confiscated after Hector was spotted by law enforcement inspecting and cultivating them.

He posted bond and was released, pending his court hearing. The State suspended his EMS license, and he retained an attorney to argue his case and to keep his job. The union negotiated for him to ride a ladder truck every day since his medical license had been revoked. They called it the ride of shame, but we all knew it was really the best place to be. There was no EMS. He only had around six months to go until retirement so they figured he could just ride it out with no license and fly under the radar until he was eligible to leave.

He had to test clean for his probationary officer as part of his sentencing. So, a month beforehand he decided to see his personal doctor just to see where his levels were at. The doc told Hector he had the highest levels of THC in his system he'd ever seen. By more than double the previous record. Hector was so proud of himself. Then he sobered up and began flushing his system for the upcoming monthly drops.

Our state had just legalized medical marijuana, and Lee applied for her patient and caregiver license. I had three herniated disks in my lower back from hauling around bodies for the past ten years and a case of PTSD, which were both qualifying conditions. We were approved for caregiver licenses and together we began learning how to cultivate cannabis.

As licensed caregivers, we were allowed to cultivate up to seventy-two plants. Patients were always calling or stopping by for some of that good ol' homegrown sensimilla. We grew Purple Haze, Super Lemon Haze, Super Silver Haze, Pure Power, Blue Cheese, Casey Jones, Blueberry, Blueberry Haze, Juicy Fruit, Acapulco Gold, Hawaiian Snow, and Grandaddy Purp.

I sold pot to fire chiefs, captains, lieutenants, engineers, and firefighters, police and corrections officers, mayors, city council members, and even state senators, too. Most everybody on the department knew that I grew, and they called whenever they needed some. They knew I wouldn't snitch on them. They knew

I had quality medicinal grade cannabis, and they preferred to buy their ganja from a trusted source.

I once had a battalion chief standing in my grow room, in uniform, on duty. He told me he never judged anyone's side hustle and encouraged me to go for mine. Hell, the chief of the whole department called me up for a delivery. Literally everybody is high. Listen to me, people. They're all high on something. If they're sober, it's most likely because at some point in the past, they fucked something up royally bad while they were high. That, or they're just good, prudent people who probably—deep down inside—wish they *were* high on something right now.

I know, I know: it's one of those sweeping, generalized statements. Not entirely true, but based on my limited view of the world, and my own sick and twisted personal experience, it held true most of the time. With the occasional rare instances of statistical anomalies present in all cross sections of large-scale test subjects.

It was common knowledge that our own married mayor was on the take for sexual favors and his son was a well-known drug dealer. The prosecuting attorney for our city was covering for, and maintaining, a human trafficking ring of prostitutes for his own personal enjoyment. The district court judges were drunk on their benches and fucking defense attorneys in their chambers during recess for favors. Dirty cops would turn a blind eye to criminal activity if the price was right and they could get in on the action.

The whole city was corrupt from top to bottom, and everybody knew about it. So, when I tell you everyone is high, it's because in my little corner of the world, they were. Everybody had their addictions and vices, and they played a game of Russian roulette with their careers. It's just the way things were then, and probably still are, to a lesser extent, today.

CHAPTER 21

Dark Times

After Hector transferred out, Mark Taylor showed up as the new boss of Station 4. He was less aggressive than Hector on the fireground and had a hands-off attitude in the station. He was busy studying for the battalion chief rank and earning his business administration degree online. Like many of his predecessors, he spent most of the day in his dorm room studying and we hardly ever saw him except for on emergency runs or at the dinner table.

Mark was a single man; a player who ran multiple girlfriends in and out of the fire station on a regular basis, sometimes two different women in a single shift. He didn't really care what the crews did. We were left unsupervised and to our own devices for the most part. Which was fine by me, as a twelve-year firefighter. I knew the routine and didn't require much supervision. I was content to do the chores, blaze smoke out in the back parking lot, and respond on alarms.

On March 28, 2010, I received my first reprieve from the ambulance rotation. I fielded a call at the morning breakfast table from Willy P in Operations asking if I'd like to be removed from the ambulance staffing list. It was the moment I'd been waiting for.

I replied with a heartfelt, "Fuck yeah!"

It had been twelve years and three months that I'd struggled to persevere on that bone box. Instead of the eight years I'd originally been promised when I hired on.

April 26, 2010, around 01:00 hours, a full alarm came in for an apartment complex in our first due. I hustled to Truck 4 along with Engineer Bruce Owens and Lieutenant Bubbles, and we rolled away into the darkness. It was blustery that night. Forty mile per hour sustained winds with gusts into the fifties. That makes fireground operations dangerous, as everything is accelerated by the wind, fanning the flames like a bellows.

I guided Bruce in with the complex guide, giving him turn by turn directions to ensure our first-in status. Upon arrival, fire was showing from the backside of the three-story, twelve-unit apartment building. The building was connected to three more twelve-unit buildings on either side of it. Bubbles said she was going to do a walk-around and told me to help Bruce set up the aerial ladder. We'd done this evolution together every morning for the past six months and went straight to work. In thirty seconds, our pads were down, outriggers extended, rear wheels off the ground, and the stick was out of its bed and in the air.

When we finished, Bubbles was nowhere to be found. I waited at the front door of the building as Engine 4's Captain Dan Cooper and Firefighter Karen Kowalsky stretched their pre-connect and made entry. I chocked the door open, grabbed their hose line, and fed it into the doorway behind them so they could advance. They disappeared into the smoky building.

Still no Bubbles. We were duty-bound by the *two-in, two-out* rule at our department, so I couldn't make entry without her there.

Just then, the garden apartment window next to me slid open. Thick, black smoke belched heavy from the opening. The screen popped out as I headed over to assist the sounds of coughing and choking. Suddenly, two arms held a crying child out the window. I grabbed hold of him and set the toddler on the grass a few feet away. Then came another child, an older girl. Then a woman, the mother, I supposed. Next, the father reached his hand through the window. We locked arms and I pulled him from the inky blackness, up onto the lawn.

Cooper and Kowalsky came stumbling out of the building's main entrance, with Dan's low air alarm on his Scott Pak going off. As he and Karen left to get a fresh bottle, I decided I'd waited long enough. With Bubbles AWOL, I masked up and followed Engine 4's hose line to the garden apartment on the far side of the building. Alone, I put the fire out there, advanced it to the second floor, put that apartment out, then climbed to the third-floor apartment and began extinguishing the fire there when my own low air alarm began to go off.

It was time to head out for a fresh bottle, and when I turned to leave, there was Bubbles, crawling on her hands and knees up the hose line to me.

"Stand up!" I yelled through my mask. "Where've you been?"

"Doing my walk-around," was her reply.

"The first, second, and third floor apartments are out. It's in the attic now and I need a tank change," I hollered. We left the nozzle for the next engine crew and exited the building.

We spent a few more hours at the scene, making a roof trench cut for a fire stop, putting out hot spots and opening walls and ceilings to check for fire extension. It just goes to show that a single good soldier can make a huge impact on the outcome of a chaotic situation. Less is more sometimes, and one doesn't always need an army to win a battle.

Cooper later said he thought his Scott bottle had been cross-threaded and was leaking air as they made entry. I just know everything happens for a reason. If I hadn't been standing on the porch waiting for Bubbles, I wouldn't have been there to help rescue that family.

It turned out they were the culprits in starting the fire. They'd cooked dinner on a small hibachi grill earlier. On the patio, the forty mile per hour winds had whipped the charcoal embers out of the container, up against the siding, and into flames. The fire burned through the siding and into the walls of the ground-floor apartment while they slept. It leapt up the balcony and into the second-floor apartment, then likewise into the third floor, extending into the common attic before finally being extinguished with the aid of a trench cut in the roof and an elevated master stream standing guard over it for the rest of the night.

Freelancing is a dangerous proposition. As a firefighter, make sure to never leave your wingman. If you ever find yourself in a situation where you're alone, stay calm and do your best to figure out a solution to your situation. If you find yourself in a scenario where your officer is chicken shit and doesn't have the balls to stand toe to toe with the beast, that's tough, but you've got to stay with them. Don't do what I did. What I did was stupid and could've gotten me killed. But it was totally worth it.

Speaking of totally worth it, Lee made the decision to get breast implants, because our son had "sucked the life out of them," as Lee liked to say. We headed off to a clinic for the augmentation surgery. A few weeks later, Lee began having health issues. She'd yell and scream at everyone in the family over the tiniest little things. Her heart would pound and race, causing her chest pain. She'd pass out when she bent over and would wake up with stabbing head pain and numb teeth.

She couldn't sleep, her hair was falling out, and her eyes began swelling and bulging from her head. She was having trouble seeing and remembering things. She was losing weight *fast*, and if we'd go to a buffet, she'd eat five plates of food and lose two pounds the following morning. Simple trips to the corner store became monumental tasks, and life in general was becoming very difficult for us. She was sleepwalking at night and was extremely hypersensitive with her personal relationships.

The doctors we saw were perplexed to say the least. Blood tests returned normal results across the lab panels. We saw our family practitioner, cardiologists, endocrinologists, homeopathic doctors, and they all came up with nothing. She'd pass out at the dinner table and fly off the handle at the drop of a hat. This went on, for better or worse, for the next three years.

One afternoon she had terrible chest pain while I was on duty at Fours and asked where she could get an EKG. I told her to run over to the closest firehouse with an ambulance, Station 9, and ask the medics there to put her on the heart monitor. Ginger McEntire was on the sled that day and she kindly placed Lee on the cardiac monitor. The rhythm was abnormal, so she immediately transported Lee to the ER and called me to meet them there. We took the engine from Fours up to the hospital. They ran blood work and determined Lee was not having a cardiac event and advised her to follow up with a cardiologist for the arrhythmia.

Several days later, in our backyard, Lee told me she felt like she was going to pass out. I tried to help walk her into the house to lie down.

She stood up from her chair and said, "Baby, I'm not gonna make it."

I reassured her that I had her. That we'd be fine. To just keep walking with me.

A few steps later she stopped and said, "Tell Banks I lo—" She'd tried to say she loved him but fainted before she could get the words out. I had a hold of her and eased her limp body to the ground.

I laid her down on her back in the yard and opened her airway. Our dog was going nuts and kept trying to lick her face. I must've shooed him away three times before finally chucking him far off into the grass. Lee wasn't breathing and had no pulse. I shook her by the shoulders and gave her a hard sternum rub with my knuckles.

"C'mon, wake up," I said as I waited for her to regain consciousness.

It had been nearly two minutes since she passed out and had taken her last breath. I was starting to worry.

"Don't you do this to me. Not now. Wake up," I yelled, grabbing her shoulders and shaking her. Still nothing.

As I mentally prepared myself for doing CPR on my own wife, I yelled, "Wake up!" and shook her violently.

Her eyes opened and she took a breath like a free diver who'd just been under water for several minutes. Her head and teeth hurt. Looking around, confused, she asked where she was.

"You're at home," I replied. "What's your name?" I asked. Trying to determine her level of consciousness.

"I just died," she said, ignoring my question. "I was here, then I was over my body, looking down on us. I remember watching you throw the dog and saying, 'Don't throw my dog,' but you couldn't hear me. Then I understood I was dead and was scared for a moment. Then I realized I was free from my body and there was no pain."

I helped her sit up.

"I was sucked upward and flew through space, past all the planets and stars, to a white light. It was so peaceful there. All the people I'd known, who'd passed away previously, were there and I met Jesus. He was big and had piercing green eyes. I recognized several people there who were pedophiles who'd violated me as a child and asked Jesus, 'How did they get here?' and he told me, 'Child—no judgment, no dogma, no creed. You are no different than these people. Only your lessons are. You are not done; you must go back.' Then I said, 'I don't want to go back,' and before I could finish, I was sucked backwards through space and crammed back into my body."

I sat there in disbelief. That was helluva story she'd just told. I was just thankful she was conscious and breathing again.

I helped Lee stand up and together we walked into the house. We sat down on the sofa. She kept going on about how fancy it was on the other side of the veil, and how she wished she could go back. She passed out another twenty times that evening. The next morning, I left our oldest son in charge of keeping an eye on her and headed off to work.

That afternoon Lee stopped by the fire station to visit. We talked while I made a plate of food for her in the kitchen. Her words trailed off mid-sentence, and I set the plate down on the countertop just in time to catch her from falling, unconscious, onto the floor.

"Hey, Joe!" I called to Captain Joe Collins, who was sitting in a brown chair across the room from us watching TV. "A little help here please," I said as he looked over and saw me holding Lee's limp body in my arms.

He jumped up, saying, "Oh my god," and quickly slid a chair into the kitchen.

We sat her down on the chair and I grabbed the blue bag from the engine while Joe assessed her. We checked her vital signs. They were normal. She passed out again, and again. Each time waking up and not knowing where she was, with a stabbing pain in the top of her head and numb teeth. Joe called Dispatch for a medic to respond to Station 4 for a cry alarm. A few minutes later Krishna and Showtime showed up on Medic 9.

They pulled into the station's apparatus bay, and we loaded Lee onto the cot and into the sled. Krishna asked me to bare her chest for a 12-lead EKG. I consented while Showtime held up a blanket so the rest of the crews couldn't see. The 12-lead showed cardiac anomalies and they transported her to the ER. I went on sick leave and rode in with them.

She passed out three more times en route, and another seventeen times in the Emergency Department before being admitted to the ICU for observation. All told, over the course of that twenty-four-hour period, she had seventy-three syncopal episodes. I kept a journal of the signs and symptoms of each one, along with what happened prior to, during, and immediately following each event, in hopes that some doctor, somewhere, could tell us what was wrong with my wife.

We spent the next two weeks in the ICU, with Lee passing out and then waking up, and telling me about all the dead people walking around the hospital ward. Not just the people who'd died there as patients, but the deceased family and friends of the living people—like the nurses and doctors. Apparently, our dead loved ones are always with us, affecting our reality.

The hospital ran a gamut of tests, including an inversion table, where it was lights out for Lee as soon as they tipped it over. She was diagnosed with idiopathic POTS (postural orthostatic tachycardia syndrome). Which basically meant they had no idea what was going on, but she was passing out a lot. Then we went home.

I had to teach our youngest son how to keep Mommy awake if she started to pass out, by getting right in her face and yelling wildly to keep her attention focused on him, on the days I was at the fire station. Black Friday was particularly interesting that year. I had to work and made the boys promise not to leave Lee alone. She had an increasingly hard time seeing after dark and was still passing out quite often. While waiting in line for the stores to open at midnight, she dropped the boys off at GameStop in a parking lot line and drove off to the other side of town to Toys "R" Us—alone.

Halfway there, she called me at the station and told me she was lost and had no idea where she was.

"Where are the boys?" I asked.

She said she'd left them at GameStop.

"What road are you on?"

She didn't know.

"What can you see?" I asked, getting frustrated and trying to remain calm and patient.

"Nothing, just farmland," was the reply.

"Why didn't you do what you promised and stay with the boys?"

She didn't know.

I stayed on the line with her until she recognized a familiar landmark and then helped her turn around and get the boys. They stayed together for the rest of the night and hit several more stops before meeting me for breakfast as the sun rose. It was a crazy time that fit perfectly with all the rest of the insane experiences I was going through at work.

It wasn't until months later, when her mother made fun of her eyes at the birth of our nephew—calling her Eye-gor because her eyes had swelled so much, they wouldn't close all the way anymore, and saying Lee looked like she had Graves' disease—that another endocrine panel of bloodwork was authorized by our primary care physician.

When the results came back the doctor advised, "Everything looks great, you're fine."

Lee disagreed and explained the lab results that *she'd* seen, and based on her own research, indicated she had Graves' disease and hyperthyroidism. Our doctor denied this and requested the head nurse bring him the lab results.

"Oh my God! I hope you don't have cancer," he said, feeling her throat with his fingers.

We left there with nine new prescriptions and an appointment with an endocrinologist and a surgeon for thyroid removal. Lee was down to eighty-two pounds, continuing to lose around two pounds per day of mass, yet consuming twice as much food as me, and her thyroid was cranking at nearly eleven times its normal metabolic rate.

I'd just about given up on our relationship. She was deathly sick, and I was miserable at home. She screamed at everyone for everything. As horrible as it sounds, I was looking everywhere for a replacement for the person I'd traded my entire life to be with. That person was gone. She'd been replaced by a maniacal tyrant who saw and talked to dead people, screamed at me for breathing wrong, and spent more time in doctor's offices and hospitals than I did at work. If someone had come along with even a remotely better offer than my current circumstances, I would've jumped at it. But there was no one. Only crickets.

Behind her back, I joined all the dating websites I could and created dozens of profiles searching for someone new. Lee's hyperthyroidism left her psychic abilities in overdrive, and she could see everything I was doing. I just lied, told her to relax, told her she was nuts—that I was there for her and always would be. Meanwhile, I was searching for an opportunity to bail on her, and she knew it.

I began an affair with a woman from an adult dating website. The only one who'd even give me the time of day. I'd meet up with her after midnight a couple of times a month at the station. I covered my tracks well, so there was no way Lee could know about her.

Yet she did. Lee confronted me with the physical characteristics of this woman in perfect detail. The color of her hair, her tatoos, her car color and type, right down to the rear window sticker on the back of it. Lee could remote view and would call me out on things she could never have known about. No one could've known.

It made me nauseated to lie to her. She was so sick, and I was such a miserable asshole for cheating on her and then lying to her about it.

One night at home, while Lee and I smoked together outside in our garage, she asked me out of the blue, "Who's Jaime?"

"I don't know," I replied. "Who's Jaime?"

"He says he's your brother," she stated matter-of-factly.

Before I'd been born, my mother miscarried a pregnancy at close to full term. My parents had told the story to me as a young boy and the name they'd picked out was Jaime. I never told Lee about it. There was no reason to. And there was no way she could have known that.

"He says he's proud of you," she offered.

It was at that precise moment that I believed in everything she was able to see and do. The magic I'd been searching for my entire life was right there in front of me and I was a terrible person for fucking it all up. The universe was *clearly* able to see everything I was doing on the sly and there were *actually* people who could tap in and see the truth. Lee was a Watcher. Like in the biblical sense. I believed in her now. And I believed in *us* again.

After months of cheating, something had to change. I ended the relationship with the woman. I just wanted to be a real hero to my family again. I told Lee we needed to talk about our relationship after her thyroid surgery. I needed her to know she was right about what was going on. That I believed in the things she could see and do. The magical things that no one else could believe. The things that made her seem crazy in other people's eyes. She deserved the truth.

She thought I was going to tell her that I was leaving, right in the middle of her illness. And maybe I was. But I held off having the difficult conversation—much to her anger and disappointment—until after her surgery. Maybe to see if things got better, or worse.

The following day, she was on an operating table, having her thyroid and pieces of parathyroid removed. A lifetime prescription of Tirosint, a synthetic hormone replacement followed, and we were golden. When she awoke in recovery, she initially thought she was dead. Her heart wasn't pounding out of her chest anymore. She was kind and loving. I had my best friend and partner back. She asked about having the conversation, and I put it off. I was waiting for her to heal up, or for the other shoe to drop before I incriminated myself in front of the jury.

It didn't take long, and she was gaining weight back, her hair stopped falling out, she was treating others with kindness, and living a healthy lifestyle again. Her meds were adjusted to get the levels dialed in perfectly and life was good. She began to press the issue of the conversation and I kept stalling. Finally, she hit me with the whole enchilada. She knew everything I'd been up to, right down to the name, photos, and social media accounts of the woman.

She'd followed up and researched what she saw in her head and found out she'd been right all along. That I was a cheating bastard. I confessed to everything and asked her to forgive me. Adding that I understood if she couldn't. I resigned myself to my fate, whatever that may be.

She found it in her heart to forgive me. She felt that even though there had been five years of lies on my part and a debilitating sickness that had potentially driven me to make those poor choices—that we were somehow meant to be together. She wanted to blame *me* for the stress on her physical body. That somehow my denial of her abilities to see every action, every position, of my infidelity had brought about her illness.

My admission and confirmation of her abilities was liberating for her and for me. We renewed our love for each other. I've been a faithfully devoted husband and man servant ever since. Attempting to prove my "undying affliction" (from *The Little Rascals*, Lee's favorite movie) for her each and every single day. Knowing that it will take an eternal commitment on my part to rebuild the trust I'd destroyed.

I learned a lot. There *is* a universal justice, and the eyes of truth are *always* watching. I can promise you that. I cleaned up my act. It's better that way. Bad choices make us lose things. Things like people and relationships. Good choices build health and wealth. The kind of wealth that nobody can take away. Like peace of mind and true love.

As it turned out, our best theory on the Graves' disease impetus was the birth of our son in 2005, potentially combined with the BII (breast implant illness) often associated with autoimmune disorders. The symptoms all fell in line with hyperthyroidism and Graves' disease, including the ophthalmopathy with her eyes as a late sign. Maybe it's genetic, but if you know anyone experiencing these signs and symptoms, have them immediately get a thyroid exam from an endocrinologist. It saved my marriage and our lives.

Now that I'd acknowledged my psychic wife and validated her abilities, it was time to help her develop them. I'd heard on the radio about a psychic fun fair coming to a nearby convention center and decided to surprise Lee with a visit to the event. We stopped at an A&W restaurant for lunch to get her favorite olive burger with cheese sandwich, fries, and some of the best root beer in the universe. In a frosty glass mug of course.

While we ate, she asked, "Wouldn't it be funny if you took me to see a bunch of psychics and I knew about it already?"

"You're a jerk," I replied. "How am I supposed to surprise you with anything now?"

"Is that really what we're doing? Holy shit!" she exclaimed.

We finished our lunch and headed across town to see the fair.

There were different psychics, intuitives, tarot and rune readers seated at tables, and we signed up for readings with several of them. They called our name and we sat with them for mini readings. We quickly learned none of them could do what Lee could. They were intuitive, but none of them were actual mediums that could see everything about everyone. There was one woman, Mother Margaret Miller, who advised Lee on a path she should take to learn more.

I began seeking a therapist who could understand the levels of PTSD I was going through at work. There weren't many around. I tried four different "thrapists" before finding a former combat medic who'd seen two tours of duty in Afghanistan. We hit it off and he set me on a path toward conquering my demons.

The best advice he gave me was to read a book titled *Wherever You Go, There You Are,* by John Cabot-Zinn. It talked about performing mindfulness meditation in everything we do. A little practice, and I was on my way to becoming a sage.

Taekwondo became an outlet for my youngest son and me, at the suggestion of my therapist, who was himself an avid martial artist. Banks and I progressed through the ranks together and participated in the local tournaments at Victory Martial Arts.

I joined Freemasonry and began my progression through the degrees, seeking enlightenment and knowledge where previously there was only darkness.

I became a craftsman and sought out technical knowledge for creating objects from wood, metal, and stone. Attempting to leave both things and people in better condition than I'd found them simply because I was there. Self-improvement replaced self-sabotage.

The destructive paths I'd traveled down earlier in my life disappeared and I was able to appreciate them for having brought me to the one I was currently on. All roads lead to the mountain top of life, but not everyone completes their journey to the peak. I was patient and humble in my dealings with others now. I sought truth and understanding. My wife was a special blessing that I leaned on heavily and confided everything in.

In June 2011, Fire Chief Rob Thompson, who'd handed me the nozzle on the garage fire while I was still in the training academy, completely gutted our department. He had to balance our budget and was tasked with eliminating a six-million-dollar funding shortfall. His solution would screw each and every one of our city's residents and all their first responders.

He decided on demotions for the bottom twenty people at every rank, the permanent closure of three of our nine fire stations, and the elimination of a battalion chief, the safety officer, two ladder trucks companies, three engine companies and a medic unit. His proposals were accepted by the city council and the firefighters union, and I was forced to choose between a layoff or demotion back to the ambulance rotation. Twenty firefighters were given pink slips; it was the first time in our fire department's nearly 150-year history.

It was a low blow to have worked so hard for so many years, and to be demoted through no fault of my own. I rejoined the ambulance rotation fifteen months after reprieve from my first meat wagon tour of duty—riding nearly every other shift on a medic for the next two years—because the ambulance rotation numbers were so low. It was a tragic time to be at work. Everybody was pissed off. It was all I could do to keep it together and stay sane.

Tony Salinas was a black shift firefighter when I joined the department. We saw each other at shift change and during trade days, and he always seemed pretty level-headed and chill. He made engineer and then the budget cuts of 2011 hit, and we were all demoted. Tony's home life was in shambles, and his side hustle of scrapping and hauling trash wasn't paying the bills. When his wife left him, he attempted suicide by hanging himself.

Another off-duty firefighter happened to be driving by his house that day and decided to drop in and say hi. He found Tony swinging from a rope and cut him down while he still had a pulse. He was rushed to the emergency room and survived his suicide attempt. He went on to be promoted to captain and eventually made it to battalion chief. I never understood why they'd put someone who disregarded their own life in such a way, in charge of other people's lives.

Pat Duncan showed up at Fours in July 2011 when Chief Thompson's budget cuts permanently closed his fire station. He'd been content to remain frozen as the captain at Station 5 for the remainder of his career, but Thompson fucked that all up for him. Without a station now, and with the extrication tools transferred to Nines where the more senior Koz had the captain's spot locked down, Fours was the next best option since it, too, had a set of Jaws. Fergie persuaded him to transfer in as our new station captain, and he took over for Mark Taylor, the recently promoted battalion chief.

Duncan was less aggressive than Mark, both in station life and on the fireground. Things quietly transitioned, and Smoothbore joined us as the engineer on Fergie's day off. He'd ditched his crazy nurse girlfriend and was now married to a local city police officer; we'll call her Officer Friendly. It was always interesting after we'd just blazed in the parking lot and a police cruiser came whipping around back of the station. Officer Friendly was cool with it and didn't really mind, and it wasn't long before Smoothbore joined the smoker's club and I supplied them with cannabis, too.

Chapter 22

Cops and Firefighters—A Seedy Love Affair

There has always been, and most likely always will be, a strange and wonderful relationship between police and firefighters. Something borderline inappropriate, that says, hey, I like you, maybe we could get to know each other better. Sort of like, I'll scratch your back if you'll scratch mine. I mean, who knows? We may be sharing a foxhole someday.

The police knew, when they were hit by an active shooter's bullets or run over by a distracted motorist on the highway while delivering a speeding ticket, that firefighters were going to be the ones rushing in and trying to save them. It went both ways, too. When the guy on PCP had just throttled six firefighters and we called Dispatch for backup, it was the police who rushed in to save our asses and neutralize the bad guy.

So, when things were done, favors were granted, returned, or passed on to others, it was expected, condoned, and understood among those who followed the code and looked out for their brothers and sisters of the badge. That little red Maltese cross window sticker on vehicles; it's the symbol of the IAFF, or International Association of Fire Fighters. That five-pointed star with the initials FOP on license plates denotes the Fraternal Order of Police. Those are the symbols of the craft. Meant to be recognized by those who know.

The police in our city were always trying to be like firefighters. We often joked with them that they all secretly wished they'd become firefighters. What do you call a person who scored a 69 on the firefighter exam? A cop. The citizens in our town loved their firefighters because we always helped them out of jams. Likewise, they hated the cops because they were always busting them for shit and hemming them up. We didn't really care if you were breaking the law. Go for it. Just don't fuck with us and we won't fuck with you.

Sometimes the cops would park right in front of the house that was on fire. We'd pull up and they'd be coughing on the porch, covered in soot and puking, having just went into the fire to search for victims. They'd attempt to transport shooting victims, or rescue people from fires, or transport a mother in labor, often dicking it up and causing more problems than they solved. And I get it. It's hard to stand there and watch people suffering. But most cops aren't licensed to provide medical treatment. Stick to the mandate. Protect and serve.

The shooting victim would often code in the back of the cruiser en route, or mom would give birth in the backseat, and then they'd have two patients with nobody treating either one of them. Just provide calming reassurance to the patient or apply some direct pressure to that arterial bleed. Don't leave the scene with them, though, unless there's a damn good reason.

After a vacation in Myrtle Beach, South Carolina, with my family one year, the highway we were on just disappeared, and I found myself on a four-lane road going 45 miles per hour for the next twenty-seven miles. With just thirteen hours to make it home before the start of my next shift, I decided to put the hammer down. As I did, a sheriff's deputy came around the bend in front of me heading in the opposite direction and promptly made a U-turn, then lit me up.

I pulled over and Lee grabbed the documents from the glove box. The deputy approached in his wide-brimmed hat and aviator sunglasses, and, through a cheekful of chewing tobacco, asked for my license, registration, and insurance. I handed him the requested papers, along with my fire department ID, so he'd know I was a brother of the cloth. He spit a fat brown gob of chaw juice on the ground and walked back to his cruiser.

When he returned, he said in a deep Southern drawl, "You got any idea how fast you were going?"

"No, sir," I answered.

"Sixty-eight in a forty-five... *Sixty-eight* in a *forty-five*!" He said it again for emphasis.

"I'm sorry, sir. I was just trying to get back to the interstate," I offered.

He handed me back my documents without a ticket and said angrily, "Slow down! Professional courtesy." And he walked away.

I thanked him, and he spit out the side of his mouth and just kept walking.

That's exactly what I'm talking about. The kind of thing that only first responders—people who have stood next to each other with a dead body hanging from an upside-down car in the center of the road at midnight, with severed body parts from a completely different stiff strewn all around them—could understand. They were akin. Alike in ways that no one else could fathom. Allies in an unwinnable war against human atrocity and stupidity.

The police would break intersections for us when we had terrible calls involving children or public service members. One time, a local cop took seven rounds in the neck, torso, and arms. We scooped him up and flew to the hospital with a police escort and every intersection had police blocking lanes of traffic with their lights on. Once we cleared the light, they'd fly past us and block the next one, like a game of leapfrog, until we made it to the hospital. The officer made a full recovery and soon returned to work. It was a powerful statement of coordination and skill, with both units working together to accomplish something that was impossible separately.

We were a close-knit family and some of the local bars would open at shift change for the cops, firefighters, and nurses who'd just finished their tours of duty. Leroy's and Corey's were on the south end, and Art's Bar was on the north end of town. The people who were single and didn't have families and young children to rush home to, usually met up and shared a few drinks over breakfast. The morning sun was always blinding when we'd leave, after sharing stories of the previous shift's highlights and lowlights with our comrades in arms.

Somewhere along the line, some genius had the idea to marry the two professions and create the PSO (Public Safety Officer) to save a few bucks in the HR department. This hybrid police officer/firefighter could do both jobs and was cross trained in both disciplines. I suppose in areas of the country with lower call volumes, PSOs could be beneficial. But in the big city, there were so many calls coming in, for both disciplines all day and night, that it just made sense to specialize in either one or the other.

In the out-county areas there are sheriff's deputies who are paramedics and respond to EMS calls. They take over patient care in the rural communities and ride to the hospitals in the Basic EMT staffed ambulances that respond.

There are also the Fire Marshals, who are like police detectives, carry guns, and can make arrests, but only investigate fire-related crimes such as arsons.

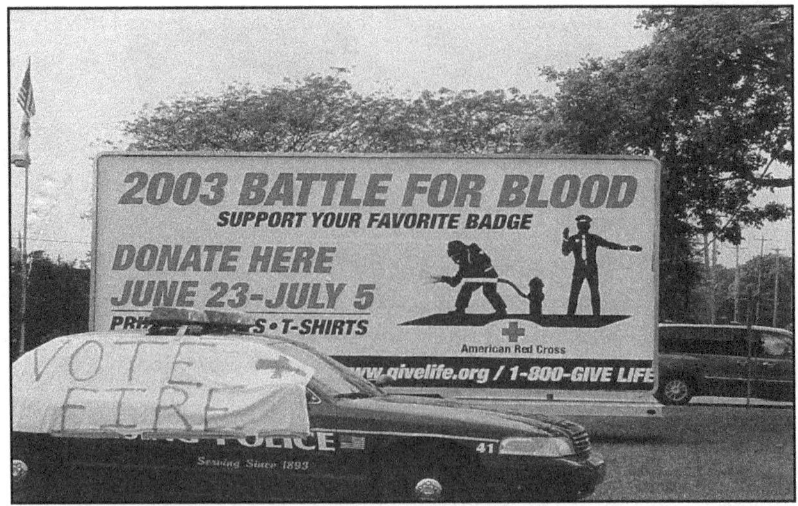

When the cops tried to influence the local blood drive in their favor, we had to respond

One evening out of Station 4, it was Brian Quagmire, Fergie, and me on Engine 4. We received a request from a county sheriff's deputy to respond on a deer in the middle of the road that was hit by a car and still alive. When we arrived, the deputy seemed perplexed at how to handle the situation.

The deer was paralyzed in its hind quarters from the impact and was dragging itself around in circles in the middle of the road. With input from Quagmire and Fergie, the deputy ultimately decided to put it down and prepared to shoot the deer in the head. When she squeezed the trigger, the magazine fell from her gun onto the pavement and her safety was still on.

"Oops!" she giggled and picked up the magazine, slamming it home into the handle this time. The deputy readied for a second attempt and aimed for the head. When she fired, her round, intended for the deer's head, missed its target, and she shot the freaking nose right off it. I've never heard a deer scream like that before. The second headshot killed it, *finally*, and she pumped a third round into the torso just for good measure.

On Engine 4 one night, Duncan, Fergie and I were called for a barricaded gunman. We arrived around midnight for the police standby and Pat spoke briefly with the battalion chief about what was going on. It turned out the suspect had robbed a pizza delivery guy for $43 and his cell phone. The pizza guy had been thumped on pretty good but managed to escape. The police then tracked the stolen cell phone to a duplex on the south side.

When they attempted to contact the suspect, he kicked through the drywall, into the adjoining home, and took his startled neighbors hostage. There was a young family: a father, mother, and an infant in the home next door. The suspect tried to slip out the back door with a gun to the infant but went back inside when he found himself surrounded.

After sitting in the engine for an hour or so, the police rolled past our staging area in their APC (armored personnel carrier). It was a tank basically, with a giant battering ram instead of a turret, and a back door that lowered like a ramp to let the officers in and out. They could drive that thing right into a house through the walls and deploy officers inside. We knew it was getting serious now. Off duty police kept driving by us, arriving in their personal cars, and dressed wearing full body armor.

After a few hours on scene, I just couldn't keep my eyes open anymore and told Brownie to wake me up if anything happened. It was 3:30 in the morning now, and there was no comfortable spot to curl up in that fire truck. I tossed around in different contorted positions, always being just uncomfortable enough to not fall fully asleep. The standoff lasted another three hours until the sun came up, and the suspect gave up peacefully at dawn. We headed back to the station tired, cranky, and ready for shift change.

One night out of Fours, the engine and medic rolled to the rows of massive power line towers that ran through the south end of town. It passed through nearly a dozen neighborhoods, and I remembered walking home from junior high school through the trails that ran beneath this particular stretch. When I was twelve, my girlfriend's older brother wanted to fight me for dating his little sister, right below one of these towers. That was a no-win situation for sure.

Sunrose was the cross street and a young man had climbed the 80-foot electrical tower and was threatening to jump from it. There were about five or six police cars with spotlights on the man when we arrived. An officer was trying to negotiate with him over the PA system on his cruiser. He was explaining to the man that whatever it was he was upset over, they could work through it together, and he'd help him figure it all out.

Julian Burke was the battalion chief who'd responded on our end. On any multi-agency response, we needed a fire department command officer looking out for our troop's best interests, so he'd been sent over by Dispatch. His Suburban's spotlight illuminated the man better than all the police spotlights combined. I stood next to Spoons and Zach Powell as the young man threw the white T-shirt he was wearing off the tower.

We all thought he'd jumped, but the shirt seemed to hesitate in the air, falling slower than a human body would've, and we soon realized it was only an empty shirt. From his vantage point, closer to the base of the tower, Burke believed the white shirt was still attached to the man, having leapt from his perch, and his mind just couldn't handle it. An awful retching noise came from his direction as chunks blew from the BC's car window.

We laughed, and Spoons went over to check on the chief. The cops ended up talking the jumper down after an hour or so of him throwing various articles of clothing down, until the guy was up there in only his underwear. He climbed down and they walked him over to the sled for a nice ride over to CMH for some therapy. Crisis averted, and the score after one was: police negotiators 1, suicide squad 0. Burke went back to Station 1 for a car wash and some clean shorts, and we headed back to Fours for an hour or two of sleep before shift change.

Chapter 23

A Necessary Evil—Medicals Pay the Bills

We can debate fire-based EMS (emergency medical services) for eternity multiplied by infinity, and I will still despise it. I might eventually be swayed into believing in the merits of a rapid response of fully staffed rigs, with rescuers standing by at the ready, possessing the knowledge, equipment, and training to spring into action and save the lives of our citizens in peril. But I will never say for *one* second that I enjoyed being a part of any of it. The only thing that made EMS worth the utter bullshit I went through as a first responder on an ambulance was the pension and the bennies. And medical runs funded them both, no two ways around it.

As my years in the rotation dragged on and the frequency of ambulance shifts increased to every other day, sometimes even back-to-back, I felt helpless and stuck. The human carnage and terrible acts of violence that people perpetrated against themselves and others around them weighed heavily on me. It made me question the extent of our human evolution and the general intelligence of our species. The following chapter describes just a few examples of the things one could expect to encounter over the course of a typical ambulance shift in our city.

In the introduction, I mentioned the intoxicated bum at the church shelter. On the medic unit out of Ones, we were called to a homeless breakfast at a church downtown, where a gentleman showed up intoxicated and was asked to leave, because they wouldn't serve patrons if they were drunk. The police called for paramedics to transport the unruly man to the hospital for detox. We met the cops and the man out in front of the church, and I greeted him politely, calling him *sir* several times while we loaded him into the ambulance.

As I took his vitals, he read my name tag aloud from my uniform, looked me in the eyes, and explained he was going to "rape and murder my family" after he was released from the hospital. I wasn't really sure how to react to that. No one had ever said that to me before. I could've beaten the shit out of the old man, or pursued a sincere dialogue questioning his reasoning for such vile conversation. But I chose to simply ignore it and called the hospital to let them know we were coming. Remember the mantra. *Pension and the bennies.* And this sack of human shit wasn't gonna fuck it up for me. Not today. Back at the station, I ripped out the embroidered stitching of my name on my ambulance jacket. Now, instead of reading B. LILLY, it just said "Y." As in, "*Why?!* Why God, did this bullshit have to happen to me?"

It was late afternoon, and we were heading home from an ambulance assist call on Engine 4 when a distress call came across the radio. Engine 6 and Medic 9 had walked into a stabbing in progress while responding on a medical alarm. A man had broken into a woman's apartment and was in the process of stabbing her fifty-two times when Engine 6 pushed open the apartment door and interrupted him. Captain Jason Hundt screamed at Dispatch for help over the radio as he and his crew fought off the offender, who was now charging them.

We were just down the road on Engine 4, and I suggested to the guys we should go help. Duncan and Fergie completely wussed out and said some shit like, "It's not our problem," and, "If dispatch wants us to go, they'll send us."

What the fuck kind of shit is that? I wondered if they would've wanted help if it was them being charged by a knife-wielding assassin. We just cruised on back to our station.

In the end, 6 Engine's crew subdued their assailant, thanks to their turnout coats being thick enough to deflect knife slashes, and their comrades being faithful enough to pounce on and restrain the madman until the police arrived and took him into custody. The lady had already passed away from her injuries, and it was ruled a homicide.

There was a lady with diabetes who lived in the Briarwood apartments with her five-year-old son. She'd trained him so that "when mommy got sick," she'd need him to call 9-1-1, and the fire department would come and help her. This usually happened a couple of times a week.

We'd show up and make contact with the boy, who'd then lead us to his incapacitated mother. We'd radio the medic unit to bring the drug box and blue bag inside. They'd start an IV and push the meds while we tried our best to befriend the little boy and hopefully make his difficult life just a little bit better. When mom came around, she'd always refuse transport. The medics were used to it and knew the routine.

Speaking of refusals, this next bit of information could be pertinent someday. If an ambulance is ever called and the patient decides they don't want to be treated or transported, there's something called a refusal competency exam that one must pass to have them leave you alone. There are certain criteria that a person must fall under to be deemed competent to refuse medical care. If not, medics can make the decision to basically arrest your ass.

(1) One must be oriented to who they are, where they are, what date or time it is, and what is going on around them. (2)

The patient is not under the influence of drugs or alcohol. (3) The patient has not experienced a loss of consciousness or an injury that interferes with their mental functioning. (4) The patient is capable of understanding the current situation. And finally, (5) The patient is not a clear danger to self or others. If they fail any of these criteria, the ambulance crews are authorized to strip them of their rights and have the police force them to comply with medical treatment and transport. An informed citizen is an empowered citizen.

Krishna was well known on our department as a shit magnet. If there was a crazy call that only one percent of all paramedics in the world could potentially get in their careers, he'd have been on five of them. He was a tall Kashmiri Indian man, and we got along famously when we rode together. In the beginning, Krishna was a stay and play kind of guy, favoring to practice his craft in the patient's home and stabilize them before transport to the hospital. I was a load and go guy and had better things to do with my life. We balanced each other out well.

I met Krishna on a carpentry job he was doing in a wealthy suburb of our city. I was bidding a flooring side job and he was the superintendent on the remodel, so we started talking and before we knew it, the fire department came up. I was on the department at the time and Krishna was in the hiring process. We hit it off and have been friends ever since. He got the job and was thrown into the fire, figuratively and literally.

We've made hundreds of calls together, but there are a few that really stand out. Out of Nines on the medic, we responded on a woman having chest pain. As we spoke with the patient in her house, she explained they were having a birthday party when she felt a sudden onset of stabbing chest pain, with no prior history. Her vitals were stable, and we administered O_2 via nasal cannula and assisted her to the cot at the bottom of the porch stairs.

As we loaded her in the ambulance, she became distraught

and said something was very wrong—that she felt like she was going to die. Her blood pressure was hypertensive. We assured her she was in good hands, put her on the monitor, and started an IV. We cleared the engine and I drove to the hospital while Krishna called to let them know we were en route.

We pulled into the ambulance bay at the hospital a minute later. Krishna was checking her blood pressure again and now it was *hypo*tensive. We wheeled her into the ER and transferred her over to the hospital bed. Almost as soon as we left the room, she fell unconscious and coded. Krishna advised the staff it could be a potential AAA (abdominal aortic aneurism).

Her husband arrived in his personal vehicle to find his wife, who, a few minutes earlier, had been walking and talking, now dead. He lost control and burst into tears as we tried to explain what happened. The patient-doctor consult room was right next to the ambulance report writing room, and it always sucked to walk past the families of the people we couldn't save. They looked at us like we were the ones who'd murdered their family member.

Sure enough, we found out later it was a triple A. She'd ruptured her aorta, the major blood vessel that supplies the heart, and was bleeding out into her chest cavity. It's difficult to detect and diagnose, but she had all the classic symptoms. That one ate at Krishna, and he felt personally responsible for a long time. There wasn't much he could've done, though; the survival rates were extremely low on these types of calls when they occurred in a pre-hospital setting.

Krishna had decided to become a paramedic after his mother passed away and he wasn't able to save her. He spent his free hours in medical journals and making rounds with doctors at the hospitals, trying to gain insight into the profession. Being a recent graduate of medic school, he was very literal on the protocols for every given situation and had them all memorized.

He would correct the senior medics if they were lax or incorrect on their patient care and some found him abrasive to ride with. I always seemed to get paired up with the funky ones. Maybe I was an odd one and Ops just wanted to see how awkward they could make it. Or maybe I was just the last one left who wasn't bitching about riding with him.

Either way, when Krishna pulled out the rectal thermometers for every pediatric patient, because they were more accurate and that's what the protocols called for, I was generally the voice of reason. Unafraid to explain how that's just creepy and that this kid would be fine until we arrived at the hospital. That an accurate body temperature wasn't going to determine their fate in the next three minutes.

We balanced each other out. I was the Yin to his Yang. Wild and crazy stoner kid meets by-the-book, doctor type. I gave him reefer to mellow out and he gave me paramedic books to increase my knowledge. It was homeostasis. We each got our first CPR save together. We had even saved each other's bacon at least once or twice. He helped me with all kinds of carpentry projects, and I did everything I could to help him with whatever projects he had going on as well. He was good people. I always say relationships are the most important thing in life, and I hope I'll always have this one.

One afternoon out of Fours I was on the engine with Duncan and Fergie when we made a call for a shooting at a car wash. A young man was lying on his side in an empty bay when we pulled up. I grabbed the blue bag and went to check on him. He said his name was James and he wanted me to hold his watch for him.

As he sat up, I could see a gunshot entrance wound in the left temple area of his forehead. While he tried to remove the Rolex from his left wrist, because he didn't want anyone to take it, I noticed a similar bullet hole clean through the center of his left hand.

"Whoa, there big guy, you hang onto that watch. You're gonna need it when you get out of the hospital," I said, "You're gonna be OK, I got ya."

He explained there was a shoot-out between two cars as they were going down Miller Road. He was in the back seat and was hit by gunfire. His friends in the car, if you can call them that, pulled into the car wash and dumped him out, then sped off. Just then the ambulance pulled up with Paul Shaheen driving. Krishna hopped out of the passenger side and walked over to us.

"Kris this is James and he's got a gunshot wound to the head."

Krishna looked astonished as James tried to stand up and do his best, nice to meet you, impression.

Paul wheeled the cot over, we loaded James up and hit the road.

James made a full recovery thanks to Krishna's expert medical care, Paul's NASCAR worthy driving skills and the trauma center hospital staff. And he still has his Rolex.

Big Daddy and I were on the sled out of Nines one day when a call came in for a naked man running down the street. We responded and found the guy sitting on a porch wrapped in a blanket, where the frightened homeowner had left him while she called 9-1-1.

In our ambulance, the man explained he was from another city and had been abducted the night before. He had no idea where he was, because the men who'd taken him hostage had blindfolded him. They tied him naked to a pole in the basement, then beat him with guns, bottles, and fists for the better part of seven hours, until they got hungry and left to grab some food. While they were away, he escaped and ran to a neighboring home, persuading them to call for help. Truth is stranger than fiction, I swear.

Few runs carried the instant repulsion of a rectal bleed. Guys would cringe and whine at the mere mention of these calls and often sulk their way over to their ambulance at a snail's pace, dragging their feet and hoping for something—*anything*—that would make them not have to go. Reluctantly, they'd fire up the rig and head out, knowing exactly what was in store for them.

Sometimes, on hot summer days, we could smell the aroma of butt bleed from the road when we pulled up. It's kind of like a diarrhea mixed with old coffee grounds. Unsurprisingly, that's what it often looked like as well. We'd grab the blue bag and head in, switching into mouth-breather mode to avoid filling our olfactories with the thick stench of bowel death.

As a general rule of thumb, if the rectal bleed was higher up in the digestive tract, it looked like coffee grounds. If the bleed was lower, closer to the rectum, it was often a brighter red. The patients were usually embarrassed and rightfully so. The smell was horrible and it's not a normal or generally accepted thing to do to call for help for a bleeding bunghole.

The treatment for these patients was to assess their vitals and give a fluid challenge if large amounts of blood loss had occurred. "*But*" typically, they were in stable condition, and after a round of vitals were collected, they rode in a position of comfort, and the EMT would take patient care. The smell would hang in the air as we traveled, and we'd have to leave the doors of ambulance open to ventilate while we transferred the patient to the hospital staff.

We had certain acronyms that served as code words for our EMS reporting—There was FDGB (fall down, go boom), TBS (total body strain), or FBS (full body strain). Chief complaints were: PAO (pain all over), FOS (full of shit), and TBS (total bullshit). The nurses all used the same shorthand, too, so it was easy to communicate back and forth with these phrases while standing beside the patient and delivering a report describing their current predicament or situation, without pissing them off.

Some of the more experienced medics would write entire run reports in these abbreviated acronyms, and anyone who didn't have the same level of licensure or higher needed a secret decoder ring to figure out what they were saying. Surely, the folks in billing had a difficult time figuring out what treatment methods had been delivered during patient care.

The experts say that only 10 percent of pre-hospital CPRs are successful and walk out of the hospital. I'd wager it's actually far less. Try closer to one percent. My first CPR save came almost five years into my ambulance career. I was riding with Krishna out of Station 9 when we received a call for an elderly man unconscious. We arrived to find the old man, lying face down in the snow, outside an apartment building's entrance. There were footprints in the snow on the sidewalk, walking both ways, into the building and out to the parking lot. Someone had walked right by the old man on the ground without stopping, twice.

We rolled him over and checked for a pulse and breathing, but there was neither. Calling for an engine company, I grabbed a backboard and we rolled him onto it, loaded him on the cot, and into the ambulance. We peeled him out of his winter clothing and began CPR. Krishna got an IV started while I dropped a Combitube and started respirations. We switched places and I did chest compressions while Krishna put the pads on him and cracked the drug box for the first round of meds.

With the meds on board, we stopped CPR to analyze the heart rhythm. "Asystole, shock not advised" was the response from the monitor. We hammered on the compressions as the engine crew drove us to the hospital. By the time we arrived, he was in a sinus rhythm, and an hour later he was conscious in his hospital bed. He had some broken ribs from the chest compressions, but he was alive. It was crazy how we'd done the same things we'd done a hundred other times, but it just worked out differently this time.

In 2010 I experienced an anomaly on the ambulance. A glitch in the matrix. Justin Stevens and I had a single run shift out of

Station 6 on the medic unit. Normally, we pulled around twenty calls in a 24-hour shift there. As the day wore on and we didn't roll out the doors, the rest of the crew began giving us shit and saying how we lived in a tree. Justin told them it was just clean living and good karma on our part, that we'd made a sacrifice to the run gods that morning before shift change of a virgin maiden and two white lambs. I knew they were both lies.

Maybe the run gods were actually having pity on our poor tortured souls and granting us reprieve from the endless cycle of traumas, if only for a day. Other stations began calling our firehouse asking to speak with us, questioning our good fortune, and doubting our reasoning for it. Some called Dispatch throughout the day and asked them to test the medical alert tones at the station, thinking maybe they were just broken. Hell, we couldn't understand it either. It was unexplainable, and we just cruised right along, enjoying our run of good fortune.

At around 01:30 hours that shift, the station opened up for a full alarm fire in our first due. We finally had our first run of the shift, nineteen hours into it. It was a fire standby, not even a medical run. We cleared when the fire was extinguished and returned to the station. As we headed back to our dorm rooms, we were certain we'd be meeting back at the rig in a few minutes. That our lucky streak had finally run out.

The wake-up alarm came in from Dispatch at 06:30 hours and we hit the head, then made our way over to the kitchen for coffee. As we entered the dining room, the breakfast table lit up with guys saying things like, "Ho-ly sheep shit," and, "What the *fuck*," and, "You two lucky motherfuckers go buy me a lotto ticket on your way home!" We just smiled and sipped our coffee. There wasn't much to report to our relief crew, only that we'd just had an epic shift and didn't use a single thing off the sled. Not one goddamn thing.

Being the son of a preacher man, I had a unique perspective on emergency calls to houses of worship. I had deep rooted questions about God, after having studied the scriptures like a monk preparing to take the helm of a monastery, in a failed attempt to earn my earthly father's love and approval. There were things in the Bible that didn't quite make sense from my point of view. Upon witnessing my father fuck up my entire life with his less than pious personal addictions and escapades with various women, putting their needs above those of his own flesh and blood, I now had a complicated view of religious activities, and the ones who proclaimed to practice its massively schismed and varied arcane arts.

Every Sunday on the medic unit, we would invariably be called out to one of the local churches. Sometimes we'd place bets on which house of worship it would be that particular day.

Perhaps it would be the First Congregational, New Pentecostal, Our Lady of the Virgin Mary, of Latter-Day Saints, New Hope of the Nazarene, Non-Denominational, Doors of Healing Tabernacle of Modern Methodist Wesleyans. Or maybe it would be the Evangelical Lutheran Reformed Calvinists, of the Presbyterian New Covenant, Church of Christ, of the Eastern Greek Orthodox Holy Cross, of Anglican Episcopalian United Brethren of Zion.

Or possibly it was the Fellowship of Baptist Fundamentalist Snake Charmers, of the Free Will Spiritualist Church of God, on the Seventh Day of the Amish Quaker's Assembly, in the Hall of Foundational Apostolic Faith. It might even be the God is Love, Prophecy of the Bible, Believer's Union of International Fellowship, of the Assembly of Mount Calvary's Christian Alliance of Catholic Scientologists, in Communion with Our Redeemer of the True Synod, of the Almighty Messianic Congregation of Heavenly Kingdom Witnesses of the Mazle Tov.

Regardless of which heavily divided group of believers we were rushing in to save, it was always awkward to respond to the sanctuary in the middle of Mass. Where hundreds of people watched, while we treated an elderly man or woman who'd suffered a heart attack or stroke during the service. We'd try to move them as quickly as possible out to the ambulance, so the entire congregation wasn't watching us as we intubated Mrs. Jackson, and then had to bare her chest to place the shock pads onto her torso, in between rounds of chest compressions. The crowded sanctuary was definitely not the best place for these techniques and maneuvers.

On Medic 11 one night, I was riding with Bubbles. We responded to Shady Pines, a "granny stacker" in the downtown area for chest pain on an elderly woman. After starting an IV in the apartment, Bubbles tried to put the needle she'd just used into a sharps shuttle and stabbed herself in the thigh instead. Worried about possible disease transfer from this sweet little old lady, Bubbles activated our exposure control policy. The lady was a widow, with one husband for 53 years, and I highly doubted her raging Hep C or HIV was a factor to consider in this matter. Sexual promiscuity just didn't appear to be on the radar for this one. Bubbles insisted on following protocol, though.

We transported the patient to the ER, where the BC met us and proceeded to have a battery of tests run on the patient to determine any contagions, while Bubbles got a double round of IV antibiotics. We were out of service all night and I slept on the ambulance bench seat in the parking lot. When the sun rose, Bubbles advised everything was fine, and we went back to the firehouse for shift change. It was always something fucked up with her around, never normal.

JT told a story about a single engine small plane crash he responded to when he was younger, where there were pieces of bodies everywhere, strewn among the wreckage. He specifically recalled stepping in a pile of organs and seeing human entrails hanging from the trees that he had to walk through, to get his hose line over to the plane that was still burning. We saw horrible things that never left our mind's eye. Things that haunted our memories.

During my demotion and ambulance reinstatement, it was always a good time when I rode the sled at Nines. Koz was the captain and Fergie was a frozen engineer there. Big Daddy and Paul Shaheen rounded out the Firefighter rank. These guys would lock the station down right after breakfast and play *Call of Duty—Zombies*, work out, and nap all day until a run came in. I appreciated the laid-back station atmosphere between all the stressful calls.

Zombies was a great escape there. I know there's no way we can ever beat the hordes coming at us increasing in numbers until we can't hold them back anymore. There's something corporeal about it that speaks to my humanity though. We all know were going to die; it's a given. One of the only certainties in life, like taxes. But we play the game anyway. Trying to see how far we can get, learning from our mistakes, and pushing on farther than we had previously.

Workouts were mandatory, and Nines had one of the best gyms in the city. Empty supplement bottles of whey protein and creatine lined the walls on top of the cabinets in the kitchen and the meatheads from Nines, pushed the powerlifting world's limits. Paul Shaheen won the gold medal at that year's Pan-American Games. At Nines under Koz's leadership, life was actually fun again, even with the chaos of emergency responses.

Joe Collins told the story of a nine-month-old baby he had to respond on who'd just been raped to death by its own pedophile grandfather. The suspect was still in the home and the police had to restrain the engine crew from assaulting him while the medics performed CPR on the infant, who had coded from his severe internal injuries. There was nothing they could do to save the poor child. The responders involved in that call were forever scarred.

There are those whose scars were in fact, literal. Many of my colleagues were disabled in the line of duty and physically unable to continue working. There was Gina Capone, Josh Porter, Tina Price, Steve Bishop, Pam Stokes, Josh Falco, Marie Rosenthal, Mitch Warner, Tiny Paws, Spike Young, Jimmy Knight, Sherry Horton, Chris Goodyear, Dan Milton, Dolph, Jeff Ludwig, RP, Julio Torres, Cowboy Dan, John Lohan, Frank Fulger, Candice Bartholomew, Hank Brooks, Chris Dunn, and Peter Coddington, that I can recall.

That's 26 out of a 250-person department when I came on in 1998. It had shrunk to just 125 total members through attrition by the time I left in 2018. I'd watched at least two dozen more simply quit the profession after a short stint in the life. So the odds were about one in four wouldn't make it through a career there unscathed. Everyone there had PTSD, in varying degrees. That was guaranteed. Who just decides one day that they want to have post-traumatic stress disorder? Oh yeah, that's right: firefighters.

I rebelled a lot after my demotion from the budget cuts of 2011. I got sleeves of tattoos on both arms and legs and refused to cut my hair. As time went on, officers started giving me shit for being a male with long hair. I searched for a justifiable reason to keep it long. Something besides: "If the ladies can do it, then so can I."

I found the excuse I was seeking when I learned of Grace Nobles. She was a fourteen-year-old girl who had leukemia and lost all her hair from chemotherapy treatments. Her story was featured at the local university basketball games, and she became good friends with the players there, who saw her as an inspiration to keep on fighting when the chips were down. Grace passed away from her disease before that basketball season concluded.

I found a hair donation company called Wigs for Kids. They were completely free for the children and served local families. I was able to make three donations of hair and cash in memoriam of Grace. Today, at least 3 lucky kids are running around with wigs made from firefighter hero hair! It's a wonderful cause and I challenge everyone to find a charity that speaks to your heart and get behind it. Every little thing you do can make a big impact in someone's life. It changes your perspective on things for the better.

When the time came for me to make rank for the second time, Willy P once again called from Ops. He said it was the first time he'd ever had to ask a person twice if they wanted to be removed from the medic rotation, that he was pretty sure what my answer would be, but he had to ask anyway. I answered in the affirmative again, with only slightly less enthusiasm, this time having spent close to fourteen years of my life on the bone box staffing list. It was September 17, 2012, nearly fifteen months after I'd been demoted by Chief Thompson's budget cuts, and I never rode a single shift on it again after that day.

For the next six years, I spent every second I was on duty riding dirty on a ladder truck. It was the most peaceful my life had ever been at the fire department. I loved *everything* about my profession. My colleagues knew they could count on me to get things done right.

Chapter 24

Mayday, Mayday, Mayday

The first ever mayday call at our department was Mary Rosenthal. Back in 2003, she was the black shift lieutenant on Engine 8, Tyrone Blake was the engineer, and Wes Freeman was the firefighter. It was a warm sunny afternoon around 13:00 hours. A full alarm came in for a house fire, just a few blocks away from Station 8. The engine and ladder truck arrived simultaneously at the two-story home, with smoke showing from the Alpha and Charlie sides.

Residents out front reported a basement fire and Wes pulled the 1 ¾"pre-connected crosslay. He stretched it to the front door, while Captain Ted Nester and Engineer Rob Osborn on Truck 8 went around back to the Charlie side and attempted to locate the basement stairway, just inside the back door. Lieutenant Rosenthal met Firefighter Freeman at the front door, and they advanced the hose line through the doorway and into the living room.

Wes recalls as he pulled the heavy hose through the living room and into the kitchen, Captain Nester was screaming at Mary about getting the hose line to the basement. From there it was a sharp left to the backdoor landing, and another left turn to descend the basement stairs. The fire crackled and popped as it free burned below them. Wes confirmed Mary was with him, and together they made their way down the stairs and into the chimney above the fire.

The stairway on basement fires is basically a chimney. Fire burns up and outward and the only place for the heat and smoke to go, is right up the stairway. We have to sit as low to the steps as we can and slide down the stairs to avoid being burned. Wes recalls that it was hot; like melt his ears through his Nomex hood hot.

At the bottom of the steps, with a fully involved basement room in front of them, Wes penciled the ceiling with his straight stream nozzle to darken the fire down, without disturbing the thermal layering. That means he quickly opened and closed the bale of the nozzle several times to cool the ceiling down. If we flowed too much water and air into the superheated gases at the ceiling level, we risked mixing the cool air at the floor with the hot air up high and it can make conditions down low at the floor unbearable.

Every time Wes put out an area of fire, it flared up again as soon as he moved to put another area out. He was confused and wondered why it kept reigniting. Maybe a partition, or some sort of room divider was keeping him from hitting the seat of the fire he thought. Just then, Mary's vibralert on her Scott Pak started going off. Her air supply was running low, and she needed to exit the structure for a tank change.

Wes checked the air level in his tank and found he still had half a bottle left. He estimates they'd only been in the fire for about ten minutes before Mary's tank alarmed. He thought about telling her to go get a fresh bottle and he'd just stay there and keep fighting. We had a two-in two-out rule at the time and he knew they both needed to leave together. Reluctantly, they agreed to leave the basement and Wes coiled the hose line and the nozzle back up the stairs and set it down on the landing. Wes worried about the next in crews coming in and taking his nozzle while he was outside getting a fresh tank.

Mary led the way, and they followed the hose line through the kitchen and crossed the living room, toward the front door. Wes turned to look for the Truck 8 crew. They were nowhere to be found. They'd continued on to the second floor upstairs to complete a search of the residence for any trapped victims.

Turning back around, Wes could see daylight through the open door ahead of him, but there was no Mary. He assumed she'd already made it out through the front door and was heading for a new tank, so he followed suit. Right before exiting the structure, he recalls tripping over something on the floor. He continued out to the front porch. Then he heard the screaming.

Wes is very clear it wasn't a "Hey, asshole—over here" type of scream. It was more like the screaming one hears when a person is being tortured to death or burned alive; the pure panic kind of howl and wail that is unmistakably human suffering. He stopped on the porch and turned around. There was no one there. He tried to listen to determine where it was coming from. He wiped away the fog and steam that coated his Scott mask. Peering back inside through the front door and the heavy black smoke rolling out of it, he could just barely make out Mary's head and arms sticking out from the floor of the living room. She'd fallen through the floor.

He rushed back inside to help her, grabbing her arms, and attempting to pull her from the hole. When that failed, he circled around behind her and put his arms beneath her armpits, trying to lift her up. Fire was blowing through the gaps around Mary. As the bottom half of her turnout coat slipped up through the hole, her screams became worse. Wes grabbed hold of the suspenders of her bunker pants to lift her out, but it was to no avail. Her bunker gear was stuck—snagged on the jagged wooden edges of the hole in the floor. She was stuck fast in the inferno as it roasted her flesh.

Out at the curb, Engineer Tyrone Blake was watching curiously. Trying to figure out why Wes was bent over in the doorway for so long, and where the tortuous screaming was coming from. When he realized something wasn't right—that there was a mayday situation—he jumped up into the seat of his fire engine and laid on the air horn to alert the other crews. Pete Howard and Matt Samuels from Truck 1, and Curtis Stanton and Ignacio Cabrera on Engine 3, along with Engineers Cynthia Frankovich and Greg Vincent, all rushed in to assist Wes and Mary.

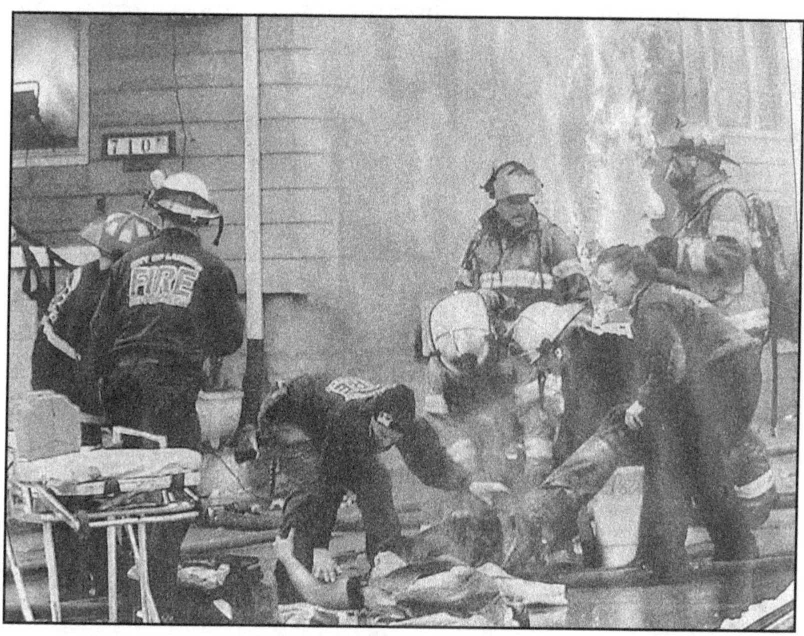

Mayday fire scene

With reinforcements helping now, Mary was finally removed from the hole in the living room floor and carried out to the driveway. The rescuers were exhausted, having spent every ounce of energy to extract her from her hell hole. Engineers and medics rushed in to assist them. Mary was still smoldering and too hot to touch. People burned themselves on the metal D-ring clips as they removed her turnout gear. Someone grabbed a water cooler from the front bumper of an engine company and dumped it over Mary to cool her down.

C-Rob and Dave Austin were on the medic and as they rushed in to help, C-Rob froze up in a panic. Her fragile psyche was unprepared to handle the sight of her colleague in tremendous pain and suffering. Her mind seized up and wouldn't allow her to proceed. Dave took over as an EMT and coordinated the rescue from there. He wheeled the cot up the drive, next to Mary, and began patient care.

At that point, BC Rob Thompson made the call to regroup and go defensive. Upstairs in the house, Osborn and Nester heard the three long air horn blasts go off and recognized them as the evacuation signal. As they tried to make their way to the stairs, they became entangled in the cordage from the window blinds, became disoriented, and were unable to proceed back down the stairs. Osborn began to panic in the intense heat and zero visibility, and against the advice of his officer, called a mayday for his own crew. Now there were two maydays on the same scene.

Out in the driveway, Dave Austin leaned over to Safety Officer Jeff Barber and suggested he should get another medic unit coming.

"Why?" Jeff asked.

"Because we have to transport Mary, and you just had another mayday called," Dave explained.

"No, you have the mayday," Jeff replied.

"Truck 8 just called another one from inside, on the second floor," the new kid advised the seasoned veteran. They threw Mary onto the cot and whisked her down the driveway to the street.

Engineer Andy Gibson was checking out Wes Freeman on the front bumper of the Engine 1 at the end of the driveway, and Dave recalls Wes appeared shellshocked and had the thousand-yard stare.

"C'mon, you're coming, too," Dave said as he grabbed Wes and together with C-Rob, they wheeled Mary on the cot down the street to the ambulance. As Wes and Dave loaded Mary into the back, a police officer asked them where they were headed.

"Saint Joe's," Dave advised.

Unbeknownst to him, the police sergeant scrambled his troops to close the streets down and block the intersections for the pair of injured firefighters.

Mary's skin was blistered and sloughing off, from the top of her neck down to her calves. She was in massive amounts of pain. C-Rob was sitting on the bench seat still frozen in shock. Unable to move, she was seized by panic and the gravity of the situation. Mary told her she needed to start an IV and administer morphine. Theresa had forgotten the meaning of words at this point. Dave applied a tourniquet to Mary's arm and placed an alcohol prep and an IV catheter in Christina's hand.

"C'mon, C-Rob, you can do it," Mary encouraged. "I need you to focus."

Dave could see where this was going and figured he was only about a minute out from the hospital. He said he was hopping up front to drive, and Wes acknowledged. Dave jumped in the cab and put the pedal to the metal. To his surprise, the police were blocking every intersection for him. As he'd pass through, they'd race by him at high speeds and close the next one down as he approached, so he never even had to touch the brakes.

He described it as feeling like a football player rushing down the field, with blockers in front picking up defenders and clearing the way to the end-zone. He says it was the one time he felt like he was winning that day. While en route, Wes cracked the drug box and assisted with drawing up and pushing morphine into the IV that C-Rob finally managed to start.

Back at the scene, Truck 8 was able to self-extricate from their predicament. Rob Osborn was getting ear fucked by his captain, Ted Nester, for having called the second mayday. Apparently, Ted was more concerned about what his colleagues would think about his moxy, than the fact that Rob had done exactly what he was trained to do.

The fire had continued to rage unchecked since Wes and Mary had gone out for a fresh bottle, and the hose line they'd left at the top of the stairs was burned through and twisting around wildly in the basement—the nozzle having been severed from its hose line by the flames. As it was shut down, another line was advanced and eventually the remaining fire crews worked to extinguish the burning house.

Wes was examined in the ER for his burn injuries and Mary caught an immediate helicopter med flight to the burn unit at a world-renowned medical center. The fire chiefs all stopped by the ER to check in on Wes, and he was cleared to return to duty a few hours later. BC Thompson ending up sending him home for the shift and getting a callback firefighter for him. He'd helped save his partner and was a true hero.

In the aftermath of the fire, it was determined that the homeowner had been running a small engine repair shop in the basement of the house. Burning gasoline and oil had been the reason the fire kept flaring up after being extinguished initially. The accelerants had served to increase the intensity and rate of the fire's advancement through the structure.

In a PIA (post incident analysis) the following shift, Mary was still in the burn unit and Wes was off duty and not even invited. The officers began talking about their roles and experiences at the event. Being first due, Captain Nester from Truck 8 explained his perspective and then chastised his crew mate, Rob Osborn, right in front of everyone, for calling a mayday when it was completely unnecessary. Rob then explained how Ted was literally punching a wall with his fists trying to escape from the heat and smoke upstairs and they were both tangled in cordage from the window blinds.

An argument ensued between the two of them and the entire event became awkward and unproductive. The remaining crews chose to say very little in hopes of just ending it faster and leaving. C-Rob admitted the sights and emotions of the day had impacted her very deeply. She claimed credit for having saved Mary's life in front of a confused Dave Austin, who recalled having done most of the actions himself, and then watched in disbelief as C-Rob attributed them to herself. No one else had been in the sled except Wes and Mary and neither of them were even there. C-Rob had more seniority than Dave did, and it was her word against his, so he decided to keep his mouth shut about it. The PIA ended and everybody went their separate ways.

Wes was very concerned that while in the ambulance with Mary, she was questioning why he'd left her in the floor. He explained he never left her side, but she was adamant he had. He theorized that after she saw him exit the front door, the pain had become so intense that she lost all concept of the events that immediately followed. Wes said after he was sent home later that day, no one ever called to check in or ask how he was doing. Not one person. Ever.

Several months later, another firefighter fell off a roof and fractured his spine at a structure fire. The rescuers on that call were invited to city hall and received Life Safety Awards from the mayor for their efforts. Wes recalls he never even got an "atta boy" from his station captain.

When asked if the darker complexion of his skin was potentially the determining factor in that regard, he acknowledged. He revealed that at the Black Firefighter's Conference later that year, he was called up on stage by the significantly lighter skin colored Indianapolis Fire Chief and awarded a plaque for his heroic actions on the fireground that day. Whiskey-Tango-Foxtrot over. No one from his own department even called to check on his well-being, but a fire chief from another department hundreds of miles away recognized his heroism nearly a year later.

Mary spent months in the hospital recovering from her injuries. Burns are some of the most painful wounds humans can suffer. After dozens of skin grafts and gallons of morphine, she received a line-of-duty disability. She didn't want it. Real heroes never do. She tried to transfer divisions into Training or Maintenance, but our Fire Administration denied it. She felt she could still do the job. Our contract stated we had to be medically cleared to return to our previous Suppression division before being allowed to transfer to another. She reluctantly accepted her only option: a line-of-duty disability pension. Then she was shuffled out the door. Tossed away onto the casualty pile.

The Chicago Street house fire in 2013 was *my* first mayday activation on the RIT team. Justin Stevens, the nozzleman on Engine 4, had fallen through the floor into the basement as his crew made entry through the front door. As we pulled up on Truck 4 and hauled the RIT equipment to the staging area in front of the house, Engine 4 called their mayday.

"Mayday, mayday, mayday, Engine 4 has mayday," Captain Jason Hundt advised.

Duncan had just handed our crew's passport tags to the BC parked in the driveway.

I howled with excitement and tossed the rope bag I was carrying onto the front porch. "Time to go to work boys," I exclaimed, removing my helmet, and donning my Scott mask. So many times, as the second-in ladder company, I'd sat outside on the front lawn with a pile of rescue gear watching everyone else fight a fire, waiting for a call to action. Not today.

Straight out of the gate we had an opportunity to shine. RIT activations were rare at our department, but when we needed them, we needed them fresh and ready for immediate deployment. So as a protocol, we always had the second-due ladder company standby as the RIT at structure fires.

I was ready in seconds and stepped through the doorway of the house to survey the situation. Duncan and Hopewell were still screwing around outside with their masks and gloves while

Justin was most likely in an unconscious heap inside a basement inferno. His crew crowded around the hole he'd fallen through, as plumes of heavy smoke rose above their heads. They were yelling his name into the chugging clouds of darkness.

Mike Rhodes from Truck 1 grabbed me and said, "C'mon, we gotta find the basement stairs."

I looked back at Duncan, and he was still dicking around on the front steps. "I'm going in with Truck 1," I hollered. He seemed unable to hear me. *Fuck it,* I thought. I'm not going to let my colleague burn to death because my officer forgot we were on the *"RAPID"* intervention team.

Mike and I headed down the hallway into the kitchen and found the basement stairs behind a door.

Mike radioed the BC that we'd found them and were proceeding downstairs. Apparently, he'd left his crew as well, because it was just the two of us descending into the smoke. I went first, calling for Justin. There was zero visibility. At the bottom, I followed the wall yelling his name repeatedly as I searched the room. I found the hole he'd fallen through, but there was no Justin beneath it. I continued searching and calling for Justin.

Just then, the evacuation tones went off over the radio and I realized I was alone in the basement. Mike had remained at the top of the stairs as I descended into the billowing blackness. Justin, meanwhile, had managed to be rescued from the hole by someone shoving an attic ladder down into it. It was just me now—alone in the basement. I searched for the stairs that I'd just descended, but they'd vanished. My arms swung through empty smoke as I felt blindly ahead of me.

The battalion chief called for a PAR (personnel accountability report), to make sure everyone was out. Maydays beget maydays, as the saying goes. They started with the crews in numerical order and when they got to Truck 4, Duncan keyed his mic and said he had a PAR—even though I was still in the burning basement. What the *actual* fuck? I thought about calling a mayday myself just to let everyone know he was a liar. How could he do that? Doesn't he know I'm not there?

Stay calm. Deep breath. If it's to be, it's up to me. It was a small house. I could eventually find the stairs and make my way out. I had plenty of air left. Remain calm. I decided to climb up the same attic ladder Jason had. I made my way up, and then out the front door. Stepping outside, I noticed the sun had broken over the horizon and its light once again filled our world.

Duncan came running up to me as I crossed the front yard, yelling and cursing as he scowled, "Don't you ever do that to me again. I had no idea where you were!"

"I was in the basement trying to save Justin," was all I said. I grabbed a bottle change and a drink of water as the medics checked Justin out in the sled. He was fine. Everyone was fine. As the other crews extinguished the hot spots, we were cleared by the BC, packed our gear, and headed home. It was shift change and I was ready for a shower and some rest. Lessons were learned that day.

Chapter 25

A Litany for Survival

There was an evening when we boated down the neighborhood streets of our city. Those who were there called it the Great Flood of 2011. It was July 27, the skies hadn't rained in over two weeks, and the earth was bone dry. A massive line of thunderstorms was approaching and when it hit our city, it dumped four inches of rain over the next two hours. Our first indication there was a problem, was at 17:00 hours when Krishna and Showtime on Medic 6 radioed in that manhole covers were being blown off along Holmes Road, as they cleared from the south side hospital and returned to their station.

Dispatch asked Medic 9 as they cleared the same hospital minutes later, to swing by a certain intersection on their way home and check for multiple reports of manhole covers being blown off by large waterspouts. When they arrived, they confirmed geysers were spouting out of the manholes and shooting ten feet into the air, all the way down the road for a half mile or so.

When Engine 9 caught a medical alarm on Willow Avenue and requested the boat from Nines to respond, the dispatcher asked to confirm the lieutenant had, in fact, wanted a boat for a run on what normally was dry ground.

Wendy Simpson keyed her radio and confirmed, "Yeah, you know—a boat. With a motor, and oars. So we can get to the patient's house."

The runoff from the storm had filled an entire neighborhood to its doorsteps from a flash flood. We were dispatched to begin evacuations of an entire section of town. We pulled people from their porches in boats and cruised down city streets at five knots. Everything was converted over to nautical speak, with terms like aft and stern, hard to starboard, and thar she blows!

We ran all evening and all night, pulling seventeen calls over the next ten hours on Engine 4. From medicals, to rescues, to natural gas leaks in flooded basements, the whole city was hopping. We worked our asses off that night, and as the sun rose, the waters receded. It was almost magical in a supernatural kind of way.

In the aftermath, it was determined by experts that the parched ground couldn't absorb the water as fast as it came down from the sky, and it quickly overwhelmed the storm water collection systems. The entire city basically drained into this one area of town that wasn't even a flood zone before the weather event. Many of the homes in that area, upon inspection, had to be condemned and demolished because of sewage overflow and severe water damage.

We'd make lots of runs to the local Motel 6 or Governor's Inn. Shady joints in Fours first due that charged by the hour. Usually, it was a hooker, or a stripper, or their John, who OD'd on heroin in the shower, or on the bed, or over in a corner face down in the motel carpet.

Around 03:00 hours, Duncan, Fergie, and I, on 4 Engine, made a run to the Motel 6. Not one, but *two* strippers were overdosed on heroin at the same time, in the freezing cold shower, where the John they were with had put them hoping to sober them up. They were butt-naked and unconscious on top of each other in a twisted heap of limp bodies.

I turned off the ice-cold water and dragged the first girl out of the tub. She was purplish-blue and not moving as I carried her to the bed. Fergie covered her up with a blanket and assessed her vitals. I went back to the tub, wrapped the second girl in bath towels, and carried her over to the bed as well.

The ambulance crew arrived and drew up Narcan for both patients. As they awoke from their hypoxic slumbers and now had to fight hypothermia as well, we assisted the nice stripper ladies down the hallways and stairs to the medic unit. The whole time I kept thinking how these kids were damn near my daughter's ages, wondering how life can get so off track they think this is their best option.

Kevin Norwood and I were on 4 Engine one afternoon when we caught a run to the local grocery store for an unconscious man in the bathroom. We'd made dozens of these calls. If any heroin users are reading this, please explain to me the reasoning for going into a public place and shooting up. I just don't get it. What? Scored in the parking lot and can't wait? So shoot up in the car, or go in the public bathroom? C'mon, man.

Listen to me. This is why you shouldn't do it, among the other obvious reasons; like it could *kill* you. Kevin and I walked into the men's restroom to find a man with his pants around his ankles, face down on the filthy bathroom floor. A young boy using the urinal beside him flushed, walked to the sink, and then stepped over his body to exit the bathroom. I rolled him over to check for a pulse and—*OH MY GOD*—his penis was inverted.

Kevin, a devout Jehovah's Witness let slip an extremely rare cuss word with a "What the *fuck* is that?"

The grocery staff standing by at the bathroom entrance consisted of three females who all began giggling at the drug addict's missing member. It was explained to me later that one of the side effects of extended heroin use was penis inversion. Now, for that reason alone, I can get behind not ever even considering using the drug that had claimed the lives of more people—some of them my good friends—than I could even count.

After the inverted penis shock had worn off, we checked for a pulse. He had one. We checked for breathing. He was, albeit shallow and repressed. We located the empty syringe and tourniquet resting on the toilet paper dispenser in the stall where he was in the process of pooping and shooting up simultaneously. Never a smart or sanitary combination in my own professional and personal opinion.

The ambulance crew rounded the corner and entered the men's room with a loud, "*Holy shit*, what the *fuck* is that?"

The grocery store manager informed them, very matter-of-factly, "It's an inverted penis."

We pushed Narcan IM, and the man had his heroin buzz cut short as the meds canceled out his street-drug bad trip. They rolled off to the hospital with a police officer in tow, almost surely to interrogate with a line of questioning that would expose the supply chain.

Doris Court was a stumper. One of the streets we'd hit new kids with during street school. There were only four houses addressed off Doris, so the odds they'd ever even heard of it were slim to none. The awkward silence that followed after that particular street was quizzed was a beautiful sound to the old-timers who'd spent thousands of hours studying their map books and contemplating various chores and punishments they could dole out to the new kids and rovers who had no clue where it was.

One night we caught a car fire on our favorite little stumper street. Duncan, Fergie, a new kid named Morris, and I rolled out of bed around 02:00 hours and lumbered over to Engine 4. This is what was so great about firefighting: we had absolutely no idea what we were about to roll up on or get ourselves wrapped up into when the alarms hit. Complete chaos awaited us, and we had no clue as we rubbed the sleep from our eyes and cruised down the dark empty streets.

I always liked to ask Fergie if he was good on a street when we rolled out onto the apron of the fire station. One cannot underestimate the value of a firefighter with a map book, giving turn by turn directions while we're trying to make it to our first-in fire address. Or better yet, attempting to beat another station into their first due area and stealing their fire. All the glory is on the nozzle. And only the first-in crew on single alarm fires is stretching a line and putting the wet on the red. Glory hounds. That's what we were.

The run on Doris simply came in as a car fire, so Engine 4 alone was responding. When we arrived, we found a car that had continued on, past the dead end of the road, sliced between two homes, then crashed into the backyard fence separating the two properties, with flames blowing from its engine compartment.

Duncan told the new kid to pull the 1¾"pre-connect up the driveway, around the back of the house on the left, through the backyard, and over to the car. Morris stretched the line and Fergie charged it. Meanwhile, I walked up to the vehicle to do my inner circle and check for patients. The car was empty, but it had knocked the gas meter off the house on the left and natural gas was roaring from the severed pipe, fifteen feet away from the car that was on fire.

The driver must've been drunk and took off on foot, I thought, as I put the car in park and removed the keys from the ignition. Duncan came around the house with the new kid dragging the hose line. I told him about the gas leak and that there were no patients in the car. He called Dispatch and requested a full alarm response while I attempted to pull the hood latch on the car. The release cable was burned through by the fire, and nothing happened. With a Halligan tool, I pierced the hood with its spike, pried up a corner, and told the new kid to shove the nozzle inside and open the bale. The gas leak roared ominously behind us.

The car fire darkened down. It wasn't out yet though and there was still more that needed to be done. I kicked down a broken wooden fence panel to access the other side of the car. Then I sunk the Halligan's spike deep into the hood's sheet metal, prying another corner up. Giving the new kid a purchase point on the opposite side of the motor to attack the fire from.

As Morris sprayed the fire in the engine compartment out, the front tire next to him exploded in a shower of sparks and flaming rubber and the new kid shit his bunker pants. That always gets the rookies good when they blow. With experience, one learned to recognize a slight whistle right before they went. I'd heard it a split second before this one popped.

One of the sparks ignited the gas line and the shadows of night burned from existence as the hissing pipe burst into a fireball of light. It was a blowout sale on explosions that morning and we'd just found ourselves with a two for the price of one deal. Everyone loves a BOGO!

The new kid dropped the nozzle and ran for cover. I shook my head and laughed, picked up his hose line, and knelt behind the corner of the car. Setting the nozzle to a fog pattern, I began to cool the gas fed fire that was burning up the side of the house now. I'm pretty sure Duncan shit his drawers too because he ran up to me and said we needed to fall back.

I hated those words. Falling back. Going defensive. It was all the same to me. It meant acknowledging we'd been defeated.

I thought about the explosions, the homeowner standing at the curb watching us, the incoming rigs that would take my glory on the nozzle and label us pusillanimous.

I looked back at Duncan and told him, "No fucking way. Not on my watch."

He said fine, that they'd be over by the engine if I needed them. Then he left with the new kid in tow.

Fucking short-timers. Something happens to certain individuals when they reach six months to retirement. They get scared as hell to take any kind of risks on the fireground. I've seen it happen plenty of times. Captains holding back on first-in tasks and letting second due companies do their jobs. They're purposely slow getting to the rigs on full alarms, so they get beat into their first due areas. They ignore the dispatchers calling for them, until another crew member acknowledges them, and then it's like "Oh, what?" Like they didn't know. They hang back at scenes and let the more aggressive officers take on the riskier assignments.

And who can blame them? I get it. They bust their ass through a twenty-plus-year career and they're at the finish line. They don't want to do anything that might screw it all up for them. I understand the logic. It's just not for me though. I want to be the guy on the nozzle, the one making the rescue. That's what I lived for, and it hurt like hell to watch someone else doing my job. I've spent a lot of time with short-time bosses, in rehab and staging areas, waiting for an assignment. Then seeing the relief wash over their faces when the battalion chief clears our rig from the scene after having done nothing. Going home in the morning is their only goal, and I can respect that. For them, but not for me.

I'm not saying Duncan was like them, not saying he wasn't either, but I wasn't falling back on this one, period. For those who haven't sat on a natural gas fed fire with a fog line before, the object is to cool everything down without putting the fire completely out. If it goes out, then we're pumping highly explosive gas into the house and the surrounding air. And with a recent ignition source still smoldering nearby, that could mean another explosion. So, I sat there, flowing water through my fog nozzle onto a fireball, as other rigs arrived and assessed the situation, with no one able to really do anything until the gas company arrived and shut off the main supply pipe at the street. I take that back. Wes Freeman came over and stood next to me for a while, just to keep me company. Everybody else stayed out at the road.

Then the fire lit up on the inside of the house, as dispatch announced the gas company had an ETA (estimated time of arrival) of one hour.

"That's not good enough, see if they can speed it up," the BC replied.

I could see the pictures on the opposite wall, through the window directly above the gas meter. The fire danced in the reflective glass of their frames, and I thought about what I would do if this was my home. What *wouldn't* I do to save all I'd worked so hard for?

Retreat was not an option. I knew Duncan wouldn't write me up for insubordination. Not after the mayday incident when he'd called a PAR from outside on the lawn, while I was still inside the fire, alone, and searching for the mayday firefighter. As I pondered the possible outcomes of the situation, the fire began to make a strange whistling, almost otherworldly, sucking sound and then with a loud *POP*, it went out. The blowtorch-like hissing was replaced by the wind-tunnel roar of the gas escaping the pressurized pipe once again. This was definitely trending toward worst-case scenario outcomes.

The great thing about fog nozzles is that we can actually ventilate with them. They draw in massive amounts of air with their rotational spray patterns, creating a vortex that pulls from behind and pushes both air and water forward. Sometimes as a prank at fires, we'd wait for the battalion chief to be doing a walk around and spray the fog nozzle out the window at them, feigning to ventilate the smoke from a room, just as they were walking past the window or door. We had to keep the short-timers on their toes.

I moved from my position by the car, over to the back corner of the house, and then to within a few feet of the broken gas line, directing the fog pattern, and the venting gas, away from the house and toward the front yard. So the fog stream was almost right over top of the roaring gas line. That did the trick. It worked like a charm until the gas company arrived and used a metal detector to scan for the shutoff valve buried in the front yard. Once they turned off the natural gas supply line, the emergency was over.

Afterward, while we were draining and rolling up our hose in the street, I was approached by the homeowner. He said he'd seen everything that happened and wanted to personally thank me for not giving up on his home.

"If it wasn't for you, I would've lost everything," he said as he shook my hand.

"That's what we here for sir," I replied.

"No, that's what *you're* here for. There wasn't anyone else on my street tonight that did what you did. I heard your boss tell you to leave and you tell him no. Thank you."

"You're welcome," I said. He was right.

We packed the supply hose into the bed of the engine and returned to the station. Duncan never said a word about it, and all was right with the world. My world at least.

There was a nice old lady who lived on Eastlawn Drive in Station 4's first due. She had ALS and as her condition deteriorated, we were often called to her place for a citizen's assist. If anyone ever falls down and needs help up, the fire department can come by and help pick them up. We'd usually see her a couple of times a week. Antoinette was a professional comedian, who'd usually be in various stages of undress, sometimes naked, and would either have fallen or been unable to make the transfer from her wheelchair to the bed.

She'd hit us with jokes like "What do you guys call a whale on the beach?"

We'd play along with an "I don't know, what?"

She'd reply with, "Tony, nice to meet you," and she'd hold out her hand as an introduction.

My personal favorite was when she said, "What do you call a cow with no legs? Ground beef... or Tony, either one works for me!" She always had sunny outlook on her condition, even though everyone knew it'd eventually become terminal. I guess we're all eventually terminal.

It was a warm summer evening when we were called out on Engine 4 for a man with chest pain. Acting Captain Smoothbore and I took the blue bag up to the third-floor apartment and established patient care, while Engineer Dave Owens stayed outside with the truck. When the ambulance arrived, he helped them bring their equipment up and then returned to his post.

Minutes later, Dave reappeared in the doorway and motioned for us to step out into the hallway and talk. He explained how some "crazy bitch" had locked herself in the fire truck and wouldn't come out.

"You're full of it," I said.

"Naw, man, come see for yourself," he offered.

We asked the medics if they were good, and they waved us off. We headed downstairs to investigate.

Sure as shit, there was a crazy lady locked in the fire engine. She was sitting in my seat and wearing my helmet. A police officer had shown up and asked if we needed anything.

"Hell yeah, some crazy bitch is in my fire truck!" Dave yelled.

The officer got out and approached the engine. "Yep, I'd say that's a fair assessment of the situation," the smiling cop said.

The ambulance crew came out, loaded their patient into the meat wagon and left. We all tried repeatedly to get the woman to open the door, but she refused. She said she'd always wondered what it was like to be a firefighter, now she was finally finding out, and nobody was going to ruin it for her. Smoothbore and the cop just laughed their asses off and poor Dave was distraught.

"You know, sitting in a fire truck is great… but you know what's better?" I yelled through the glass. The crazy lady stopped sniffing Dave's turnout coat and looked over at me. "Visiting the fire station. If you open the door, Dave here will give you a personal tour of it," I said, figuring it was worth a try.

She looked at Dave and said, "You'd do that for me?"

"Just open the damn door," he replied.

"OK," she said, leaning over and opening the firefighter's door.

We helped her down the truck steps and onto the ground. "You know what's even better than the fire station?" the police officer asked. "The backseat of a police cruiser. Let's go," he said as he grabbed the lady and stuffed her into his cruiser.

Dave breathed a sigh relief, and we headed home.

Dave Owens and Zach Powell were both from the same hometown, and I swear they taught shit-talking to the kids there as a primary subject in public school. These two would go at it for hours on end just ripping each other apart, yet they were the best of friends. If a game of dominoes was popping off at the table after dinner, we'd have to cover Banks's ears.

After a while, Banks began picking up on the fine art of talking shit and we'd join their banter as they slammed bones on the table and yelled, "Domino motherfucker!" Banks and I'd been honing our favorite *yo momma* jokes on each other at home, and when he asked Dave and Zach if they knew any good ones, it was on like Donkey Kong.

"Yo momma so ugly they had to tie a pork chop around her neck just to get the dog to play with her," Dave began. A timeless classic.

"Yo momma so fat she stepped on the scale, and it said 'to be continued,'" Zach replied.

"Yo momma so ugly she made a happy meal cry," Banks joined in.

"Yo momma so fat, her car got stretch marks," I added. It was round two and we were all belly laughing now.

"Yo momma so ugly she threw a boomerang, and it refused to come back," Dave razzed.

"Yo momma so fat, she's got her own gravitational pull," Zach retorted.

"Yo momma so fat her waist size is equator," Banks quipped.

"Yo momma so old she was a waitress at the Last Supper," I said, ending round two.

Lee was crying from laughing so hard and begging us to stop.

"Yo momma so fat, her blood type is Ragu," Dave zinged.

"Yo momma so ugly, her birth certificate is an apology letter," Zach declared.

"Yo momma so hairy, when she pushed you out, you got rug burns," Banks slammed his hand on the table, and everyone laughed so hard they cried.

"Last one, last one," I yelled. "Yo momma so short, you can see her feet on her driver's license picture." The whole crew fell out laughing, except Zach, who was five feet six and refused to laugh at short jokes as a matter of principle.

Dave lost his keys at the firehouse one day while I was on the phone with Lee. She had this thing she'd do, where she'd ask Saint Anthony, the patron saint of lost items, and then he'd tell her, or show her, where the item was.

"They're on his desk in his dorm room," she told me to tell Dave. I relayed the message to a frustrated Dave.

"I've already looked there three times," Dave said.

"They're on his desk, under some papers," she said again.

Dave came back outside a minute later swinging his keys. "How the heck did she do that?" he asked.

"Magic!" I answered him. "Nah I'm just kidding. I don't know man; she's got the gift of sight, bro."

Dave was confused. "Yo, is she a witch? I'm scared, bro. How'd she know that shit?"

"You're a dork, just be thankful she helped you find your keys." And he was.

On March 26, 2012, Chad Carter hung himself. He was inseparable from his best friend Seaboy. They partied everywhere together. These two could get us cocaine or ass anytime we wanted it.

Chad had a penchant for over-the-top antics and when he bought a bright yellow Chevy Camaro and whitened his teeth (that another firefighter had recently knocked out at the Christmas party) to extra bright white, the fakeness just oozed from him.

No amount of toys, drugs, or women could cover up the emptiness Chad felt inside. His father had been murdered in a motel cocaine and hooker deal gone bad when Chad was just a little boy. His personality progressively became more extreme as the years went on. When he started calling his friends and selling all his personal possessions, we started to worry.

It was too late, though. Over the weekend, Seaboy found his best friend swinging from the rafters in his garage and was permanently scarred. Chad's girlfriend was pregnant with his child, and they'd been going through a nasty breakup. Chad dipped out on this life, the burden of fixing and living with his many terrible choices apparently too much for him to carry on. Another funeral, for another firefighter.

On Engine 4 one sunny, summer afternoon, Duncan, Fergie, and I made an explosion at a used car dealership. We were third-in because the other members of my crew drug their feet getting out the door. Upon arrival, we headed up to the garage to investigate. As we entered to search the burning building, I crouched low under the thick black smoke to find my way along. Duncan was right behind me and standing up slightly higher when he slammed his head into something hard, knocking his helmet off.

After making sure he was OK, we examined what exactly it was he'd run into. It was a car elevated on a hoist, and we were directly underneath it. That was typical of the crazy shit we got into in zero visibility conditions. As we moved out from below the car, the first-in crews yelled that they'd found a victim. We headed deeper into the shop and Duncan and I each grabbed one of the man's legs, while 9 Engine's crew lifted him under his arms. We four-pointed the man through the shop and out the door to a waiting medic cot. He was alive and conscious still.

Outside in the sunlight, we could see the man was severely burned. His hair and face were singed, and the skin on his arms and hands was blistering badly. His blue jeans and shirt had large burn holes on them. The medics whisked him away and we made entry back into the garage to finish extinguishing the fire.

It turned out; the man had been using a torch to cut the straps from a gas tank. When they'd been cut through, the tank fell to the floor, spraying gasoline all over the mechanic and his shop, with the torch causing the ignition and explosion. He ended up making a full recovery.

There was a tricky intersection in town where a four-lane boulevard crossed a five-lane main drag street. The lights were timed funky, the signage was poor, and the logistics were awkward for drivers to understand. At around 02:00 hours one morning, it was just one drunk driver who failed to hit his brakes and slammed into the rear of the only other car on the road, stopped at a red light.

We awoke at Fours when the lights popped on over our beds. The dispatcher directed us to a PI accident at the notorious intersection. Duncan, Fergie, and I, dragged our tired asses to the truck and rolled out into the darkness. A few seconds later we arrived at the scene of pure devastation. Besides the two *completely* destroyed cars, however, we were the only other vehicle I'd seen on the way there, the roads were barren and empty.

The driver, who'd been stopped at the red light, was pushed forward through the intersection and his trunk was in his back seat now. Duncan went over to check on him, and I never even got to see that patient, because my guy was pinned in his vehicle and unconscious. He had massive damage to the front of his car and there was hardly anything left of the engine compartment. The front rocker panels were sitting on the pavement, both front wheels had been torqued upward and rearward, and were completely off the ground.

The smell of booze, blood, and antifreeze wafted through the warm night air and kissed me gently on the cheek as if to say, "hello again." The man was buried beneath the dashboard and moaning his last agonal breaths. His doors were stuck shut and I yelled over to Duncan that we had a pin-in. He radioed Dispatch for an extrication response, a second ambulance, and we set to work. I grabbed the Jaws from the cabinet on the rear of the engine. Fergie pulled the pump and hoses from their cabinet and set them down in the hot zone.

I hooked the hoses to the spreaders and cutters, while Fergie started up the hydraulic pump, and Duncan yelled, "Door pop, roof removal, dash roll!"

"Got it!" I hollered back.

Grabbing the spreaders, I stuck the tips in the gap between the door latch and the B pillar. Twisting the handle, the spreaders opened, and I could hear the second stage of the pump engage as it pushed against the increased resistance. The sheet metal began to tear, so I backed off and repositioned the tips for a better bite. They wedged against the frame and then bit hard and fast. The door latch popped away from the Nader pin, exposing its hinges.

I closed the tips of the spreaders and placed them just above the top hinge of the driver's door. Giving the handle a twist, the tips spread open, splitting the door from the A pillar, and ripping the top hinge apart. Closing the tips again, I positioned them just above the lower hinge this time and repeated the process. The door broke free from the car and was only held on by the wiring harness. A quick snip with the cutters and it was free. I swung the door by the top of the window frame, heaving it from the hot zone to the boulevard curb.

Fergie dropped off the rams and the rocker braces for the dash roll.

"I feel like I'm doing everything by myself," I yelled, cutting the pillars on the driver's side.

"That's because you are!" Fergie hollered back.

Duncan returned from helping the medic crew with packaging and loading the other patient, and I passed him the cutters over the car's roof. He went to work on cutting the passenger side pillars, as I swapped the hoses over from the spreaders to the hydraulic ram.

When I stood up, Duncan was finished, and we flipped the roof over the windshield and onto what was left of the front of the car. This was always easier and less messy than cutting through the windshield. Those tiny little glass shavings got everywhere when we fucked around trying to saw it open with the Glass Master or a Sawzall. I positioned the rocker brace on the door sill panel and laid the ram's piston cleat down on top of it.

Twisting the handle, the hydraulic ram extended to meet the dashboard at the curve of the A pillar, right where the fire wall met the roof pillar. We rolled the dice on just one of the big-daddy rams on the driver's side and it worked out fine. The ram bit into the pillar and raised the dash, freeing the trapped patient just as the second medic and next engine crews arrived.

"Sorry boys," I said to the other engine company extrication crews who'd just walked up, "were all done cutting here."

I let the medics and fresh engine crews take care of the patient, who'd severed both legs just above the ankles. That was always a treat when we rolled the dash up to find the lower appendages hanging on by a thread of flesh. Not for the faint of heart. Many a new kid has passed out carrying a dangling foot, as the patient was moved from the car, to the backboard, and then the cot. Usually, the little bugger held fast to its owner, swinging wildly by the connecting sinew as the person carrying it hit the ground and dropped the ball, so to speak.

This guy had some old salty sea dogs who'd been through the fire carrying his feet for him so there were no dangly bits to be found tonight. The man did moan a bit, though, as they rotated him onto the backboard and slid him onto the cot.

"Dude probably didn't even touch the brakes," I said to Fergie. "Look, no skid marks," I added, pointing to the pavement behind the car.

"Probably doing like seventy or so from the damage," he replied.

We stayed on scene for the wreckers and swept the pavement clean of debris, putting our HyDry absorbent on the road and scrubbing it into the oil and antifreeze with our stiff bristled push brooms. It was dark and quiet on the street again. No cars were driving by, and the big city seemed to stop everything and stare at us, under the light of the streetlamps. We were like tiny little helpers in a world full of trauma.

On the highway one night around 02:00 hours, 4 Engine was called for a head-on vehicle collision. The freeway had already been shut down when we arrived, and we made our way across the wide median to the southbound lanes, by means of the emergency access turnaround. We met with state and local police who assured us it was a double fatality accident. They just needed an official time of death.

As I approached the first vehicle, the front of the car was gone, crushed into the firewall, which itself was crushed into the back seat. An arm stuck up from between the engine and trunk, with a purple hand hanging limp-wristed and motionless. The rest of the arm's body was now one with the mangled, smoking wreck.

Just ahead of the first car was the second, in a similar state of wreckage, with only the driver's head visible, rising slightly, from between the engine and the rear seat of the passenger compartment. The four-door sedan had been converted, in an instant, into a two-door coupe. The second driver, it was explained by the police, had entered the off ramp, going the wrong way at a high rate of speed. Several other drivers had successfully dodged the oncoming slaughter and called 9-1-1, while the victim in the first car wasn't so lucky. We stood by the devastation until the medics and wreckers came and then cleared the scene.

On Truck 4 one night, Duncan, Fergie, Hopewell, and I were called on the second alarm to respond to a north end fire. Three houses in a row were on fire, with the center one fully involved and having caught the two on either side of it on fire, by the time the first-in companies had arrived. Our crew was tasked with staffing the RIT team and we watched from the curb as the crews struggled to make headway into the middle house. One by one, they came out to rehab exhausted and frustrated.

They were losing the fire and had gone from offensive to defensive tactics twice by the time we finally got the green light to join the operations. Everyone had evacuated the structures and I climbed up onto the ladder that had been placed at the front of the house and ran a nozzle up to the second story gable window. After locking a leg into the rungs of the ladder, I opened the bale and put out the entire second floor fire, then advanced into the structure, through the window, with Duncan and Hopewell right behind me.

We continued to make headway into the house and opened windows to ventilate as we cleared the rooms of fire. When the entire house was extinguished, we headed to the curb for a bottle change. This shit was easy. I struggled to understand why the other crews had such a difficult time with it. We overhauled the middle house while the other crews extinguished the exposures, and as the sun rose over the battlefield, I was content with my life.

Chapter 26

MMA (Mixed Martial Arts)

At Station 4 one afternoon, Captain Pat Duncan and Engineer Smoothbore, both martial artists, were making fun of me as I practiced for my upcoming Taekwondo exams. They were both Karate black belts at Charlie Peters's school. Pat was saying something like, "Taekwondo, eh? I think I stepped in that once, smelled terrible." Smoothbore giggled and agreed, offering to teach me some *real* moves when I was ready to get serious.

There are subtle differences to each martial discipline. Some of them teach grappling, some emphasize striking, some reveal pressure points, and some disclose ways to incapacitate an opponent immediately. Taekwondo placed a premium on kicks—especially to the head. When Duncan suggested a sparring match on the apparatus floor, I flatly refused, not wanting to be the guy who either beat his captain up, or on the other hand was bested by his captain. It was a no-win situation. And so it was, after being called several derogatory names of emasculating demeanor by my colleagues, that I reluctantly agreed.

Pat did a warmup that reminded me of some Bruce Lee Kung Fu shit. Then he came at me. He stepped in close, and I tapped his left cheek with the toes of my right boot. It was a perfectly placed round kick, with a size twelve to the face and Duncan ate it.

"Oh my God, I'm so sorry. Are you OK?" I asked.

Holding the side of his face, Duncan said something about not expecting that and I continued to apologize, hoping not to get written up for the incident.

In the end, his pride was wounded more than his cheek meat, and no more jokes were made about Taekwondo. On a side note, my all-time personal favorite kick is the spinning heel kick. Almost indefensible, if that puppy lands, it's like tapping the easy button. Your opponent is going night-night and you'll be standing over top of them like the famous photo of Muhammed Ali, standing victorious over an unconscious Sonny Liston.

Charlie Peters was the red shift captain at Twos and a sensei at his local dojo. One day at the breakfast table, John Lohan was talking about how Karate doesn't work in a street fight and Charlie calmly took offense to it.

"Do you think you can hit me?" he asked.

John began to backpedal. "Aww, naw, Cappy. I-I don't want to," he said.

"I'll bet dishes for the day that *you* can't hit *me,*" Charlie offered.

John, who'd just lost at poker and won the dishes, hesitantly agreed.

As they stood and faced each other beside the kitchen table, Captain Peters, his hands down by his side, casually told John to take his best shot. John, his hands raised like a boxer's, fired out a left jab. Charlie caught the punch between both hands, then wrapped his forearm around John's wrist, torqued it backward, and placed John in an uncomfortable arm bar.

In an instant John was on the ground screaming in pain, yelling, "OK, OK, OK!"

"You've got the dishes," Charlie said, as he released him and walked away, sipping his coffee.

Donny Kowalsky was a black shift captain when I hired on. He too, was a master of Taekwondo and was nicknamed "Killer." Killer Kowalsky had, as the story was relayed to me, stopped at a convenience store on his way to the beach one afternoon. Upon exiting the store, he was confronted by four drunk men who surrounded him and demanded his wallet and car keys.

Donny simply said, "Not today." Then he calmly removed his flip-flops, standing barefoot in the parking lot gravel.

"What are you some kind of *Kung Fu* guy?" one of the drunk men asked.

"You see this foot?" Donny replied. "I'm gonna take this foot and put it right there," pointing at the man's head, "and there's not a damn thing you're gonna be able to do about it."

He did. And there wasn't. In a few moments, the attackers were rendered unconscious. Donny asked the store clerk to call the police and an ambulance, then waited for them to arrive. Two of the men ended up in critical condition in ICU and barely survived. Killer was a new kid in the training academy at the time and was placed on probation for the incident. Search up a video of Billy Jack's right foot to see a rendition of exactly what happened that day.

Engineer Felonious talks about a time when an unruly citizen blocked the way of the fire engine he was trying to back up to leave an emergency scene. After a few moments of sitting still, Captain Killer kicked open the officer's door and approached the belligerent man who had delayed his crew in their mission.

"You looking to get your *fuckin'* ass kicked?" Donny bluntly asked the civilian.

Shocked, the man declined the abuse that was offered to him that evening and kindly allowed the engine crew to depart accordingly.

Killer's daughter Karen Kowalsky ended up hiring on at our fire department sometime after me. She was one of the toughest lesbians I've ever met. It was just like talking with the boys when shootin' the shit with her. I knew, without a doubt, she could rescue me from any incident if need be and wouldn't stop until the job was done.

At Fours one day, Stan Clemens decided to bucket Karen as she was returning from ACLS class. Her laptop was in her hands when he let it fly, and when he descended from the roof, he met the full fury of Killer's kid.

"You're gonna buy me a new computer, Clemmy," she calmly stated.

"No way. That's not my problem, it's yours," he retorted.

"Well, it's your problem now because your reckless horseplay has caused me monetary damages in excess of $1,000. So, you're going to replace my damaged property, or we can get the battalion chiefs and my attorneys involved and see whose side *they* take. Especially heinous is the fact that you specifically targeted me because of my gender and sexual orientation."

Clemmy saw where this was going and waved the white flag. He agreed to pay the price for his iniquities, and we all marveled at Karen's ability to take on injustice, kick it in the balls, and walk away victorious.

Chapter 27

Kozmo Kramer

Duncan decided to retire in July 2013 and planned a small gathering at a local restaurant for family and friends to celebrate. In his place, Koz came over from Nines to wrap up his career and study for his master's degree online, hoping to write literature as a second profession after the fire service.

It was good to have an old friend as my new boss and we welcomed him into the crew and family. He wasn't the same guy I'd met on my second shift back in 1998. He was weathered and haggard—a shell of his former self. On the fireground he could still kick it into gear and perform like a soldier. However, in the station, he was angry, defeated, and solitary. Preferring greatly to disappear into his dorm room and pop out occasionally for cigarette breaks and coffee refills.

Koz came over to Fours at the twilight of his career. He was a miserable old bastard at this point who spent most of the shift sleeping in the captain's room, smoking weed (which I supplied since he was a licensed patient of ours) and popping pain pills for the ruptured disks in his back. We saw him when the tones went off and at dinner time and that was about it.

After arriving there, his leadership role in my life resembled that of my absentee father, and within three months he decided to burn off the remainder of his sick time until his retirement eligibility date. The city only gave us credit for one third (eight hours per every twenty-four) of our accrued sick time balance when we retired, and Koz was determined to get his full payout for the days he'd earned by burning through it all. Use it or lose it he'd say.

Koz was tall and lanky, and uncannily resembled the *Seinfeld* sitcom character Cosmo Kramer, played by comedian Michael Richards. His jerky movements and eccentric personality, his upright hairstyle, even the intonation and inflections of his speech were like the TV show personality. Like Kramer, Koz was sometimes caring and kind-hearted, yet could be neurotic and high-strung a short time later. He even decided to become Jewish one day and joined a synagogue. We all encouraged him to go for it and follow his interests.

Out of Fours, the alarm opened up for a house fire on Compton Circle. This was in Station 9's first due with Station 6 as the second-in company. We were third-in, and after 6 Engine blew past the hydrant, the BC from Nines was screaming for a water supply, and we obliged. After wrapping the hydrant and giving the engineer the signal, Natalia pulled away and the five-inch supply hose flipped out of the bed and onto the street. I opened and flushed the pipe, hooked the steamer connection to the fittings, then waited at the hydrant for the word to charge it.

When the other end was connected to the first-in engine's intake, the signal was given, and I opened the crank. Water flowed through the big yellow hose, and I made my way to the scene, kicking the five-inch over to the curb as I went, so the other trucks could get by.

At the scene, Koz was itching to make entry and already had a top-shelf assignment to get our asses in there and end this fire. The BCs knew who the fireground ass kickers were and gave them special assignments that normally wouldn't have been done.

We grabbed our tools and Scotted up at the door. Following

the hose line inside, we found Ginger on her knees in the hallway with her new firefighter doing the same in front of her. It wasn't even hot in there and we were standing up with no hoods on. Koz must've got tired of waiting in the hallway because he kicked Ginger in the Scott tank then stepped on her to get by. As she was getting back up to her knees, I did the same thing. Hey, we've gotta stay with our wingman.

Joining back up with Koz in the bedroom down the hall, we began putting the fire out with our axes. We smashed everything burning, and the fire was reduced to embers and ashes. We opened the windows to vent the smoke, then had the new kid in the hallway with the nozzle spray water on the cinders and we were finished. On our way back down the hall, Koz kicked Ginger, who was still on her knees, right in the chest, knocking her over again. He laughed like a crazed hyena as we exited the structure. Like a *fucking* animal!

"Done!" Koz yelled to the BC, collected our tags, and we cleared the scene.

There was a young man on Hollywood Avenue who decided he was going to commit suicide. He placed two LPG grill tanks in the back seat of his car, opened them in his garage with the car running and the doors closed, and then decided to smoke his last cigarette. The car and the garage exploded with him in it, and a call came in for a full alarm fire response.

It was in station Nine's first due and Engine 9, Truck 9, and Medic 9 all rolled up together. The explosion had blown the garage door out into the street, burnt off all the gas that accumulated from the LPG tanks, and stalled the car out. So, all that was left was a well-ventilated and barely smoldering garage, and a shellshocked man in his driver's seat, still alive and in tremendous pain because his skin was now melting off him.

We pulled up on Engine 4 just in time to see Ginger McEntire walking the man down his driveway to the waiting medic unit, the skin gone from his face and dripping from his bloody hands. We watched in sympathetic shock as the poor guy was loaded into the bone box.

"Damn, why would he choose to go out like that?" I asked.

"Then fuck it all up and live through it, too," Koz added.

The BC snapped us out of our stares and told Koz and me to check on exposures and put out any hot spots we found.

Everything around the exterior of the garage was fine. The building itself was barely standing, and the blast had lifted it off its foundations. After everyone exited the structure, Koz and I gave one of the walls a well-timed kick, in the direction it was leaning, and it toppled right over. At least now it wouldn't fall on any of us. There was still plenty of room for the Fire Marshals to get inside and investigate. We cleared the scene, and I told Koz to remind me never to attempt suicide like that guy did. Now he was even worse off than he was before.

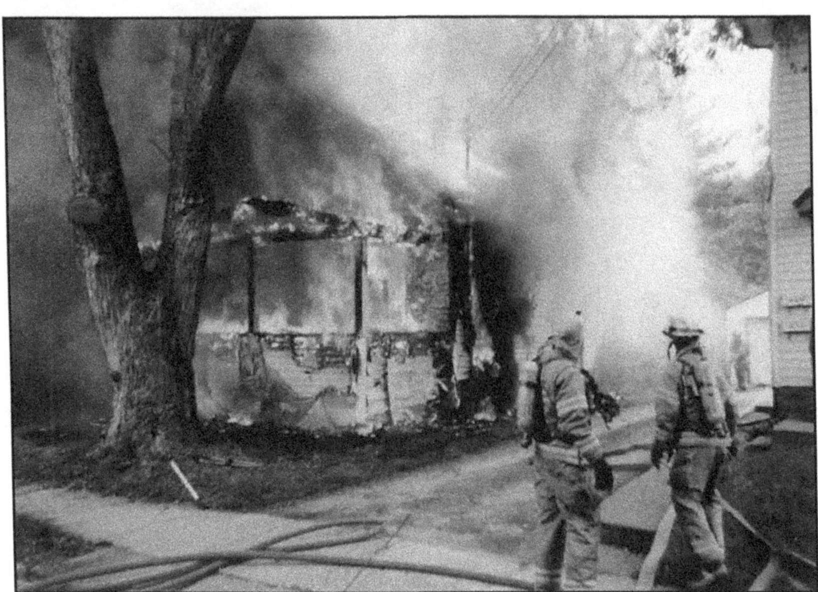

Robert Avenue fire

CHAPTER 28

Cooking is Alchemy

Cooking on duty in the fire station was extremely difficult for me at first. What was this sorcery where a magician took various ingredients and combined them together to create a completely new substance? Why, it's alchemy of course! I'd never been trained in this strange new firefighting discipline.

Every firehouse meal was expected by our superiors to be a two or three course masterpiece. There must be a meat cooked to perfection. A starch like rice or potatoes, done right, not "boney" as the old-timers would refer to it if underdone. A vegetable cooked *al dente* and properly seasoned. A fresh garden salad. A handcrafted beverage like fresh squeezed lemonade, iced tea, or Kool Aid. And a delicious, mouth-watering desert.

This is a difficult task to pull off at home, with help. Now try doing it at work, in between emergency calls, alone, and in a random kitchen where you have no idea where anything is. I was *bad*. Awful even, in the beginning. I was twenty-one years old and my own mother, God bless her, had not yet risen to these culinary standards of excellence.

The old-timers seemed to take a special pride in cook-shaming the young firefighters. They ate the innocent souls of new kids for lunch and had a double helping of probationary pride for dinner. It was both hilarious and heartbreaking. The young cook's fear and lack of confidence seemed to leech directly into their food, as if it was overly seasoned with insecurity and everyone at the table could taste it.

For certain, there were plenty of awkward moments in my first forays into the kitchen. Like when Captain Russ Jackson threw his whole plate of food right in the trash, and then the plate on top of it for emphasis. That was right after JT told me how much Russ loved olives, so I put that shit on everything. Kalamata olive tapenade for the garlic toast, a pasta salad with sliced black olives, and a delicious cheeseburger with sliced green olive sauce. The man absolutely hated olives. Jerome set me up to fuck with Russ, who'd been giving him a hard time lately.

Or there was the time when Dale "Mercury" Morris tied the steaks I'd just cooked to the bottom of his shoes because they were so tough. Then proceeded to wear them around the station for the next couple of hours. Everyone dodged the greasy boot prints and hunks of fallen beef all over the station, and I had to clean up after him. But the beginner was learning. Watching the pros at work and helping them prepare their own culinary masterpieces. I was taking notes and creating my own style. Borrowing from the masters.

There were legends of firehouse cooking in the ranks at my department. People had their signature dishes named after them. Timmy Dall's chicken casserole, Don Pablo's stir fry with egg rolls, Greg Mason's Red-Hot chicken, Spike Young's chicken and dumplings, Koz's bean soup, Damyon's cabbage and bacon, and Leno's fried chicken. They were kitchen gods. Their dishes were sought after, requested even.

The local newspapers and TV channels would come in from time to time and do a write up or a live interview piece on these heroes and their delicious firehouse cuisine. They won awards at chili cook-offs and bar-be-cue festivals. Trophies and blue ribbons hung in the dining halls of the stations they frequented.

On the flip side of this, there were some legendarily awful cooks whose meals went down in fire department history and subsequently got them banned from kitchen duty altogether. Connie's bloody chicken, Mulders 9-hour roast, Nelson's still-kickin' chicken, Krishna's Stoup—not quite stew and not quite soup.

Whether by accident or purpose-driven, these cooks were not allowed by their peers to continue along their culinary paths. Engineers or captains, upon seeing these names on the running chart for the shift, made it priority number one to secure a quality replacement for them in the kitchen that day. Lest they be poisoned or suffer from starvation due to the inadequacies of their lower seniority chefs that day.

Fortunately, I was never demoted from my kitchen duties and was allowed to continue in my culinary endeavors. One of my favorite meals to prepare was roast beef tacos from the leftovers of the Sunday roast. I'd learned most of it from Hector Garcia and Dan Martinez at Station 5, so it was fairly authentic. I was relatively proficient, at least in their eyes, to cook their mother's family recipes from south of the border. I just knew it tasted *really* good and I could whip it up easily for the troops.

I'd slow cook the Sunday roast for at *least* four hours at 350 degrees in a Dutch oven with a little water in the bottom. Use a packet of onion soup mix or some beef bouillon for added flavor. Sprinkle it with garlic, salt, and pepper or some Canadian Steak seasoning, sear it in a skillet, and throw it in the oven. Don't even think about trying to serve it before it's gone for at least four hours, or they'll all be gnawing on it like Clark Griswold with the turkey, in *Christmas Vacation*. I found if I picked the roast up on my way in to work, then got it seasoned, seared, and put in the oven right at shift change, I could serve it right on time.

Add potatoes, carrots, onions, and mushrooms with about an hour and a half to go. Then with fifteen minutes left, drain the water and drippings into a saucepan. Mix up a little corn starch and cold water, bring the saucepan to a boil, add the corn starch slurry while constantly stirring, bring it back to a boil, and make a gravy. A perfect gravy is the glue that binds all firefighters together at the dinner table, and it provides more *flavor*.

Flavor can be elusive for the beginner chef. I recall many new cooks asking the crew if their meal needed anything, and for advice on how it could potentially be improved. The old-timers would say things like, "It could use some flavor," or "Hey, Jim, pass the flavor," or "Hey, new kid, are we all out of flavor, because mine didn't get any on it." Flavor was a strange and fickle thing it seemed. Sometimes too much—sometimes not enough. There was a fine flavor line to be walked, for certain.

Serve that roast with a nice salad and some dinner rolls and voila! The cappy is happy. It was the cook's job to keep the cappy happy and the path to the captain's heart, it seemed, led directly through his stomach. I'd deliberately try to put the old-timers into food comas so they'd pass out in the brown chairs, and we wouldn't have to do their bullshit in-house ropes and knot-tying schools or two-hour street schools. It actually worked most of the time. Finish it off with chocolate chip cookies or a frosted brownie for desert and we've just tipped them over into food coma territory. Lights out.

After lunch, while the rest of the crew is snoring and twitching in the brown chairs, shred the leftover beef and simmer it for another hour in a bit of water and seasonings. Some garlic, cumin, chili powder, salt, and pepper were my go-to spices. Truthfully, we want a mostly salty meat with just a hint of spice. Let the real flavor come from the fresh ingredients.

Make a fresh salsa with diced tomatoes, cilantro, onion, and jalapeno, all finely chopped, then add lemon juice, garlic, salt, and pepper. If they enjoy guacamole, now is a great time to slice the avocados and mash them. Add some fresh salsa or pico to it, a dollop of sour cream, and some lemon juice to keep it green. Pro tip: leaving an avocado pit in the guacamole until we serve it keeps it looking fresh for longer. Cover the guac and keep the pit in it until show time.

Make a Spanish rice, for a side dish, by frying two cups of rice in a skillet with four tablespoons of vegetable oil and four chicken bouillon cubes. Add garlic, salt, and pepper and stir constantly until the rice turns white and just starts to brown on the edges. Add 3.5 cups of water and 1 cup of the salsa. Bring to a rapid boil, turn off the burner, and cover the skillet. Wait thirty minutes and enjoy the perfection. Garnish with a sprig of cilantro for visual effect.

Now take the Corn tortilla shells and lay them one at a time in a skillet of hot vegetable oil, fry one side for fifteen seconds and then the other for fifteen seconds. Remove and place on a paper towel to cool. Cut a stack of corn tortillas in sixths and fry them up crispy for chips after making the tortillas, adding a sprinkling of salt as they come out of the hot oil.

Next, add a jar of whole pinto beans to a saucepan, without draining them. Coarsely chop some cilantro. Add garlic, salt, and pepper and ¾ of the cilantro to the beans. Cover and bring to a low simmer. After ten minutes or so, use a potato masher to crush most of the beans, so a nice, chunky, pintos refritos (refried beans) begins to take shape. Sprinkle the remaining cilantro over the top as a garnish and we're almost ready to serve.

Slice a fresh lime into wedges for sprinkling over top of the finished plate. Finely chop a head of lettuce and place it in a bowl. Shred a block of Colby or Monterrey Jack cheese and place that in a bowl. Walk over to the PA system and inform the entire crew that "Chow's on!" *Bon Apetite!*

As a firehouse cook, we learned the intricacies of our crew's eating habits. We already know about Mean Dean's penchant for Zesty Italian chicken breast, and Jackson's disgust for olives.

Factor in that Jenna's a pescatarian, Koz says he's allergic to onions (although I think they just give him heartburn), Mumbles puts ketchup on everything (so we'd better damn well have at least a half a bottle of that), Wes is on a lemonade diet so he's not eating today (but he did throw in three bucks to help cover contingent thank God), and Butler is off the mess entirely so that means we'll have to stay up past midnight if we wanna bust him picking through the leftovers and then shame his ass for double fucking his crew out of both mess money and food.

This was like rocket science, and there were a lot of variables to consider if we wanted to pull off a great spread. And the reward? The personal satisfaction of a job well done, maybe getting out of in-house training for the afternoon while everyone napped, or eating food the way *we* liked it prepared, not fucked up by some fresh-out-of-training probie? Please. None of it really seemed worth the rigmarole that we went through to make it happen.

As time went on, these gather round the table, the family that eats together stays together dinners and pretty much all the other old firehouse traditions seemed to die off. We stopped playing poker for dishes. More people began to bring their own food and declined to be "on the mess." This made it more difficult to cook, with less money for food, and the meals became less extravagant as a result. I recall some of my favorite firehouse meals toward the end of my career being simple chili-cheese dogs with potato chips and dip. Or a nice soup and sandwich combo like grilled ham and cheese with homemade chicken noodle or beef barley soup.

Sometimes the crew wouldn't even show up to the meal because they were either working out, or washing their car, or writing reports, or playing an intense game of ping pong, or any number of excuses to get out of sitting down with their colleagues and breaking bread. Or maybe it was to get out of doing the post-dinner chores like sweeping, mopping, and doing the dishes.

Whatever the reasons, it made for a frustrating experience to put that amount of effort into making a great meal and to have to eat it all by myself. I began inviting friends and family to my station dinners, just to have someone to share it with. Things were changing. The traditional ways of the firehouse were beginning to disappear.

At my department, when I hired on, the bosses expected certain foods on certain days of the week. There was Taco Tuesday, Fish Friday (especially during Lent), Steak Saturday, and Sunday Roast, but the rest of the week was pretty much up to the chef. Everybody eating at the station that day would kick in $7 for mess money. We'd check the ads in the morning paper for sales, and plan a menu based on the budget. God forbid I went over budget and had to take a special assessment from the crews because of my fiscal ineptitude.

Meals were to be prepared and served at precisely twelve noon. When the meal was ready, we were to call over the PA system "Chow's on, chow's on." If we were late, people would start hovering around the kitchen, asking if, "everything's OK," and, "Do we need any help?" We'd better have a *fucking* salad, with at least three ingredients; iceberg in a bowl was just lettuce. Put some chopped carrots and cucumbers in it for Christ's sake. If we were really good, we'd leave a few strips of skin on the cucumber and rake it with a fork lengthwise before slicing. Put some real panache into it. Cooking, I've learned, is all about presentation. If it looks and smells good, they'll eat it.

Make some Kool aid too, the old-timers loved that shit. JT was a master of mixology. He'd take orange and grape Kool Aid and mix them together to make Mississippi Mud, or lemonade and grape for a Purplesaurus Rex. The key to great Kool Aid he taught, was making it early, and with hot water. Use slightly more sugar and slightly less water than the recipe calls for. He'd even put hot water in the empty packets to get all the flavor out. The hot water mixing helps the sugar and powder dissolve better. Put it into the freezer for a few hours until its slushy. *Perfecto!*

Desert is the meal saver, period. We could fuck everything

up, burn the meat, have bony potatoes, mushy vegetables too, but if we had a solid desert, we were golden. That's why they called it the meal saver. Bake some brownies or cookies and make sure they're soft. Set a fucking timer so we don't end up with hockey pucks. I've literally had guys get hockey sticks out and play with my cookies. Slapshots across the station and all, just to shame me. That's always fun to clean up after.

Some of my favorite firehouse deserts were homemade apple crisp with vanilla ice cream, or a nice fruit pizza. The latter could throw our budget way off, with the sugar cookie crust and the blueberries, raspberries, and strawberries (sometimes a kiwi or two). So, I only made it on days when we had an overtimer on shift. If *we* were on overtime, we were expected to ante up twenty dollars for our mess money for the day, instead of the usual seven. We were making the big bucks and it was customary to share the wealth with our crew that day.

The old-timers had some god-awful nasty foods they'd whip up when I came on the department. Cracklins was one of the more peculiar of these. One morning, I'd finished trimming the fat from the meat I was preparing to cook for the day and was about to throw it in the trash. Charlie Zamora stopped me and taught me about cracklins. He chopped the fat into tiny squares and fried them in a skillet until they were golden brown on the outside. Then he took a slice of white bread, spread a bit of softened butter on it and filled it with the fried fat, like a taco. They were called cracklins because they cracked and popped in our mouths, bursting open with warm, fatty goodness as we chewed them.

Shit on a shingle was another classic that soon fell out of favor with the younger crowds. They'd make a nice sausage gravy by frying ground sausage in a skillet, then prior to draining, add milk and cornstarch, stirring continuously until golden brown and thick. Toast an entire loaf of bread well done and spoon that sausage gravy all over a couple of pieces of toast on a plate. *Voila!* Shit on a shingle.

After freezing my rank at firefighter and having, in my opinion, the best job in the world; stationed at Fours and riding the ladder truck every shift, I volunteered to cook every day. The bosses knew they were getting quality chow, and the ladder truck was less likely to roll out on bullshit alarms, so the meals could be prepared and served on time (usually).

After three years of cooking every shift though, I was getting bored, and the bosses were getting tired of the same rotating meals in my repertoire. I'd ask everybody what they wanted to eat that day, and no one would offer any suggestions. So, my good buddy and fellow Capricorn, Dave Austin suggested we go on a world tour. He proposed we cook two dishes from a different country, each shift, for the next twelve days. I thought it would be a disaster, but agreed to go along for the ride, just to "spice" things up a bit.

His random country selections were initially too difficult to procure the ingredients. The national dish of Iceland for instance, Hakarl, was a fermented shark that was cured for four to six months. Scottish Haggis was not appealing to the officers as it contained sheep organs and blood mixed with suet, oatmeal and seasonings that are boiled in the animal's stomach.

Ultimately, we settled on a simple American dish of burgers and beef franks with grilled sweet corn for the inaugural meal. Next, we traveled to Cuba for ropa vieja and a *delicioso* Cuban sandwich. Then we ventured to Ireland for colcannon, boxty, and soda bread, then a Guinness beef stew. We hopped over to Greece for some gyros (pronounced YEE-ros) with tzatziki and a Greek salad. Then it was off to Switzerland for Swiss steak and roesti. Next, we "stoemp-ed" into Belgium for waterzooi, and breakfast-for-dinner with fruit-and-cream-topped Belgian waffles, rounding out the first six shifts.

Word spread around the department and people began asking at the breakfast tables where we were traveling to next, offering suggestions. It was becoming a culinary adventure for everyone, both chef and gastronome alike. Poland's classic pierogis and golumpkis showed up on the menu, followed by China's chow mein, wonton soup, and General Tso's chicken with egg rolls and fried rice. Have you ever seen the corn starch slurry used to batter those pieces of chicken? Is it a liquid or a solid? It's both—talk about alchemy!

Italy was next with olive stuffed chicken breast, bruschetta, and pizza Napolitano. Then we headed to Mexico for chilaquiles and my favorite roast beef tacos, salsa, Spanish rice, and pintos refritos. We traveled to the Caribbean for Jamaican jerk chicken with fried plantains, cornbread, and red beans and rice. Mother Russia completed the final shift with a beef stroganoff and fried cabbage. It was a hit with the whole crew and a great way to mix things up in the kitchen by experimenting with new and tasty dishes.

One of my all-time favorite meals was Dave Austin's fish tacos. He'd bake fish fillets brushed in olive oil and seasoned with garlic, salt, pepper, and paprika on a cookie sheet, while I chopped fresh red and yellow peppers, pineapple, mango, cilantro, and jalapenos for a mango salsa. There's a recipe for wickedly good fish taco sauce on soupaddict.com that we'd whip up. I'd fry corn tortillas for the taco shells and a little shredded asiago cheese for a topper. A rice pilaf and a garden salad completed our sacrificial offering to the fire gods.

I'm a firm believer that we become good at what we practice. In Taekwondo I learned the saying, the master has failed more times than the beginner has even thought about trying. Pay attention to what the masters do. Learn from them and adapt it to your own style and tastes. I cooked everywhere I could. I'd help the other cooks when I wasn't in charge of the meals, just to pick up little tips and tricks from them.

Chapter 29

Truckie for Life

As Koz rode out the final months of his career on sick leave, a young lieutenant was just making the captain's rank. With all the other stations locked up with senior captains who'd frozen their rank, declining to advance to battalion chief, Fours was the only option for Damyon Wallace. Damyon had a reputation for training relentlessly—yet relevantly—at his craft. Making certain his troops were prepared for battle.

When he arrived on the red shift at Fours, we had a veteran crew with Fergie as our twenty-three-year frozen engineer, and me as the seventeen-year frozen firefighter. We all knew what we were doing on emergency scenes and in the firehouse. My classmate Spoons transferred in as the new lieutenant, Dave Austin came over from the black shift upon making the engineer's rank, and firefighters Zach Powell and Matt Baker transferred in from Nines along with Damyon. We actually liked being around each other. Nobody was a fuck-up or an asshole and station life was *really* good for a change.

I think of the X Ambassadors song "Nervous" when things start going well and I start feeling content with a certain situation. I've seen way too much shit to know when I get that feeling, thunderheads are forming just over the horizon, or the tectonic plates beneath our feet are about to shift. I knew something big and ugly was coming. Call it a healthy skepticism. Like Obi-won Kenobi, I could sense a disturbance in the Force.

One frozen morning in February 2015, a call came in for a house fire on Maple Street. I was on Truck 4 with Damyon as the boss, Zach Powell was the engineer. We were the first due truck company and pulled up just behind Captain Bubbles on Engine 9. The house was unassuming: a small, one-story bungalow. The walls were made of cinderblock and the interior crew was calling for a roof vent almost as soon as they'd entered.

We pulled the ladders from the truck and jumped over the chain link fence surrounding the front yard because the gates were blocked by huge snow drifts. Zach fired up the saws and passed them over the fence to us. We climbed to the roof and discovered it was extremely slippery under the snow and ice.

It turned out to be a metal roof, so we switched to our rotary saw with a metal blade. In hindsight, and for those currently employed as firefighters, stick with the regular chainsaw, and just burn the fucking blade right off it. Plunge that puppy right through both the aluminum and wood, just like we normally would for a regular wooden decked roof.

After cutting through the metal sheathing, we switched back to our chainsaw to plunge cut through the shingles and roof decking. It was slow going and the saw kept bogging down in the sub-zero temperatures and smoky conditions. Underneath the metal roof were *three* layers of shingles and decking, one over top of the other. With the interior crews still calling for a vent, we worked our asses off to pop thru the roof decking and finally did.

When Damyon took the pike pole and tried to punch through

the ceiling drywall, it just bounced off. We each took turns pounding on the ceiling with all our might, but it simply wouldn't budge. I dropped into the attic through the vent hole we'd just cut, to get a better idea of what we were up against. Through the thick attic smoke, I could see that on top of the ceiling joists were two by twelve planks screwed in. It was a fucking bunker that our traditional vent techniques were woefully unprepared for.

I yelled up to Damyon to pass me the chainsaw. He handed it down and I began cutting through the massive planks. I was right above the fire and standing in what would soon become the chimney. I cut alongside the rafter joists with deep plunge cuts that zipped right through the ceiling drywall as well. Soon, several strips of two by twelves had been removed and the attic filled with intense heat and smoke.

I passed the saw back up through the hole to Damyon. Then he extended his hand and pulled me up onto the slippery roof. Back on the roof ladder, we made our way down to the eaves and onto the extension ladder. We dropped our tools into the snow drifts below, removed the roof ladder and climbed back down to the ground, exhausted.

Smoke and heat flowed from the vent hole in the roof and the crews inside pushed forward to extinguish the fire. After it was out, we discussed our tactics, given the difficult circumstances. Damyon mentioned he was impressed that I never gave up in the face of adversity. We rode together almost every shift for the next three years after that.

Words fail to adequately describe the horrors we come across as firefighters. I'd like to bury them deep and never think about any of them again for as long as I live. They're scars. Wounds that time has covered with a thin layer of skin, but the marks and memories they leave behind remain and torment their captives for eternity. The afternoon of September 9, 2015, was one of those days that ripped the soul of our fire department wide open and left a gaping wound that will *never* heal for those of us who were there.

They tell us this is a dangerous job when we apply. Everyone knows the obscenely high divorce rates and shortened life expectancies in our profession. The numbers aren't good. The shit we see has a definite impact on our psyche. It's unavoidable.

Darren Richardson was a Marine who'd carried a light machine gun through Afghanistan for two tours before he hired on at our department. The Taliban couldn't kill him, but a mentally deranged civilian who was pissed off about a traffic jam did. Darren's engine crew was helping to raise money for muscular dystrophy during the MDA fill the boot charity campaign. They were collecting donations at a busy intersection in the south end of town.

My wife had been saying for years how someone was going to get killed doing that shit and today, she was right. I was off duty when we decided head to the pharmacy to pick up her prescription. As we sat in our car at the intersection waiting for the light to change, traffic was backed up. We were unaware Darren had just been hit and lay dying in the road ahead.

Emergency vehicles came screaming into the intersection. I watched from our personal vehicle as my friends—Krishna, Eric Howard, Mike Rhodes, and Mitch Lang—jumped from Truck 4 and ran at a full sprint, rushing to help. I'd never seen Krishna run in my life and knew right away something terrible must've happened. There were only two firefighters on our department who'd been killed in the line of duty in our department's 150-year history, and I'd just been in proximity to one of them.

While collecting for Fill the Boot, a nationally backed program where firefighters raised public donations for MDA, both Darren and Bruce Allen had nearly been struck by a vehicle when a motorist—angry at the traffic backup—had flown around the stopped cars and zipped down the open left-turn lane. He proceeded straight through the light instead of turning left as required. Then he made a U-turn into oncoming traffic and slammed on the accelerator.

Bruce dove out of the way as the madman swerved violently attempting to run him down. With his tires squealing and now coming from the opposite direction, the driver lined up Darren in his sights and plowed straight into him, at around 45 miles per hour, without ever touching the brakes. Darren's fire boots, paper money, loose change, and MDA stickers flew up into the air and rained down on the horrified motorists that were stuck in the charity traffic.

When the stunned fire crews realized what happened, they yelled for help over their handset radios and rushed in to assist. Darren was unrecognizable from massive facial swelling and the deformation of multiple skull fractures. The crews were struggling to save him, just as my wife and I pulled up at the intersection. Enraged motorists called 9-1-1 and took off in pursuit of the offender, following the maniacal murderer as he fled the scene just as lawlessly as he'd entered it. The civilians stayed on the phone with dispatchers, giving them location updates, as police closed in and finally cornered him at his parents' home about a mile away from the scene of the crime, where he surrendered and was taken into custody.

Darren was a load and go as soon as the sled rolled up. He was intubated, multiple IVs were established, and he coded several times on the way to the hospital. Krishna took over as the lead medic on the scene, being the most senior one there, and delivered perfect patient care in the ambulance. As they arrived at the hospital, Darren was transferred to the Emergency Department staff, of which his own wife was a member. Darren didn't make it. Despite the best efforts of police, fire, and hospital staff, he succumbed to his massive internal injuries. The vessel that was his body was broken beyond repair and unable to house his beautiful spirit any longer.

There was nothing anyone could've done to save him—we all knew that—but Krishna took it personal and particularly hard. The next morning, I was contacted by Fire Administration, who'd assigned each of the responders a close personal friend for suicide watch shortly after Darren passed away from his injuries. We were told to contact our assigned partners twice a day and to advise them if we required more resources. I checked in on Krishna regularly and religiously. Ironically, he'd be tasked with doing the same for me years later.

Darren's LODD (line-of-duty death) funeral was one of the saddest days I've ever experienced. His mourners filled the local college basketball arena to capacity. There wasn't a dry eye in the place. Firefighters and Marines from all over the world came to pay their respects. The honor guard was flawless. The bagpipes wailed their mournful sound.

The funeral procession was over fifteen miles long, and some bystanders remarked that it took two hours for all the vehicles in the procession to pass by them. The roads were closed, and people were lining the streets and overpasses for over thirty miles as we proceeded from the funeral to the cemetery. Darren's pregnant wife received the flag that draped his coffin, as it was lowered into the Earth. The Marines fired their Three-Volley salute. Everyone bawled their eyes out...and the sound of bagpipes still fucks us all up something terrible to this day.

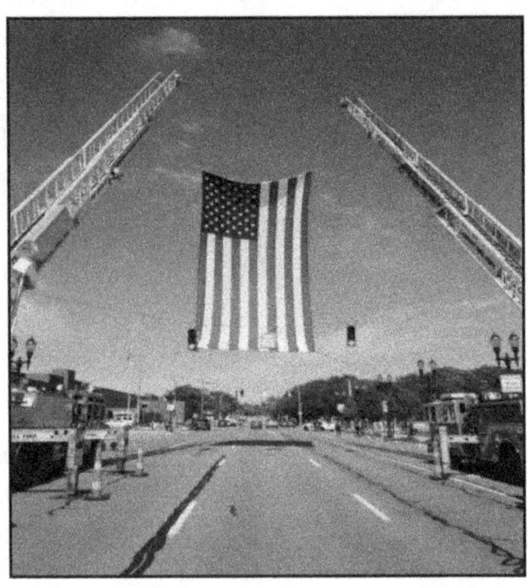

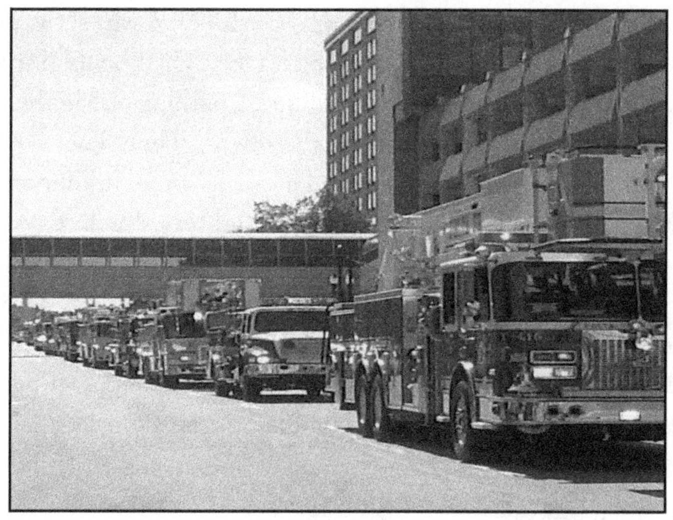

A few days later, when Krishna didn't respond to my phone calls one evening, I decided to head over to his house and do a welfare check on him. At shift change the following morning, I went to his home on the north end of town and pounded on his door. There was no response. I called his cell phone for the fourth time that morning with no answer and started peeking inside his windows to see if he was OK.

"Krishna, wake up, fucker," was the voicemail I left. "I've been up all night and I'm standing on your porch. C'mon, man."

The door opened a crack and Krishna stood there, disheveled.

"You look well," I said sarcastically, pushing my way past him and into the house. "Put the coffee on, honey. I'm home!"

We talked for hours about the things he'd seen and felt. Then we talked about the weather, sports, the Bible, the fire department, anything else rhetorical I could think of, and we smoked weed. A lot of weed. That shit has true medicinal value. If only to calm the nerves and numb the pain.

He thanked me for showing up, and I continued to do so for the next few weeks, just to make sure he was flying straight. We became good friends and to this day we still check in on each other. He says I saved his life that day. But all I did was show up and be there for him. Sometimes that's all it takes. Just being present in the moment. Letting a person know there's nothing else in the world that matters other than just being there with them. That we value them and the relationship. Some call it quality time. It's important.

When things like this happen, firefighters don't really have time to grieve proper. I was due back at work the day after the funeral, and the emergency runs and traumas just kept piling up. There's no time for decompression. We all jumped right back into action and kept grinding. Each of us hollow inside, numb, and heart broken. As another hero lay dead in the ground.

Out of Fours, we made a full alarm early one morning around 03:00 hours on Buffalo Avenue. Damyon was the boss, Zach Powell the engineer, and Matt Baker and I were riding dirty on Truck 4. Damyon mentioned this was his grandparents' house when he was growing up while I approached the BC for an assignment. We were tasked with the vent job since Truck 1 was busy with the interior search and rescue.

We threw ladders and climbed to the roof. I'd been cutting plenty of holes lately and decided to let Matt have the opportunity on this one, thinking he could use the experience. Zach started the chainsaw on the ground, and I ran it up to Matt on the roof ladder. He stepped out to cut, and I held on to his belt with one hand and the roof ladder with the other.

Matt revved the saw to full RPMs and plunged the blade into the roof deck. He made his first cut closest to the ladder, which was a big mistake. We didn't ever want to stand over a compromised piece of roof decking. Then he did the farthest cut and the top one next. As he was feathering the saw blade over the roof joists, the fire lit up underneath him. Flames were blowing from his initial cut, right beneath his legs. I tapped Matt on the shoulder to alert him and he changed position. The fire was right below us in the attic now and we needed to pick up the pace.

Finishing off the top and then the bottom, Matt sliced through the middle of the square he'd made and stepped back onto the roof ladder. I passed the saw down to Zach and he traded it out for a pike pole and sledgehammer. I pounded the louvers open with the hammer and Mike popped through the drywall ceiling with the pike pole. Flames and smoke roared through the vent hole. The fire had extended into the attic and was raging through the void spaces.

Damyon radioed the BC that the vent job was complete, and they needed to advance a line into the attic, or we were gonna lose the roof. We climbed down and took our roof ladder with us so it wouldn't get burned up. The interior crews went to work pulling ceiling and knocked the fire down with their hose lines. The beast was stubborn and tried to hide, but soon it was out. We rolled back home for shift change as the sun leaned in close and kissed the horizon.

Sometimes when we pulled into work for shift change, the rig we were assigned to was already gone. Sometimes it was out on an EMS run or a citizen assist, and it'd be back shortly. In which case, we just set our gear down and grabbed a cup of Joe. Taking it easy and waiting for our ride to get back.

Other times, our rig had been out all night at a cock knocker, and they weren't coming back anytime soon. In that case, we waited for our full crew to arrive at the firehouse, then drove to the scene, and relieved them there. Then they'd take the ride we'd driven there, back to the station, get cleaned up, and head home. Hopefully before it caused any overtime. They'd say, "a minute equals an hour," as in, one minute past 07:30 hours, the start of the next shift, and we got an hour of overtime pay per the union contract.

One summer morning as dawn broke, Damyon, Zach, a new kid named Otis, and I drove the Suburban (or red car as we called it) from Fours to the scene of a fire at Mike's Party Store.

We arrived to find one of our favorite ghetto party stores with the roof completely burnt off it. A lone ladder truck (now our ladder truck) still had its elevated master stream pouring water onto the hot spots remaining beneath the collapsed roof.

We relieved our crew and received an assignment to enter the adjoining building to check for fire extension in the attic and roof. As we entered the video rental store, the water on the floor was several feet deep, and I was reminded precisely where that hole in my left boot was as it filled with the cold, sooty water. We sloshed through the store, popping ceiling tiles with pike poles, and looking for fire extension. Finding none, we returned to the BC for another task.

The BC cleared the scene for his own shift change, and left us in command with another crew, Engine 9. We were tasked with putting out hot spots and overhauling the scene. We laddered the roof of the video store and made a trench cut for a fire stop. The new kid and I ran two chainsaws right next to each other and we both ate a lot of putrid, yellow smoke doing it. Otis was visibly winded, so after mocking his personal exercise routine, I suggested we exit the roof for a break.

Back on the ground, we grabbed a drink from the water cooler. It was warm. If there was one thing Damyon hated more than anything else, it was warm water in the cooler. There was no excuse for it as far as he was concerned, other than being a lazy engineer. He spat it out.

"It's piss warm!" he growled.

Otis and I chugged that shit, though. It was wet, and our throats were dry.

"I think I took a snootful up there," Otis said, "I feel kinda woozy."

"Did you just say a snootful?" Zach asked, laughing and shaking his head. He tossed Otis a towel as he leaned over and ralphed. "Hmmm, what'd you have for breakfast, huh new kid? Looks like, what's that, bananas, and maybe… oatmeal?" Zach continued.

Damyon headed back over to the fire, and I told Otis to c'mon. As a truckie we always stick with our wingman. Never let our boss do the work that we should be doing. For the next hour we overhauled until the Fire Marshal showed up and the last of the embers were snuffed out. Then we packed the ladder back into its bed, closed the outriggers, and headed home.

When I was new, Steve "Showtime" Hitchcock was a Fire Dispatcher who had a stellar voice for radio and always added a certain panache to his alarms. When new kids would call for their run report times, he'd ask them if they knew what time it *really* was. Then, in an homage to Jim Carey's *The Mask*, he'd explain to the new kid that it was... in fact... "showtime!"

Showtime's career with the city's Dispatch was obliterated when they decided to combine services with the county. He was close to fifty years old and all his seniority and pay rates were destroyed—erased by the stroke of a pen and a bureaucrat's decision to save a buck. Showtime was given the choice to either hire into Fire Suppression as a new kid or start over at half the pay and zero seniority in the county's new Dispatch.

He chose the prior, and along with fellow Fire Dispatcher Keith Michaels, was hired in the following recruit class. He immediately became the *OMASWA*—the Oldest Man Alive Still Working the Ambulance. Showtime was always happy. He was 150 pounds soaking wet and would always give us 100 percent. He was like a kid again, doing a job he'd always dreamed of.

Things started to wear on him, though, after ten years of near constant ambulances shifts. He became salty and would pop off at his patients and crew members when things didn't go right. This was a young person's job, and at sixty the grind was too much for him to bear. The always bubbly Showtime dispatcher I'd grown to know and love had changed, jaded by the carnage and overwhelming volume of trauma and sleep deprivation that came with the job.

He didn't ask new kids if they knew what time it was anymore. Yeah, he knew it was showtime, but not the way it was for him back when he was the voice behind the radio. Now it meant *he* was the one hauling bodies around. Picking up the broken pieces of people's shattered lives and trying to put them together again in an endless cycle of death and destruction. He was no longer the guy calling for rigs to respond and guiding the heroes to where they were needed. He was in their shoes now, and after a while it was hell for him. For all of us.

Showtime was diagnosed with stage 4 lung cancer shortly before he made it to retirement eligibility. He withered away to skin and bones in a hospital bed, and Krishna stayed by his side night and day. On February 3, 2016, less than six months after Darren's murder, Showtime passed away. His wife received his pension with a posthumous line-of-duty death award, and Krishna presided over the funeral ceremonies for yet another close friend. He ended the funeral with Steve's trademark phrase: "Hit 'er two, Showtime. You know what time it is." Dispatch rang out his last alarm over the radio, and we buried another brother.

Nothing says hero more than a person snatching a soul from the clutches of certain death. It's the very essence of what we as firefighters do and why we do it. The perfect rescue is the culmination of endless training, doing the right thing at the right time, and being luckier than a leprechaun with a four-leaf clover in one hand and a rabbit's foot in the other, on St. Patrick's Day, at the end of a rainbow, with all the planets aligned in their heavenly orbits.

Station 4 was the water rescue focus station. We were supposed to be dispatched on every call that required a boat in the water. So when a call came across the radio one afternoon for a man stranded on a rock in the river, we waited for our alarm to open up. It never did, though. Station 1 and Station 9 were the only ones dispatched. They had boats, but never really practiced working with them. They were too busy with other disciplines to bother with water rescue.

Damyon called out over the station PA that Truck 4 and ATV 4 with the boat trailer attached, would be responding normal traffic to the scene in case we were needed. I led the way driving the ATV, and the ladder truck followed close behind. There seemed to be a lot of confusion when we arrived at the low-head dam area. Neither Ones nor Nines had a boat in the water yet, and a soaking wet man was still clinging to a large rock just upstream of the dam. Ones was trying to get the park's entrance gate open with bolt cutters and Nines couldn't figure out how to get the ratchet straps off their boat and trailer.

I looked at Damyon in the rearview mirror and he gave me the thumbs-up. I jumped the curb and drove the ATV and boat straight through the middle of the park to the boat launch. Swinging it around, I backed the trailer into the water and was met by the crew of Engine 1.

"Man, it's good to see you!" Lieutenant Juan Ortiz said as we launched the boat with the rescue gear and donned our life vests.

"I'll be your coxswain bitch. Let's go!" I quipped, slapping him on the shoulder.

With the fuel supply hooked up, primed, and the motor choked, I pulled the ripcord and the outboard motor roared to life.

"Hang on," I yelled as we backed out of the launch ramp and zipped off at full throttle downstream toward the victim.

There's a certain pride we get when we come in and steal another station's glory. Knowing we'd just done everything right and saved the day, while some other idiot was about to fuck everything up and get somebody damn near killed.

We pulled alongside the victim, who was inebriated, and pulled him aboard our boat. Ralph put a life vest on him, and we headed off. The drunk man asked if we could swing by the shore and snag his cooler of hooch on the way back.

"No!" Juan and I both said in unison.

Back at the boat launch, we were met by BC Julian Burke and Damyon.

"Good work, boys," Julian said as we secured the boat to the trailer and helped the victim to shore.

"Damn right!" Damyon said, as we packed up our gear and headed back to the station.

Juan Ortiz was one of the most intelligent men I've ever known. A fucking sage—nay—a wizard who'd hired on shortly after me. We rode countless shifts on the medics together and shared strategies and maneuverings that would make other people's heads spin. If there were two ways of doing something, Juan and I would've come up with twelve. If there was a plan of attack, we'd have a half dozen. He was my confidant and my guru and always gave it to me straight. When I needed advice on procedure or contract interpretation, Juan was my go-to guy.

On a four-lane bridge one night, a truck crossed the center line and hit an oncoming car head on. The car careened into the guardrail and the front wheels hung precariously over the side of the bridge, above the river below. Extrication crews were dispatched for a family of four trapped in the car. We rolled up on Truck 4 to assist and upon arrival, began to crib and secure the car so the crews could begin cutting it with the Jaws.

I placed step chocks under the front of the car to stabilize it, on both sides, and a winch cable from 5 Engine's bumper was hooked around the frame of the car. The valve stems of the rear tires were pulled, to lower its center of gravity and prevent rocking of the vehicle. I stretched a booster line from the closest pumper in case the car caught fire. The medic crews stood by as the doors were popped with the spreaders and removed at the hinges.

The A, B, and C pillars were cut, and we removed the entire roof. The kids in the back seat were C-collared, backboarded, and removed first. The parents up front were still trapped under the weight of the collapsed dashboard. When a frontal impact is severe enough, it can cause the dashboard to roll down onto the occupant's legs, trapping them.

Next came the dash roll. Relief cuts were made where the firewall met the front rocker panels. Hydraulic rams were placed in a rocker panel brace on one end, and against the curve of the A pillar on the other. The rams were extended, and the dashboard was forced up and away from the patients. This was done on both sides simultaneously and the hydraulic rams were left in place while the parents were packaged and extricated from the car.

The patients were transported to a nearby hospital, and all made full recoveries from their injuries. In a PIA (post incident analysis) everyone was lauded for their coordination and teamwork. We headed home feeling good about a job well done.

Back at the station, I noticed my shoulder was sore when I removed my turnout coat and hung it on the fire truck. Rubbing it, I could feel my collarbone sticking up through my shirt. It had separated from my shoulder during the call. A grade three separation was the Occupational Health doctor's diagnosis and she said that while I might have some discomfort, it was largely superficial, and I'd have an ugly bump there on top of my shoulder for the rest of my days.

After a second opinion, I ended up having it surgically repaired a few months later. On my own dime of course, I'd seen it happen too many times: that shitty, line-of-duty injury system had left dozens of my colleagues disabled and never able to return to work. I'd rather be on my own sick leave, see my own personal surgeons and doctors, rehabbing and returning to work on a proper recovery timetable.

When Battalion Chief Pat Hopkins called to ask why I was on sick leave and in Jamaica, I explained how it was all part of the rehabilitation process. See, in our climate, it was cold out, which aggravated the arthritis in the joint. Being in a warmer climate helped me endure longer rehab sessions, hastening my return to work. In addition, I was rehabbing with scuba tanks on my back in the ocean, slowly easing back into wearing a Scott Pak on my recently surgically repaired shoulder. Everybody knows it's too cold right now to do scuba where we lived.

It was all very high-level and cutting-edge surgical recovery shit, 100 percent planned and executed by my team of personal surgeons and doctors, and I assured the BC that they'd all be happy to write an excused absence if he required further explanation on the healing benefits of my physical therapy. I reminded him this *was* a line-of-duty injury, and that I'd be returning to work in two weeks, at the exact time my team of doctors had previously established. Pat said that wouldn't be necessary, that he agreed, and understood completely. That was some more Obi-Won shit right there: "These aren't the droids you're looking for..."

There was a house on the west side of town that burned for three days straight. Nestled at the end of a dead-end road, behind a park, and at the edge of the river, it was extremely secluded. It was an AirBnB destination and was being occupied by a group of a dozen or so friends when a full alarm came in for a structure fire.

Darkness had fallen when we made it as the second truck company and assumed RIT operations. Damyon gave us the green light to help with some of the exterior operations, so we threw a few ladders and helped Truck 1 get set up for their roof vent. The fire raged for a couple of hours and was finally extinguished around 02:00.

Karen Kowalsky was the other firefighter on our rig that night, and I recall looking over at one point and seeing her pissing in the woods. When those early morning alarms come in, we don't have time to visit the restroom before rushing out. It was just one of those things. On the big ones, we'd always walk in on a firefighter pissing in a bathroom toilet or rifling through the refrigerator looking for a beer or some stupid shit like that.

The following day, the incoming black shifters had to put out a rekindle at the fire scene. A rekindle is when the initial fire suppression crews don't do a good enough job putting it out, and an ember or two stick around and decide it would be fun to get the party rocking all over again. So the black shift returned to the scene and put it out for a second time.

The following day, as the red shift returned for duty, the black shift proceeded to rub it in that they'd put our fire out, *again*. That sort of thing has been going on at firehouse tables for hundreds of years and probably will for hundreds more. As they stood up to leave, a fire alarm came in for another rekindle at the same house.

"Oh, who's putting out whose fire now?" we all joked. We headed over and the place looked like a bomb had gone off. It was a crater.

There was almost nothing left to the structure as we pulled up. The frame dwelling had completely collapsed into the basement and piles of rubble were smoldering here and there. The only thing left standing, were two walls of the garage, though the roof had collapsed. We pulled hoses and sprayed it down for the next couple of hours. We mingled with the Fire Marshals, who had their hands full with determining the cause and point of origin on this one. The evidence was pretty well destroyed by now.

There was an enormous, old, three-story, heaver timber and brick factory called the Jim Beam building in our city. It was a cutup maze inside, with all kinds of hazardous materials being stored and used by subleasing tenants. The short-timers dreaded the place, and if a fire alarm came in there, they'd try anything to ditch the call or remain outside the structure.

I always thought it was an interesting place. Think *American Pickers* warehouse, then multiply it by twenty. There were old private car collections being stored on the top floors, giant ramps and freight elevators, welding shops, custom car fabricators, lawn care businesses, concrete companies, storage units, and the whole place was a potpourri of anything goes. We never knew what we'd pull up on or walk into.

It was always fun to jump a fire as we were rolling through another fire company's district. Dispatch would usually call the trucks that were on the road in radio service first and ask if they could clear for a full alarm before they sent the actual alarm out to the stations. This gave them a huge jump on the rigs still in-house.

Truck 4 was just around the corner from the Jim Beam, at the city garage, when Dispatch asked if we could clear for a full alarm there. We pounced on it. Arriving to find light smoke coming from a side door, we grabbed our tools and headed in to investigate, knowing the next engine company was still a few minutes out. The air in the dimly lit hallway was filled with a hazy, light gray smoke. We followed it for a few hundred feet to a garage door that was belching thicker, darker smoke from its edges and seams. Smoke always becomes heavier the closer we are to the seat of the fire.

Beside the paneled garage door was a smaller service door that we unlocked with the master keys we'd pulled from the Knox Box upon entry to the building. We masked up and used our TIC to navigate the open floor plan. It was a motorcycle garage, and we started to feel the heat from up ahead of us. This was good, we were locating the fire. Unfortunately, after wandering around in the building's smoky atmosphere, I had no idea where we were anymore.

Damyon's TIC had a compass, though, and he radioed out to the first due engine to pull up about midway down the south side of the building and pull a pre-connect. He could see an exterior garage door to our right, and we opened it to find the nozzle crew waiting outside with their charged line. With visibility improving, they made entry and extinguished the motorcycles that were free burning. After it was out, we learned that some stray welding sparks smoldered and ignited the fire while the staff left for a lunch break. There were some sweet choppers and Harleys in there, and we chatted with the owners a bit about them before we left.

Seaboy was deeply disturbed by the loss of his best friend. Having found him hanging and cutting him down was more than he could take. He fell headlong into a deep depression that no amount of therapy (or drugs, or sex, or adventuring) could pull him out of. He was tail-spinning into the Earth at breakneck speed. He took time off from work to enter rehab for drug and alcohol addictions. When he came back one morning at shift change, he called all personnel from both shifts to the breakfast table and gave his AA speech to us.

I remember Zach getting up and walking out at one point because it was so awkward. "What the *fuck*, Seaboy," he said and exited the room.

Seaboy reached out to everyone seeking help and therapy recommendations. We tried to offer support and steer his ship back on course. It wasn't enough, though.

On June 4, 2017, after his wife told him she was leaving him, Seaboy went out to his garage and joined his best friend in the afterlife by hanging himself from the rafters. Another funeral, for another firefighter. It was horrible. The whole department grieved for its fallen soldiers. Something big was brewing on the horizon and the men and women of our fire department were suffering terribly inside. Something needed to happen.

The wheels were falling off the party bus that had been our fire department, and a change to a more sustainable, long-term way to deal with all the trauma was in order. Mental health became a priority and programs were established to help members deal with their suffering. A functional program was still a long way off, and it was still easier to talk to the bottle than to sit down with our supervisors and talk about how we just couldn't cope with the stress of the job.

Eric Fisher was one of the single funniest human beings I've ever met. He was a short, skinny man who had lightening quick wit and a sarcastic view of the world that made for some amazing days of laughter and hilarity. One day as he arrived for his shift on Medic 11, an alarm came in for a possible SIDS baby not breathing. When he went to crack the drug box for CPR meds to treat the infant, the entire drug box was missing.

The previous crew had failed to replace the drug box after their last call, for whatever reason, and had left Fisher with no course of action. The infant, who most likely was not going to make it anyway, had its fate sealed by the folly of another crew. And Fisher lost his mind.

He felt personally responsible for the infant who'd just died in his arms. He suffered from massive depression and PTSD. He couldn't come to work and burned through his sick leave and vacation days trying to claim a duty disability. He had panic attacks whenever he'd stop by the station to drop off doctors' notes or to check in with his captain.

The city denied his line-of-duty claims and crushed his soul. They claimed his mental issues were not a result of a line-of-duty injury. He hired an attorney and settled out of court for remuneration of lost wages and sick time, and begrudgingly returned to work. But he was never the same. He was the funniest man I'd ever met, and after that single event, he became the most cynical. It was heartbreaking to witness.

My youngest son, Banks, was practically raised at the fire station with me. Lee would bring him by every day that I worked, and he'd pick out a fireball from the candy store, lift weights with me in the workout room, pretend to drive the fire trucks, and climb all over them. He had his birthday and holiday parties in the firehouse community room and would climb the crabapple trees in the back of the station while his mom and I talked about our day.

When Banks started school, Lee and I would chat on the phone every morning after she dropped him off and was driving home. I'd be slinging a mop around the station for the morning duties, and we'd touch base on what we had planned for the day. At night, we'd put our phones on speaker and sleep together. Sometimes she'd wake me up snoring, or I'd catch a run and the tones would scare her right out of bed. We did everything together again and I had my best friend back. I'd ask her before bed if we were going to catch a fire that night, and get all excited when she'd say, "Yes; two in fact." Or sometimes she'd say we were going to sleep all night; those were good, too. She'd be right every time. I'd ask her if I was going to make it the full twenty-five years or retire early, and she'd say I'd leave about three years ahead of schedule.

When Banks was eight years old, he asked for and received permission from Damyon to ride along with us for a few hours while his mother ran an errand. After she left, we caught a mutual aid response on a second alarm to a shuttered restaurant fire. Banks rode in the jump seat of the ladder truck, right beside me, while we rushed to the scene lights and sirens. Damyon, Matt Baker, and I headed off to slay the beast, while Banks stayed at the rig with Engineer Dave Austin and watched us through the cab window.

As we grabbed our tools from the truck and headed to the fireground, we set up at the curb while Damyon made contact with the BC and assessed the scene. We had angry brown smoke pumping from the gable ends of the roof and lazy white smoke coming from adjoining sections of the structure. We could tell a lot about the intensity of the fire by the volume of smoke coming out and how fast it's moving. The color of the smoke would let us know what type of material was burning and how involved with fire it was.

The part-time township firefighters were on air, going hard from the yard with 2 ½" hose lines and our crew walked right past them and started breaking windows right under the heavy brown smoke pumping from the eaves, trying to vent the structure before a flashover could occur. There was a charged 1 ¾" hose line that had been advanced to the locked front door of the structure then abandoned. We commandeered the hose line and I kicked in the front door. Heavy dark smoke rolled out from the top half of the opening. We made entry and found no fire visible in the room.

"It's in the attic!" Damyon yelled, and Matt Baker began punching holes through the ceiling and pulling down drywall with his pike pole. I located an attic skuttle hole and opened the smooth bore nozzle stream right into its panel, blowing it off and away into the dark smoke that poured from the opening in the ceiling.

As I sprayed water into the attic, the smoke changed from a dark brown and black color, to a lighter, grayish white. We were beating it back and the beast was nearly defeated because of our aggressive tactics. A few minutes later, with most of the ceiling pulled down, the majority of the fire was out, and we spent the next half hour or so chasing hot spots and flare-ups. Then we cleared and left the township guys to do the overhaul. That was always the best part about mutual aid fires; coming in and taking over the best jobs, then leaving when it was cleanup time.

About six months before the incident, Lee began asking me to stay away from the police.

"What for?" I asked.

"I don't know. I just see some something really bad happening with you around police." She was vague, and her forecast was cryptic.

"Baby, I love you. I'm not gonna bang a cop," I said, joking.

"Just promise me you'll stay away from police," she replied, unamused.

I promised her. Not having the slightest idea what she was alluding to.

Rob Hughes was a black shift engineer when I first met him. A funny, somewhat awkward portly man with a great personality and a strong faith in God. When he became our battalion chief, he'd swing by every shift and chat with the troops about how they were doing and what they needed. He'd always say how it was impossible to be angry when we were grateful for the blessings we had. He talked about showing others "eight seconds of humanity" and how that's all it took to learn someone's name and show them we cared about them. Everybody was worth eight seconds, he'd say.

It came as a shock to everyone when he announced, a month after retirement, he'd been diagnosed with pancreatic cancer. Because it was caught at stage 2, the hopes were high that with surgery, chemotherapy, and radiation, it could be beaten. Tragically, a few months later it had spread to his lungs. As Rob withered away to a veritable skeleton, he kept his spirits high and asked everyone who cared anything for him, to practice eight seconds of humanity toward others. He was fifty-one years old when he passed away.

On a hot, steamy afternoon in the summer of 2017, we were called to respond mutual aid on the initial alarm, to a structure fire in Delphi Township, out of Station 4. It was Damyon, Dave Austin, a new kid named Eric, and me on Truck 4. Then Spoons, Powell, and Baker on Engine 4. We arrived first and took the address. Fire and smoke were showing from the living room and front porch, and fire had extended into the eaves and attic as well.

While the engine crew stretched a line through the front door, we were informed by the residents that everyone was out, so we prepared for a roof vent. Eric and I threw an extension ladder against the eaves, then slid the roof ladder into position, latching its hooks over the peak. We gathered an eight-foot pike pole, a pick head axe, and a chainsaw, then headed up the ladder to the roof. Damyon was already there with the TIC and was searching the roof decking for the hottest point.

"There," he said, pointing to a section of roof.

"Give me a 4' x 4' hole right at the top of that dormer," he ordered.

Eric was too green and scared to step foot off the roof ladder, so I fired up the saw and made the cuts. The farthest vertical one first, then the top—feathering the blade over the trusses—next the bottom, then the louvers between trusses beginning with the farthest, then another down the middle, then the last vertical cut, and I was back on the ladder. Damyon popped open the louvers and as we turned around for the pike pole, Eric was scurrying down the ladder, right off the roof with it.

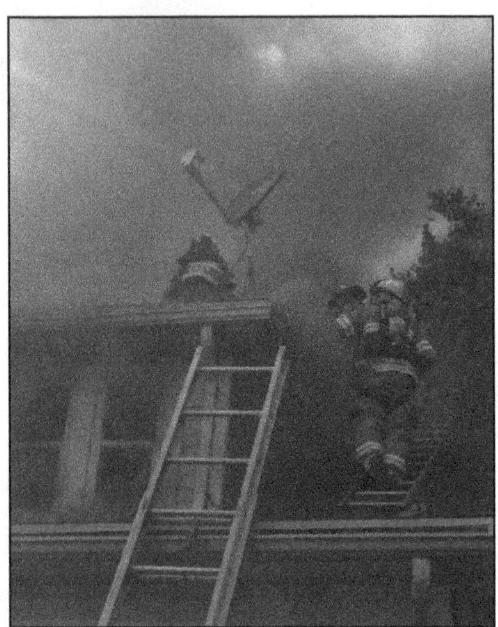

The author performing a vent job on the Delphi fire

"Hey!" we yelled after him as he disappeared over the edge of the roof.

Zach saw that bullshit from his pump panel and met Eric on the ground.

"The fuck you think *you're* going? Get your lil' bitch-ass back up there. Don't you *ever* leave your crew!" he said, blocking the new kid's retreat from the ladder.

As Eric climbed back up, the fire began blowing through the hole I'd just cut. It was impossible for us to stand over the inferno and punch through the drywall ceiling now. The new kid had screwed up the whole vent operation. Interior conditions were too hot for the engine crew to continue and as they bailed out; evacuation tones sounded from the radio and the trucks.

"I'm not getting off this roof, or we're gonna lose it," I told Damyon.

Smoke obscured his face as he replied, "I know; me either."

Eric ran for the ladder and Damyon dismissed him with a wave of his hand.

The two of us stood on the roof, with the fire free burning beneath us, discussing strategy, and how we could get back ahead of it. We smashed the dormer windows and had the engine crew pass us a nozzle up the ladder. We sprayed through the dormer windows as the shingles began to boil under our feet and the roof became spongy. Damyon said it was time.

We climbed down the extension ladder and helped Dave Austin set up the aerial. We positioned the elevated master stream nozzle directly over the house about thirty feet above the roof. Zach hooked a water supply line into the truck's pump intake. Dave pulled the gate lever, and I scaled the ladder, toggling the nozzle to a fog pattern and flowing thousands of gallons per minute, until the entire house was water-logged and physically unable to burn any longer. We lost the house, but the fire was contained, and eventually went out. After we terminated defensive operations, the township crews made entry and extinguished the hot spots. We packed up and returned to the station while they finished the overhaul.

Security is all a state of mind. At any moment, it can be shattered by someone who knows how to breach it. As firefighters, we're highly trained professionals at breaching locked and otherwise impenetrable areas. We turn windows into doors, breach walls, destroy locked doors, breach basement foundations, turn floors into basement access and basically have our way with any type of building construction.

Professionals call this *forcible entry*. Climbing in windows, popping doors, punching through walls, defeating locks, ventilating roofs, cutting security bars, taking bolt cutters to chains and such. The whole premise is to find the weak link release. How is the place built and where are the weakest points to attack? Avoid the strong spots and exploit the weak ones. That deadbolt lock in a wooden door frame? Weak. A poured concrete wall? Strong. Get the picture?

We'd study the layouts of the buildings in our response area. We pre-incident planned the construction type, occupancy, when people were there, where they were in the building and how to tell if they were there or not. We'd have at least three plans to complete our task and if one failed, we were immediately on to the next. We always wanted the best firefighters on our RIT teams, because if it was us that went down in a fire, we knew they weren't going to stop until we were safe and heading back home to our families.

RIT teams carry all kinds of tools to get firefighters out of jams. Rope bags, carabiners, chainsaws, rotary saws, axes, Halligans, sledgehammers, door controls, knives, pliers, vice grips, webbing, wire cutters, pry bars—the list goes on and on. If it could potentially be used it to get through the impassible, our RIT teams carried it.

We could zip out a piece of floor and shove an attic ladder down it in thirty seconds for access to the floor below. We could bust through drywall and be into the next adjacent room in fifteen seconds. Got exterior hinges on that door? Use a hinge-pin puller and the door is off in ten seconds. Have a steel door with a metal frame? A flat head axe and a properly placed Halligan tool will have it open in a jiffy. Believe me when I say, security is all a state of mind.

Our RIT team could grid search a warehouse in zero visibility with ropes or by using a thermal camera. We could whip up harnesses with our rolls of webbing and use ropes to drag, raise, or lower an unconscious victim. We laddered second story windows for bailouts, slid down the ladders on the rails, upright and upside down, and could even perform flips on them in case we had to bail out a window headfirst.

We were masters of our craft and could make magic happen on the fireground. We were Truckies. A group of the best and most senior firefighters, engineers, and captains who rode with each other damn near every day. We knew each other's *modus operandi* and trained daily on every potential fireground task. Damyon Wallace, Dave Austin, Zach Powell, and I were the Truckies at Station 4. We had a combined seventy-five years of experience on our department and knew exactly how to make things go our way on the fireground and in the station. It was everything I'd ever dreamed of in a career.

While the other firefighters around town were napping in their brown chairs, we were sitting in ours, blindfolded, buddy breathing off each other's Scott tanks, in case one of us ran out of air during a rescue later that night. Or studying Higbee notches, blindfolded, with our thick fire gloves on, so we could find our way out of a fire in zero visibility, with poor dexterity, by feeling the lugs on the hose couplings.

In addition to helping thread the couplings together faster, the Higbee notched lugs could tell us which direction the nozzle was. The female side of the hose coupling always had a shorter lug and led outside, while the male end had a longer lug and led toward the nozzle. Little things like these could make the difference between being a hero and being dead, so we put extra time and effort into practical training methods every day.

On a 99-degree summer afternoon around 16:00 hours, a full alarm fire came in for an abandoned, turn-of-the-century high school building in the center of town. We rolled over, lights and sirens on Truck 4 and, upon arrival at the old school, observed heavy brown smoke showing from the three-story roof of the building. We set up the truck on the charlie side, and I helped Dave raise the aerial while Damyon checked in with command.

As we laddered the roof, Damyon returned, and I climbed up to discover a roof hatch had been opened over the gymnasium. That's where the smoke was pouring out from. We exited the roof and cut the chains on the gymnasium's double doors, then made entry. This was a dual court basketball gym that was over three stories high. The thick smoke was banked down to the floor and chugging out the doors. We used the thermal camera to search the gym and found that it was empty. There had to be another area that was burning and causing all the putrid brown smoke.

From the opposite side of the building, Engine 1 and Truck 1 were working our way. They'd entered the locker rooms and found an Olympic-sized swimming pool that had been filled with foam blocks for gymnastics classes. After the gymnastics company had gone out of business, renovation crews had covered the pool with plywood. A stray spark from a grinder had found its way into the foam pit and the entire pit had burned away, leaving the floor over it precariously perched above a long fall to the bottom of the empty pool.

All of this became apparent during overhaul operations, but with the place still heavily charged with smoke, crews were searching all over for the seat of the fire. After our team's *fourth* air bottle change, and subsequent foray into the smoke, I was midway through the search of a room in zero visibility when I just couldn't move another step. I was beyond exhausted and felt like I could die. My muscles wouldn't work. I grabbed Damyon to tell him I was in trouble.

He said to stay right there. That he was going to finish searching the room and come right back for me.

I couldn't have moved if I'd wanted to. It was all I could do just to keep breathing.

He returned, helped me to my feet, and we made our way out of the structure. I collapsed on the ground, and the medics peeled the snowmobile-suit-like turnout gear off me to cool down.

The seat of the fire was eventually located in the pool and quickly extinguished. The foam in the pool had burned away and smoldered until almost none remained. It filled the entire high school with toxic hydrogen cyanide gas. We were all poisoned with it, and a few of our crew were even transported to the hospital. Their blood gasses later showed near lethal doses, and they were administered cyano-kits to counter the effects of the poison gas.

Our gear had to be deconned twice because it was so contaminated with cyanide that even after the initial cleaning, it still registered toxic levels on our four gas chromatography monitors while hanging in our floor lockers. The combination of the heat and exertion, coupled with the cyanide, severely limited my body's ability to transport and deliver oxygen to my organs and muscles. I'd never felt that way before or after, and it was the only time in my life I *ever* felt I could've died in a fire.

Chapter 30

Hurt in Holt

On December 10, 2017, a full alarm came into the station around 02:00 hours for a structure fire at a home in Delphi Township, known locally as Holt. Engine 4 and Truck 4 rushed off into the chilly winter night, toward the mutual aid scene. We arrived first, beating the part-timers and volunteers into their own fireground.

Heavy smoke and flames were visible from the charlie (or back) side of the three-story home. The homeowner met us at the curb and advised everyone had evacuated the structure. Captain Spoons and I, on Truck 4, walked around to the back and discovered the chimney chase at the rear of the house had completely burned away, down to the framing members. The fire had moved into the attic, from the chimney all the way to the peak of the roof.

The smoldering, thirty-foot-high, framing members of the chimney were teetering precariously. Spoons said to try to pull them down, to avoid a collapse injury to the incoming units. I pulled hard on one of them with my pike pole and it came crashing down to the ground in a flurry of embers and flames.

Firefighter Donny Hurt and Captain Bubbles on Engine 9 came around the back corner of the house. Donny began attempting to help me pull the second burning chimney spire down. It teetered precariously in my direction, so I told Donny to wait for me to move out of the way before pulling it down. He acknowledged.

I turned and walked away opposite from the direction it was leaning—toward Spoons and BC Julian Burke—up the hill and away from the house. The whole world shook as a tremendous weight crashed into my head and surrounded me in a flash of brilliant light. Donny had pulled the beam down right on top of me, sending my helmet flying across the yard.

Spoons and Donny both rushed over to help, and as I picked my lid off the ground, Spoons yelled, "Oh my god, are you OK?"

They were patting my turnout coat, trying to put out the fire from the burning beam.

"What the *fuck*, motherfucker!" I yelled at Donny.

He apologized. I shoved him and took a swing as Spoons restrained me from behind.

"What the hell is wrong with you *asshole*? I told you to wait so I could get out of the way, and you dropped it right the *fuck* on me!" I yelled.

I should have known when Bubbles walked up shit was going to go south in a hurry. What were the odds that beam could have fallen right on my fucking dome? There were at least 180 degrees it could have toppled over and slammed to the ground. But it had to fall directly into the path I was walking.

My helmet was still smoldering and burned from the beam's impact, and my shoulder was blackened from burning soot. BC Julian Burke was standing a just few feet away when the incident occurred right in front of him.

Spoons asked again if I was OK, could I continue?

"I'm fine. Just pissed off," I replied.

"Let's get the roof laddered and run a trench cut to stop the fire then," he suggested.

Together we returned to our truck at the street. I pulled an extension ladder, while he grabbed the roof ladder. We set them up as Engineer Powell left the saws and hand tools on the ground next to the ladder. On the roof I went about zipping out the trench cut with the chain saw. We both struggled to stay vertical on the snow- and ice-covered surface of the shingles.

When the trench cut was complete, the interior nozzle crews located an attic scuttle hole and sprayed the fire out from there. Soon the flames were extinguished, and we packed our gear and headed back to the station, leaving the township rigs to handle the overhaul of their scene. Before we left, the BC ordered Spoons to write up the incident in an injury report when we returned to the firehouse—due to the severity of the impact he'd witnessed. Back at the station, we showered and fell into bed for an hour or two of sleep before shift change.

Over the next twenty-four hours my behavioral and cognitive abilities declined rapidly. I forgot my close friend's names, couldn't finish thoughts and communications, had memory hiccups, developed Tourette-like symptoms, and was extremely combative and confrontational. Though my life was the best it had ever been up to this incident, I became suicidal.

The next morning, I ran a few errands with my son, and everything just felt off. I was angry at everyone for the slightest things and popped off at them with flurries of cuss words. I told my wife a beam had fallen on me at a fire. That I had a headache from the incident, but that was it. I was fine. That evening we had our whole family over for dinner and they all said I seemed quiet, withdrawn, and unusually contemplative.

The following day I was back at work and things went normally, for a slow, quiet day on the ladder truck. We had a couple of fire runs—nothing too crazy. My colleagues said that I seemed agitated and kept asking me what was wrong. The next day was my son's birthday, and he says I yelled at him all day. We went out to dinner at the Old Chicago restaurant, and I argued with my wife and son. He told me it was the worst birthday ever, and my wife said she just wanted to be with someone who was happy. What does that even mean? I couldn't understand.

The next day they left for work and school, and I sat on my bed with a pistol in my lap having suicidal thoughts. I text them they'd be better off without me. Lee called Dave Austin and asked him to check up on me. A few minutes later I got a phone call from Dave as I was sitting there about to blow my brains out. I talked to him for the next forty minutes—just bullshitting—never once mentioning anything about my emotional state.

I put the gun away after we hung up, but I carried it everywhere I went for the next three weeks, even to work. I suffered from uncontrollable crying (lability), increased impulsivity, anger, nausea, lack of appetite, headaches, neck pain, slurred speech, and was just waiting for a somewhat worthy opportunity to kill myself. I was a ticking time bomb.

I crashed my brand-new Jeep Wrangler into a tree while backing out of my own driveway because I forgot which pedal was the brake and mashed the gas. It happened a second time while backing into my driveway the next day, and I plowed into my wife's vehicle with mine. I kept forgetting my best friend's names and couldn't finish sentences because I had trouble recalling the words I'd wanted to use.

On December 28, I booked a $10,000 Disney vacation for the upcoming spring break without talking to my wife about it first. The 29th was my birthday, and I adamantly refused to celebrate. It was a difficult day, I cried a lot, and argued with my entire family. My wife pleaded with me, telling me something was seriously wrong and made me promise to talk to my supervisors about my head injury symptoms. I agreed and just blew it off.

When I returned to work on January 2, 2018, Lee called me at 07:30 and begged me to put her on speakerphone with my officers, threatening to call them herself if I didn't. We talked with the captains; she explained the situation and walked them through her last two weeks of emotional struggles with me. They agreed I hadn't been my normal self and removed me from duty. Battalion Chief Jughead took me to emergency for an exam. They ran a head and neck CT scan, with a blood draw and urinalysis.

As we sat in the room together waiting for the test results, I wondered what Jughead would do if he knew I had a loaded gun in the duffle beside me. All those sleepless nights on the ambulance together, and here the two of us were, in the fucking ER, him now a BC, and me still a dumbass firefighter with a gun, getting checked out for a concussion. How had we ended up here? I just wanted to be cleared for duty and get back in the game.

The nurses and doctors we knew from our ambulance days kept coming in and offering condolences and ways to help if we needed anything. It was sweet of them. When the test results came back, the CT showed negative for brain bleeds, positive for bulging discs in vertebrae C5, C6, C7, and all the labs came back within normal parameters. I was diagnosed with concussion syndrome and released right back to work. They referred me to PAR Rehab for concussion grading and advised me to follow up with my PCP. Jughead dropped me back off at Station 4 and took copies of my discharge paperwork back to Operations with him.

I finished the shift at the firehouse and had the next day off at home. I worked another quiet shift on the 4th of January—just a couple of fire alarms, nothing too crazy—in what would end up being my last shift ever as a firefighter.

All hell broke loose on January 7.

That morning I argued with my wife. She threw the mistakes and misdeeds of my past at me, suggested our relationship was over, and that was all it took. It was the moment I'd been waiting for. I pulled out my pistol and chambered a round. I raced from our bedroom, down the stairs, with Lee screaming behind me. I flew out the back door thinking, if I shot myself on the surface of our frozen in-ground pool, it would be easier for everyone to clean up the mess.

As I stood in the center of the pool, I looked up to the sky and said, "Here I come."

I put the barrel of the gun to my head, squeezed the trigger past the halfway point and waited for the hammer to strike the firing pin. My wife ran outside and screamed in terror, "Baby *NO*! Our son is watching!"

Time seemed to stop as I paused for a moment and thought about him—witnessing his father's blood and brains sprayed across the white snow and ice on our pool, and the trauma and horrible life he'd have to suffer through in the aftermath of it all. Possibly following in my footsteps and killing himself, too. The odds were that he would, you know.

In that brief moment, I thought of all the future moments I'd miss. His graduation, his wedding, his children. Their weddings and their children. I took a deep breath of crisp January air, came to my senses, and lowered the gun. I went to go find my son, who'd witnessed the whole event and had taken off running down the snow-covered street in his pajamas and bare feet as he cried uncontrollably, unsure how to handle the flood of emotions drowning him in sorrow.

"Banks, come back! It's OK," I yelled after him.

When he returned to the end of our driveway, I could tell he was skeptical of my offer.

"Come inside," I said.

"No! Why did you do that?" he asked me through the tears.

"Mom said she wants a divorce," I answered.

Lee was standing in the driveway behind me and vehemently denied that was the case, through sobs of her own.

I heard sirens approaching as I stood at the end of the driveway. I asked Lee if she'd called the police, and between hyperventilating breaths and tears, she confirmed, yes. I ran back into the house and out the back door, racked the shell from the chamber of the gun, and put the round into my pocket. I stashed the gun in the rafters of the garage and jumped the back fence onto Liberty Road to go for a walk until things cooled down. As I walked down the street, police cruisers passed by going lights and sirens. I waved at the ones I knew from seeing them at training events and emergency scenes. Some waved back, some didn't. None of them recognized me as the person they were rushing in to secure.

I made a big circle around the perimeter of my neighborhood and as I was coming back home, I passed the street my captain, Damyon, lived on. Surprisingly, at that very moment, he happened to drive by. He pulled over and rolled down his window.

"What up B?" he asked.

"Just out for some fresh air," I replied.

We exchanged greetings, and he asked if I was all right.

"Of course. It's a good day for a walk," I said.

He was on his way home from church with his two sons and I asked him what the message of the sermon had been. The boys couldn't recall. Damyon mentioned it was something about friendship and brotherhood among Christians. *How perfect,* I thought.

He said the cops had the whole neighborhood blocked off over by my house; he was worried it was for me, and asked again if I was all right.

I lied to him and denied knowing anything about it.

We said our goodbyes, then he went on his way and so did I.

I walked past the park and approached my street. At the far end, I could see a dozen or so police cars surrounding my home. The BC's car, Medic 9, and Engine 9 were staged a block away. Farther down the street, a police cruiser was blocking the entrance to the neighborhood. I decided to head back to Damyon's place until it all blew over.

I rang the doorbell and he invited me in.

After confessing the situation, he said people had been calling him. Chase Powers was the BC on the scene for a barricaded gunman at my house, and they were trying to contact me. My wife and son were in the back of a police car. He still hadn't told them he'd seen me.

Damyon advised that sooner or later I was going to have to face the music.

He was right. I'd become somewhat of a fugitive and was jeopardizing his kindness by being there. I thanked him for his hospitality and advice, then headed back out into the cold January morning. I walked down my street and straight into the scene. Nobody even noticed me.

I was standing in the middle of the road in front of my house and could see the START team readying to break through my doors. They were dressed for battle, wearing body armor, with riot shields, and semi-automatic rifles at the ready. I'd left my cell phone inside the house, and they'd been calling and pinging it, thinking they had a barricaded gunman, and that I'd most likely killed myself when they received no response to their calls over the past hour or so. I could see my wife and son in the back seat of a cruiser a few houses away. As the police were about to swing their battering rams and break down my doors, I called out to them.

"Hey!" I yelled from the middle of the road. "You guys looking for me?"

Everyone turned and leveled their AR-15s, shotguns, and pistols at me. "What's your name?" the commander asked, training his gun on me.

"You all know me. I'm Brad Lilly. This is my house."

"Stay right there, show me your hands," the sergeant ordered.

I raised my arms with empty, open palms.

"Turn around. Do you have any weapons on you?"

"No sir," I replied.

"I'm going to pat you down, don't move," he replied. He told his squad to cover him while he frisked me.

"All clear," he called out. "Where's the gun?" he asked.

"I don't have a gun," I replied.

"Is it secured? That's all I need to know."

"Yes," I answered.

"I'm not going to handcuff you in front of your family," he said. "You know we have to take you to CMH, or to the hospital for a psych eval."

"I know. Which car are we going to?" I asked.

"Right over here," he said, leading me to a cruiser and Jane Berry, a female police officer I'd known for years.

In the car, she asked if I had a preference of CMH or the hospital.

"CMH. Then I can just walk home when I'm done," I replied, and we were off.

We passed BC Chase Powers standing at the curb. He wouldn't even look at me.

It was a short ride across the street from my backyard to CMH. As we entered the lobby, an intake nurse asked me what type of insurance I had.

"PHP," I replied.

She coldly advised they didn't accept that insurance and that it would be five hundred dollars out of pocket to speak with a therapist there.

I laughed and said something witty and sarcastic to Jane about our quality city health insurance. She didn't appear to find it amusing.

"Y'all really know how to kick a man when he's down," I said to the stone-faced intake nurse. "I don't have five hundred dollars to waste on a bad day." And we headed off for the hospital next.

We arrived and I was placed in room four, right next to the entrance. They put me on suicide watch and removed all the medical equipment except the bed from the room, with a mandatory open-door policy. My coworkers on ambulances kept coming in and out, waving hello as they passed by, dropping their patients off in other rooms, then coming in and out of my room, asking about the situation. There was zero privacy. Engine 9, Medic 9, and Battalion 1 had all been called to the barricaded gunman scene earlier, and by now, the whole fire department knew.

I explained to the doctors about my head injury and the previous hospital visit. That I'd suffered a concussion at a fire and just needed treatment for that. The doctors ordered the same tests the other hospital had. I explained they'd find nothing new, respectfully declining all further tests, adding that they were completely pointless.

The doctors called the battalion chief to let him know I was non-compliant. Chase sent a couple of new kids—Francesco Russo and Javier Longoria—the Medic 9 crew who'd been at my house earlier, over to coerce me into following the doctor's orders. They were allowed into the room along with other fire department employees who had no business being there.

The lead physician, Dr. Warrant, attempted to empathize with me by leaning in close and explaining, in a whisper, how he'd just caught his wife in bed fucking another man, and would've killed them both if he didn't have children with the woman. He said he sympathized with me, and he just needed me to allow them to do their job and run a lab panel. Did he really think his confessional was going to make me consent to giving them blood draws and urinalysis? The man was both creepy and crazy.

Speaking of crazy, the ER psychologist came in next and asked me several questions regarding the day's events. I was honest and told her the truth about what happened. Then she and the PA signed a clinical certification committing me to a mental hospital. They believed I was a danger to myself and others.

Krishna and Dave Austin showed up and stayed by my side with me in the room. After seven hours of observation, I was told by Probationary Firefighter Russo that if I consented to the blood draw, they'd let me go home. When I agreed, all the labs came back normal again. However, instead of going home, I was denied release and committed to a psychiatric hospital. I'd been lied to by my coworkers, and I was furious.

I contemplated walking out. What could they do? Security was preparing to stop me, and more guards were assembling outside my room.

"What are you guys gonna do?" I yelled. "You really wanna fight me? You all *fucking* know me!"

I knew the $10 an hour they were paid to provide security for the hospital was far less motivation than I had to leave the facility. I could take them all. The betrayal of my colleagues enraged me to the point of superhuman strength. My head was pounding, and I was beyond combative.

Damyon walked in and joined Krishna and Dave in attempting to calm me down.

"Just roll with it, bro. You'll be back in no time. The three of us will look after your fam until you get out," he said.

I couldn't fight both my brother firefighters and security now, and I was despondent.

A private ambulance arrived to transport me to the psychiatric hospital.

As security personnel came in to return my possessions, they asked me to sign a release, stating everything they'd taken away earlier had been returned to me.

"How can I sign a legal document when I've just been certified insane?" I asked.

They seemed perplexed and had no answers. I threw my engagement and wedding rings across the floor of the emergency department as the private ambulance crew wheeled me out to their meat wagon. I wouldn't be needing them anymore.

I was grief-stricken and rode to the psychiatric facility in silence, refusing to speak. At the intake exam I was treated like a criminal. I told them I shouldn't be there and requested immediate release. They said everyone says that and denied my request. I asked to call my attorney and they denied that, too. I requested treatment for my head injury and was told they weren't capable of that at this facility. They asked me the same hundred questions the previous hospitals had, and I refused to answer.

They had me strip naked, shower in cold water, then performed a skin check and body cavity search for contraband. My possessions were confiscated, and I was involuntarily placed on medication. It was like a prison, and no one seemed to care that I was acting this way due to a head injury. It was the exact opposite of the care I so desperately needed at the time.

I was put in a facility with the mentally insane and the clinically psychotic. I refused to eat or drink anything and was prescribed anti-seizure medicine to control mood swings. I'd hide them in my upper gum line and spit them out after I walked away, tucking them deep into the dirt of the community room plants, where the surveillance cameras couldn't see. I didn't sleep a wink. Every fifteen minutes the techs would stand in the doorway and shine a flashlight on me to make sure I was still breathing. I simply held a thumb up in the air, so they'd leave.

The next morning, I met with the facility director. She threatened to keep me there for up to ninety days if I didn't comply with their treatment program and sign a voluntary admission intake form. Again, I asked how my signature, while clinically insane, held any legal gravity.

"Just sign the document or you'll have a much harder time fighting to be released from here in court," the director told me.

Apparently, if I signed a voluntary admission, I'd be released faster, and the director would request the court ordered certification be dismissed. If not, she threatened to keep me for up to thirty, sixty, or even ninety days.

I signed that shit on the spot, legal signature or not. Later, I found out by signing it, I'd agreed to personally pay for my five day stay there, which totaled over ten thousand dollars.

I went along with the program, attended group therapy, and participated in activities just to get released. I spent my free time doing push-ups, sit-ups, and dips on the community room furniture, trying to stay fit in case one of the psychos in there attacked me. I didn't sleep, eat, or drink and it was one of the absolute *worst* times of my life.

The chairs and tables in that joint were freakin' heavy. They were specifically designed with a ballast inside, to make them less likely to be used as projectiles, and were all one molded piece so no parts could be broken off and used as weapons. Every table, planter, entertainment stand, or desk, even the pictures on the walls were bolted down to their surfaces and immovable without special tools, which we didn't have access to. The place was designed like a prison, with checkpoints and access card approval for entry and exit of certain areas. I had to request a toothbrush and toothpaste, then return them after supervised use. I had to request a drink of water from the staff, and they'd give me a tiny paper cup full.

I was a crazy magnet. The certifiably insane patients were always flocking over to me, and in a room full of twenty chairs, they'd find the ones right next to me every time. They'd copy my activities and follow me around the facilities everywhere I went. Even the doctors, nurses, and techs began to agree that I probably didn't belong in there. I didn't quite fit the mold of their typical patient.

I met Ali, a twenty-year-old habitual cutter who'd been incarcerated at the facility for six weeks. And Trevor, a sixteen-year-old manic depressive whose own parents had him committed because he told them he'd heard voices telling him to drop out of school and then attempted suicide after they told him he was crazy. Stephanie was a middle-aged woman who'd been in and out of the facility for numerous anxiety and paranoia spells. Later that night, a new inmate was admitted around 02:00 hours and he immediately caused a stir.

Lunatic Nick, as I affectionately called him, started screaming obscenities and slamming things around 03:30 hours. He screamed, sang songs, and threatened the staff at the top of his lungs until around 05:30 hours. The open-door policy there really sucked ass. Especially when a psychopath was standing in the doorway of my room, six feet away from my bed, threatening to kill everyone in the joint.

I remembered my Krav Maga lessons from Victory Martial Arts. If my hands were still free, I could cup them and slap my attacker's ears, rupturing their ear drums and eliminating their sense of sound. Then take my thumbs and drive them into my attacker's eye sockets, eliminating their sense of sight. With my left hand, hold their head and with my right elbow, drive it into my attacker's left temple, hopefully knocking them unconscious. Grab their head with both hands and send a flying knee into their face to finish the job. Then get away fast and find help.

That was my three-second plan of action, as I feared for my life safety in a place that was supposed to help me recover from my injuries and restore my sanity. My concussion symptoms were still as bad as ever, and I struggled with headaches, depression, and anxiety. I was in survival mode and just trying to make it through the moment.

I ate my first food the morning of the third day. Pancakes and bacon, a banana and water. After breakfast we had group therapy. The patients all sat in the community room with our instructors, answering questions about how we felt today, and were we having any suicidal thoughts. Through the half wall Plexiglas window that ran the length of the room, we could see and hear the new guy, Nick. He absolutely lost his mind at the nurses' station. He slapped a stack of papers from a tech's hands up into the air and then ran over to a metal open door and began slamming it repeatedly. "Code grey" blared over the PA system on repeat, and soon close to thirty staff members surrounded Nick while he rampaged.

The group therapy class watched in horror as he slammed the heavy steel door over and over, for what seemed like fifty times, until the *entire* metal door frame just fell right out of the wall and onto the floor. Apparently, that was the isolation room they'd locked him in the night before and he was just making sure they couldn't do the same thing to him again tonight.

The entire staff just stood back and let him rage, doing nothing at all to stop him or to protect us from him. They just stood there and watched. When Nick was done, he screamed at the staff and stormed off to another part of the hallway out of view of the class, and the crowd of employees followed along behind him. This was the exact opposite of therapeutic rehabilitation.

After filling out our daily intentions sheet, we had free time. I was advised my wife was on the phone for me and I could take the call if I wished. Lee said one of the nurses there had called CPS (Child Protective Services); they were meeting with my sons and daughters, and had just finished speaking with her.

Lee had a meltdown and bawled her eyes out on the phone, saying she hadn't slept or eaten since the incident. I knew the feeling. She was so stressed out, handling everything for her business and the whole family while I was incarcerated. We agreed to meet at visiting time the following evening and said goodbye.

Brenda was the nurse who'd called CPS after the intake exam. When I hung up the phone and confronted her, she apologized. She explained she was required by law to report all incidents with guns and kids. I get it; she was just doing her job. Whatever. The hits kept coming.

After lunch, during the afternoon group therapy, Lunatic Nick lit it up again. This time screaming and yelling as he pounded a Plexiglas window repeatedly until it shattered from its frame onto the hallway floor.

The "code grey" alert was again broadcast throughout the facility with its annoying alarm tone. As our instructor left the group to tend to Nick, he asked me to lock the door behind him and keep track of the other patients while he was gone. Great. Now I was a babysitter for the insane patients. It was kind of like making the officer rank at the fire department, I thought.

The facility director, a tiny, frail old woman, walked right up to Nick, a giant young man, in the middle of his tantrum and handed him a small paper cup with meds and another with water. He stopped his raging and looked at her for a moment, then took his meds and calmed down. What the *fuck*, man? This place was like the *Twilight Zone*, I swear.

We made strength trees in the evening group therapy with a male therapist named Leslie. We had to list all our perceived strengths on the branches of the tree and then color the page with crayons. Toward the end of the session, Leslie stepped out of the room and left the door open. Nick walked by screaming, "FUUUUUUCK!" and then yelling, "AAAAAHHH!" in alternating sequences at full-roar volume. I closed and locked the door just as he walked up to it. Once again, I was protecting the looney bin crew, who scurried off into opposite corners of the community room and began rocking back and forth, chanting inaudibly on the floor.

At physical therapy that evening, I talked with Ms. Sarah one of the nurses, about filing a request for immediate discharge if Lunatic Nick went on another rant all night again, screaming up and down the hallways and pounding on the walls. I told her it was the exact opposite of therapeutic there since he'd arrived. She said that only the director could approve it, otherwise I'd be leaving AMA (against medical advice) and the CERT would be re-filed. Damn.

Nick flipped out in the hallway outside of the gym as we spoke, pounding his fists against the walls and screaming his patented, "FUUUUUUCK," and then, "AAAAAAAHHH!"

"How come you guys don't do anything to stop him when he does that?" I asked.

"We're a strictly hands-off facility, low security, and not licensed for physical restraint. He does fine when he takes his meds, and it's just a matter of dialing in the right dosage for him," she replied.

"Yeah, I'm gonna recommend you guys double that shit right now," I advised.

Ms. Sarah laughed and agreed.

Back in the dormitory after PT, I requested permission to get cleaned up, then took a cold shower and brushed my teeth before bedtime. Why was there no warm water here? There were no doors on the bathrooms and a tech had to stand outside while you washed. As I showered, the tech asked me if I'd had any suicidal thoughts today, what my anxiety and depression levels were, and if I felt that I was ready for discharge.

I answered, "None for the first three questions and you're goddamn right for the last."

Don't ever fucking tell them the truth. You are absolutely in tip top mental health and you've never felt better in your life. If you breathe a word to the contrary, they will incarcerate your ass and strip you of all your basic human civil rights. I'd learned my lesson; they don't give a fuck *who* you are *or* what you've been through. You're just fresh meat and a paycheck for them if you say how you really feel about things.

After returning the toiletries to the nurses' station, it was lights out. It's not very restful, though. Not when every fifteen minutes someone walks into the room and stares at you through the darkness. It's quite unnerving. I'd wake up every time and at this point say, "Hi, Carl," or "Hi, Laura," or "G'mornin, Scott," because we were all on a first name basis by now. That way, I'd let them know I was breathing straight away so they could go carry on with the rest of their rounds and let me catch a few winks. At least until the next set of rounds fifteen minutes later.

Nick was back at it again that night. Apparently, Ms. Sarah didn't relay my advice on the medication adjustment. Tonight, it was Scott and Jesse on night watch duty, with both techs standing in my doorway at 03:00 hours.

"Wide awake, guys!" I shouted.

"Damn, man, we thought you were asleep," Jesse said.

"Who can sleep with a madman banging on the walls and standing in my doorway screaming, 'I'm so fucking thirsty!' or with you guys sprinting past my room to try to calm that idiot down from pounding on shit," I replied.

Just then, Nick snuck up behind them both and screamed, "FUUUUUUUUCK!" and then, "RAAAAAAHHH!" The two techs jumped out of their skin and hurried off to return Nick to his room and sedate him with more tranquilizers.

I jumped up and slammed the dormitory door behind them as they left. A few minutes later Scott came in and asked why the door was closed. It was a rhetorical question; he knew exactly why it was closed. Sitting on the radiator in front of the window, I explained that nurses Sarah and Brenda told me that if Nick popped off again and I felt unsafe, I was allowed to close my door. This was the third night with no sleep, and I'd been up for seventy-two hours straight.

I laughed and wondered how the fuck this could be happening to me. *This* was the therapeutic treatment we gave our heroes and emergency responders who were injured in the line of duty? No wonder so many of our soldiers were coming back home and ending their lives. The care we need as heroes is nonexistent at best. Not only that, but it's the exact opposite of helpful and only exacerbates the problems we're having in the first place.

At 04:15 hours, Scott came in, and I gave him the thumbs-up and said, "Still awake."

"Damn, man, why?" he asked.

"Outside of the door slamming, wall pounding, and yelling, I'm a firefighter. I'm used to sleeping light and popping straight out of bed when the alarm goes off."

Jesse came into my room midway through the conversation. I guess this was the hangout spot for now.

"I used to be an EMT for a private ambulance service," Jesse said, "Then I had to do a goddamn cricothyrotomy on a little kid and promptly quit that shit right after."

I could sympathize with that. "They bleed a lot from that procedure. Way more than you'd expect," I offered.

This place sucks, I thought. How was I supposed to get better here? Do the people at the hospitals even know what this place they'd sentenced me to is like?

"What's the worst thing you've ever seen on a call?" Scott asked me.

Yep. There it was. Here we go again.

We stayed up all night talking about horrific runs and the crazy things we'd seen, until the day shift arrived, and it was time for morning vitals. They'd take our vital signs at 06:15, so we were pretty much up for the whole day at that point. I was usually 115/60, 60 strong and regular for a pulse, with a 93 percent SpO_2 on room air.

Breakfast on the fourth day was scrambled eggs and bacon with a banana nut muffin. The cafeteria was definitely my favorite thing about that place. If there was any good thing to be gleaned from that shit show, it was the food.

We had morning group therapy next. The therapist was an older gentleman named Bill, who said he knew my wife and was a regular client of hers. Great. With a double extra creamy helping of super juicy sarcasm right on top. Bill turned off the low-volume background music I'd put on the TV earlier to try to calm the crazy patients' nerves, and now it was just awkwardly quiet in the room.

I swear I could hear Bill's heartbeat as he asked Trevor and the other Brad about their anxiety levels today. They just sat there in silence, refusing to answer him. They knew the routine. If they said how they really felt, they were fucked. Only now they were double fucked at the same time because they refused to lie about it. They just sat there not willing to participate, which only served to increase their intolerable length of stay at the *Hotel California*.

The facility director asked to see me in her office and when the tech knocked on the community room door, I jumped at the chance to leave the group. She mentioned she'd spoken with my

PCP, my wife Lee, and my *brother* Krishna (he told her he was my real brother), and she'd agreed to release me tomorrow morning at 10:00 hours. I thanked her and returned to the group therapy just as it was finishing up. As Bill left the room, crazy Nick sauntered in and sat down right beside me. Twenty other *fucking* chairs at the table, and he sat right next to me.

After a brief moment of silence, he said, "Nice tattoos. Watch this."

He stood up and took the basket of crayons, left on the table after group therapy, and walked out into the hallway. Looking back at me he yelled, "Oops!" and dumped hundreds of crayons onto the hallway floor right outside of the nurses' station. He snagged an apple from the fruit basket on the nurse's desk and returned to his seat beside me at the table.

He was staring at me. "Don't you want to know why?" he asked.

"Why?" I said, unamused.

"Because I'm bored, man! Everyone around here is so stuffy and uptight. I just bring a little spice into their lives and make it exciting!" he stated.

"So, you're an anarchist," I replied.

He stood up and threw the apple against the wall across the room, exploding it into a hundred pieces of pulp and juice, and then sat back down.

"Naw, man. I give them purpose and meaning to their lives!"

I leaned in close. "Don't fuck with me, Nick," I said, looking him dead in the eyes. "I'm going home in twenty-four hours. You mess that up for me and I will end your miserable fucking existence. Are we clear?"

"Crystal," he said, sitting back in his chair.

Ali came in with Stephanie and we all played a nice game of UNO, until Nick got bored right in the middle of it and walked out without a word. Undoubtedly, to wreak havoc somewhere else in the facility.

I spoke with my oldest son on the phone later that day. He reminded me of a poem he'd written back in junior high about me being his angel and savior. It was good to hear from him. I was looking forward to seeing my family tonight and going home tomorrow.

Nurse Rene gave me some advice on forgiveness and for meeting with my wife and son for the first time since the incident. "Just let it play out, no expectations. Listen to what they have to say and accept it. You fucked up. If they want to forgive you, that's up to them. If it's meant to be, it'll be," she offered.

Hah! I recalled Hector Garcia telling me that in the parking lot of Fives when we'd first smoked pot on duty together. What was it, damn near twenty years ago now?

Music therapy that afternoon sucked balls. The therapist played her favorite country music songs and asked us to explain the stories and how the music made us feel. Pretty sure I was the only one who went along with the game. Most were too concerned with Nick out in the hallway ranting at full volume.

"This place is pointless! All I do is sit around and sleep, eat, and shit, and the staff here does nothing to help me! You're all worthless!" he yelled.

He wasn't wrong, and none of the staff members chastised him for making a scene. He kicked open the door to the community room. As it slammed off its backstop, most of the class scurried off to their corners and began rocking. He walked over and sat in one of the recently vacated chairs right beside me. I ignored him, and the therapist welcomed him to the class. Midway through one of her next sentences, he got bored and walked out of the room, pretending to throw a punch at one of the techs standing in the doorway, just to see him flinch.

After group he was following me everywhere and copying my actions. He'd sit right next to me in the cafeteria now and order the same foods I would. In the gym he'd watch me from the opposite side and copy all the exercises I'd do. He was actually fairly respectful to me now, but I didn't trust him enough to take my eyes off him for a second. I just hoped I'd make it out of there alive before he tried something stupid.

Dinner that night was ribs, mac and cheese, corn, and a cheddar biscuit. I'd made friends with the food prep staff, and we'd kick around recipes and kitchen tips when I'd go through the line. Their breakfast bacon was always perfect, and we discussed using the oven to make it that way. Nick filled his tray up with food and then dumped the whole thing on the floor on purpose, refusing to clean it up. What a crazy, stupid motherfucker.

On the fourth night, I was allowed to meet with my family after dinner, in the cafeteria. Banks sprinted across the room when he saw me and jumped up into my arms. Lee joined us and we embraced for a long time, with no one saying a word. We sat at the cafeteria table. It was great to see them. We'd missed each other tremendously. We apologized and forgave each other, promising to work on our issues and not let things happen that way ever again. They said they knew it wasn't my fault, it was the firefighting head injury that caused it.

That night, I slept for two hours straight, between Nick's temper tantrums, of course. After breakfast I said goodbye to the staff, and they wished me well. Krishna met me at 10:00 that morning and signed for my release into his custody. He immediately noticed and questioned the glaringly obvious lack of *any* continuum of patient care and requested to speak with the facility director.

I loved this dude. He called them out on their shitty substandard of care and was exactly right. He asked why my PCP's three phone calls per day went unreturned for three days and why I was held for forty-eight hours longer than required by law, when they knew full well that they were completely incapable of treating my TBI (traumatic brain injury) at their facility. They had no excuse.

He absolutely grilled the director and questioned why there were no appointments scheduled for my continued head injury treatment, when their own discharge paperwork listed the clinical diagnosis as depression and suicidal ideation due to head trauma. My warrior brother was lambasting my captors with the legal ramifications of their negligence, and I just sat back and smiled while they scrambled to book follow-up appointments and cover their tracks.

The discharge took two hours longer than expected, but I was finally released and given my personal belongings back. Oh, the joys of wearing shoelaces again! Of having cherry Chapstick on my lips! And my leather jacket on my back again! It had been five days of sensory deprivation and all the little things were magnified to the extreme. Krishna pulled the wedding rings I'd tossed across the emergency room from his pocket.

"You're gonna need these, too," he said matter-of-factly.

When the facility doors opened to the parking lot, the fresh air of freedom smelled amazing! It was the first time I'd been outside in five days. Everything was so crisp and vibrant, like I was experiencing it all for the first time.

The road conditions on the way home were beautifully treacherous. A snowstorm had raged all night into the morning and huge drifts encroached onto the pavement. Krishna drove to our favorite Mexican taco bar, and we ate like kings, my treat of course. I went to the restroom and was never so thankful for a door on the bathroom. I didn't even mind the piss all over the floor and the scent of urinal cakes. It was all perfectly beautiful to me.

It was surreal. I could feel the emotions of all the people in the restaurant. After not having those sensory experiences for a while, I could see and feel everything going on around me with increased vibrancy and intensity. I was hypersensitive to it all.

Grateful for my freedom, I paid for lunch and filled up Krishna's truck with fuel. He dropped me off at home and then left.

I made some coffee and shoveled the snow from the driveway. Simple things carried with them strong emotions of gratitude.

Lee arrived home from work a short time later. We made up for lost time and spent the rest of the night in each other's arms. She hadn't eaten since I'd left, so we ordered food and then fell into bed together.

She woke me up crying at 06:15. She was still asleep and having a nightmare about me pulling the trigger and that she couldn't revive me. I shook her awake and she cried in my arms. She was in rough shape, and I realized the full extent of what I'd put her through. She'd lost seven pounds in six days from heartache and suffering.

In the morning, I played a video game with my son, enjoyed time in the hot tub and sauna at our house, and took an *actual* hot shower. The showers at the psych hospital were freezing cold, and there was always someone standing in the bathroom asking if I felt like killing myself today. It was good to be home.

I was having concussion symptoms still. Feelings of anxiety, being overwhelmed in the heavy traffic, and having difficulty articulating thoughts into words. I utilized deep breathing techniques and calm, patient decision making. I was quiet and contemplative about life and the value of things I'd previously taken for granted. Lee says I was withdrawn; that I was still mentally in lock up and not fully present.

Over the coming days, we'd occasionally stop by the firehouse and have breakfast or coffee with the crews, and they'd offer their support and assistance if I needed it. I was on duty injury leave and checking in with the officers was required. There was an uncomfortable feeling in the air when I'd visit; a sort of, elephant in the room that no one wanted to talk about. Was I coming back to work or was I going to duty out? I'd always thought of the line-of-duty disability people as weak and sissified, and now, here I was on the other side of the table with the active-duty guys looking at me in the same light. It was difficult, to say the very least.

In the weeks following the incident, Lee was still having trouble sleeping and suffering from severe anxiety and depression. I was attending follow-up appointments at Therapist's Lair, but CompOne, the workers' compensation subcontractor for the city, wasn't paying the bills. The union president, Felonious, called and said he'd heard the city had terminated my duty injury, and I needed to get my hospital discharge paperwork to the chief.

I gathered the documents and turned them into Operations. The following day, I received a call from Human Resources apologizing for the confusion and saying my duty injury had been reapproved. I was suffering from intense negative emotions, and it felt like a heavy anchor was pulling me down. Nothing ever really got to me before. Now, the smallest things could make me intensely frustrated, and I had difficulty letting them go.

All the doctors were saying I shouldn't go back to work. That concussions were cumulative, and with the extent that this one brought me to the brink of self-destruction, the next one could likely be my last. That I should just walk away while I could and find a new career. I'd sworn while watching others go out on duty injuries, that would never be me. I'd never be a burden to my city and not earn a wage. Even disabled, I'd find a way to be relevant and do a job for my city. My doctors, however, were convinced my career as a firefighter was over and refused to grant return-to-work clearance.

On January 18, 2018, I met with Mr. Williams, the investigator from CPS. After meeting with my family and me at our home, he agreed the complaint was without merit and decided to close the case. One step forward.

The following day, Felonious called to say the city had once again denied the duty injury claim and was disputing benefits. All my treatment and rehabilitation appointments had been canceled due to billing issues with the city's workers' comp provider. They wanted my private insurance to continue with treatment, there were significant delays in care, and my calls and emails to the city's human resources department went unreturned. Two steps back.

The next day, while shoveling *more* snow from my driveway, I received a call from Bobby at PHP, my personal health insurance carrier. Bobby said he was checking in on me and wanted to let me know he was personally advocating for my care. I found out he'd been following my case and calling my care providers, to coordinate my appointments after CompOne denied them. He assured me all appointments would be paid on their end. That he'd see to it personally I received the care I needed.

It'd been six and a half weeks since the injury, and I'd had zero diagnostics done to determine the extent of my cognitive concussion symptoms. The idea of proceeding with my personal insurance so I could get better seemed appealing. There was finally a light ahead, and I was determined to reach it.

On January 29, 2018, I met with my primary care doctor to evaluate the disk damage in my neck. He suggested waiting for the neuro-psych eval from PAR Rehab before discussing any return-to-work options. PAR Rehab called me later that day to say CompOne had denied paying for the neuro-psych eval and they could schedule it within the next two weeks on my private insurance. I was so frustrated with the ups and downs of this broken system.

The next day, I received a phone call from Kelly in HR to say they were dropping me from duty injury status and disputing all medical claims from January 7, 2018, forward.

I asked her, "When are you going to start taking care of your heroes? I know dozens of other firefighters you've done this to."

She said she just had "a job to do and it was nothing personal."

Well, it was personal for me. I hung up and called the union president, Felonious, who referred me to a workers' compensation attorney. I called and scheduled a consult for a lawsuit. I was feeling litigious and still suffering from multiple concussion symptoms.

Word came down the chain of command from HR, to Fire Admin, to Operations, to switch me from duty injury over to my personal sick leave. None of the doctors I'd seen would grant me return-to-work clearance, and I began to search for one who would. I just wanted to go back to work and finish my career. It was important to me. My wife fought desperately to keep that from happening, and at times we were on opposing sides of the issue.

I was on a trajectory that would use up all my sick leave, exhaust my vacation and personal leave time, and I would need to request administrative leaves of absence to protect my family's health care coverage. After four months, when I'd run out of paid time off, the city would stop paying my wages, and my family would be solely dependent on my wife's income. But I'm getting ahead of myself. We all knew that was coming. Here's how it played out.

On February 2, 2018, I received a letter from the city with a "Notice of Dispute" from the city's HR department stating they were denying my workers' compensation claim after a review of the medical documentation from my emergency room visits on January 2 and January 7. Additionally, they were removing me from duty injury status and placing me on retroactive sick leave from January 8, 2018, forward. This decision was based on "not enough medical documentation that your behavioral issues were directly or causally related to the workplace injury on 12/10/17." Even though every hospital's diagnosis read: "suicidal ideation and depression as a result of a head injury while at work on the fireground."

More specifically, they were saying my behavioral issues were "not causally related" to being hit in the head on the fireground. My attorney and I located a force calculation algorithm developed by the tree cutting industry, that could determine how hard a felled tree impacted an object on the ground, based on the diameter of the tree, the length, and the distance the impacted object was away from it. When the data was input with my specific scenario, it worked out to nearly 2000 lbs of force at the impact site. Which, when taken in context with the denial of responsibility by the city, proved absolutely false and egregiously wrong.

On February 23, 2018, I visited PAR Rehab and Dr. Robert Napolitano for my psychological evaluation testing. While being administered the WASI-II psych test, Engine 4 and Medic 9 pulled up for a medical alarm right outside the window I was sitting at. I just shook my head and laughed. What were the odds of that happening?

I scored well on the test and "Big Bob" Napolitano—his nickname in the medical community because of his powerlifting hobby—set about reviewing the results. I remember the terms *extirpate, mollify,* and *panacea* were the only vocabulary words I didn't know at the time. (If *you* happen know those definitions, congratulations. You're a fucking genius.)

I continued to see Dr. Mangina at Therapist's Lair on a weekly basis to discuss recovery techniques. She apologized on behalf of the entire mental health community for the terrible standards of care I'd received at CMH and Anarchy Acres. She also refused to clear me for a return to active duty and suggested I find a new career.

I met with my PCP, to review the range of symptoms I was still having after the accident. He too, declined to clear me for a return to active duty. Based on the symptoms I was still experiencing, and the high risk for another concussion associated with firefighting.

On March 15 I met again with PAR Rehab and Dr. Napolitano, to follow up and review the results of my psychological evaluation. I'd placed in the 99th percentile for intellectual acuity, with underlying major depression and PTSD. He also did not recommend a return to duty. He asked me what I loved to do, and suggested with the test scores I had, the sky was the limit.

That I should consider other careers. Specifically, less physically dangerous ones.

Nearly a month later, I met with my PCP again to review the psych eval results and fill out my FMLA paperwork in order to keep my job. He recommended I *not* return to emergency situations and was in agreement with Dr. Napolitano. This was not what I'd wanted to hear. I could still do the job just fine, and there had to be a way to stay in the fire service. Maybe in a different division where I didn't have to respond on calls anymore.

I signed a job posting for the Training Captain III position and was the most senior person to do so. According to the union contract, I had one year from entering the Training Division to obtain all the necessary credentials. Lee and I met with Assistant Chief Bruce Owens, in his office.

"You've earned your pension Brad," he explained, "Twenty years of service is an honorable thing. There's no shame in applying for a duty disability."

"No fucking way. I'm not disabled." I didn't understand it then, but from a fire service liability standpoint, I was damaged goods. They were just trying to ditch me in the least painful and litigious way for everybody. They didn't give a flying fuck about me or the brotherhood.

As Lee pleaded with Bruce to push a duty disability through, I thought back to the incident at my home with the police. The police... *Holy shit!* That's what Lee was talking about nearly nine months ago when she told me to stay away from the police. And it's why she kept telling me I was going to retire three years early. Holy shit. Definitely not how I wanted to retire.

The Training Captain position was offered, and I accepted it the following day. Then Dave Owens in Fire Administration called me later that day and said I didn't qualify for it and was being passed over for the next candidate. They said I had to be physically capable of returning to the Suppression division in order to transfer divisions and then vetted me for a Training Captain IV position, based on their interpretation of the union contract.

On April 25, I emailed the promotional committee in advance of their meeting regarding the contract language discussion. I urged them to find me qualified and to vet me for the position that was posted, Training Captain III, which afforded me a year to get the credentials. They denied my transfer and promotion at the promotional committee meeting, and I was officially screwed. My family was going to have to suffer through me losing my wages due to a workplace accident, and my career was in jeopardy, if not over.

I turned in my FMLA paperwork to Human Resources and was placed on unpaid medical leave for next twelve weeks. I filed a grievance with the union and the city for breach of contract, stating I was passed over for promotion based on not having met the qualifications when the contract clearly stated I was fully qualified for the Training Captain III position they'd posted; however, I'd erroneously been vetted for a Captain IV, a fully accredited spot.

On May 1, 2018, I had my pretrial hearing for the workers' compensation case, and neither the city nor their attorneys showed up. A control date for a status hearing was set for July 10, 2018. The following day, Fire Administration denied my grievance.

I met with Steven Veritas, Esq., my workers' comp attorney. He recommended I file an ADA (Americans With Disabilities Act) and EEOC (Equal Employment Opportunity Commission) complaint, and to seek representation for discrimination and breach of contract lawsuits. We determined the goal for the workers' comp case was a restoration of duty injury status, a restoration of my personal time, and that my medical bills and lost wages be paid by the city.

The firefighters union requested, and was granted, a ten-day extension to file a response to the grievance denial. On May 9, I had a meeting with the city's HR department to discuss the duty disability application process. Lee went with me and together we filed the application.

On May 16, I spoke with the union president, Felonious, on the phone regarding the union requesting to advance to Step 3 of grievance. Unbeknownst to me, he was playing both sides and had no intention of fighting for me. He'd told the promotional committee to stand united against me, and this would all go away.

Two of the committee members questioned him and said, "Don't you have a duty to represent him?"

Felonious replied, "He hasn't paid his union dues in three months. I don't have a duty to do shit for him." He told the city to deny my grievance and gave them information and instructions on how to do it so everything looked proper. It was all smoke and mirrors. He'd completely shirked his duty to represent me.

I'd been betrayed by a childhood friend, a brother firefighter, and a union president I'd trusted to represent me. My family was suffering because I'd given everything to do a job for my city, and now I'd been committed to an insane asylum, stripped of my dignity, had my wages taken away, and none of my doctors would return me to active duty. When people ask me: "What's the worst thing you've ever seen as a firefighter?" *This* is it for me.

At the advice of my attorney, I contacted the EEOC about a possible disability discrimination case. They investigated and determined the case had potential merit. The statute of limitations for issuing a right to sue arrived before the investigation concluded and the EEOC referred the case to the US Justice Department who issued a right to sue based on the length of time the investigation had taken.

I filed the cases with the ADA and the EEOC. But they both stalled out in procedural bullshit. The city's position on the matter was that I'd never actually requested reasonable accommodation for my disability. At no time was I advised by anyone at the city, to do anything other than apply for a line-of-duty disability.

Medical bills were piling up to the tune of $30,000. Aflac denied all my claims, stating behavioral issues were not covered under the family accident rider I had faithfully paid for, every two weeks, for the past eight years. Everyone had left my side except my wife and a handful of close friends—namely, Krishna, Dave Austin, Damyon, and Dave Owens.

I felt liked William Wallace in *Braveheart* when Robert the Bruce betrayed him. The throes of deep depression followed me everywhere.

A medical leave of absence was requested and approved for ninety days to secure my family's health insurance. Since May 2018, I'd received zero wages, as my attorney sought to resolve the matter in court.

The workers' comp status hearing took place in July 2018, and another was scheduled for September. That one took place, and another was scheduled for November.

The Police and Fire Pension Board took up my line-of-duty disability case in October 2018. I submitted the necessary documentation for review and began the process.

Still making no money, I applied for a second ninety-day leave of absence and a COBRA health insurance continuation and it was granted.

At this point, eight separate doctors were denying a return to active duty for me. The workers' compensation company that denied my care and benefits, requested a second psychiatric evaluation from their independent doctor. It was scheduled for January 7, 2019.

Meanwhile, the Pension Board requested their independent doctor review my disability case and render a determination on whether or not to grant a line-of-duty disability. This would have a tremendous bearing on the workers' comp lawsuit, and the appointment was set for December 5, 2018, with Dr. Rothchild.

The city continued to send me biweekly paychecks in the mail that read: $0.00. That was always a kick in the balls to open those letters.

The November workers' comp hearing came and went, and another hearing was scheduled for February 6, 2019.

On December 5, 2018, I headed off to meet with the city's independent doctor, with all my medical records in tow. Dr. Rothchild was a small man with gray, Einstein-esque hair and thick round glasses that magnified his eyes. He took my vital signs and asked me about the incident and the days that followed.

I explained in painstaking detail what I'd been through. Everything hinged on this medical interview appointment, and I answered all his questions honestly and to the best of my ability. I gave him all the documentation from previous medical exams and the opinions of the examiners. He thanked me for the information and said his report would be sent to the Police and Fire Pension Board for review. They would convene again on January 22, 2019, and I had to wait until then to learn the results of Dr. Rothchild's recommendation.

The New Year came, and I still was off work and unpaid.

I attended CompOne's independent, second opinion doctor's psych eval on January 7, 2019. It was the exact WASI-II psych test I'd taken previously at PAR Rehab six months earlier. Unsurprisingly, he found I was completely fine and recommended an immediate return to work. Especially so when I explained during the vocabulary portion that *extirpate* meant to completely eradicate something, *mollify* meant to appease someone, and *panacea* was a cure-all for everything that was wrong—acing that particular category of the intelligence quotient test.

My attorney advised me to do my best on the exam and explained to me how this was par for the course. That independent investigators were paid by the opposing counsel to render an opinion that countered the preponderance of clinical evidence we'd assembled. It was anticipated by the court and was rarely found to hold significant value.

Everything hinged on the recommendation of Dr. Rothchild. If he granted the line-of-duty disability, CompOne had to pay all expenses and the court case was essentially won. Their denial of benefits would be deemed as without standing, and they'd be ordered to pay the full amount of wages and medical bills. On January 22, 2019, I received word the Pension Board had voted unanimously to approve my line-of-duty disability. From that date on, I'd receive 66 percent of the wages I was earning at the time I was injured.

The February 6 hearing came and went, and another was scheduled for April 4, 2019.

On February 28, I received the first paycheck in nearly a year from the city. In March, my attorney and I calculated the exact number of payable benefits under the Workers' Compensation Act and submitted a request for settlement of $87,500.

The April 4 hearing came and went, and the trial was set for June 11, 2019. That date came and went, and a hearing date was set for August 8. That date came and went, and another was set for September 26. That date came and went, and another was set for November 27. That date came and went, and another was set for January 16, 2020. That date came and went, and another was set for March 17, 2020. A new settlement request was submitted by my attorney for $67,000 in hopes of speeding things up.

COVID hit next, and all the courts closed. The hearing was rescheduled for April 28. Then for July 21. Then for September 8. Then for November 10. The city attorney requested, and we agreed, to settle for $50K. A phone conference for settlement was scheduled with the magistrate on October 19, 2020, and the city's attorney was a no-show for a second time. My attorney accused the city of deliberately stalling the case to avoid paying out the settlement. The next hearing was rescheduled for November 10. That hearing was rescheduled for January 12, 2021.

Then March 9. Then April 16. Then May 4. Then June 9. Then August 10. Then October 19. Then November 23. Then January 27, 2022. Then April 21, 2022.

And here we sit, still waiting to settle on the wages and medical expenses that should have been paid back in 2018. Four years later, it's not even a question of whether or not they're due. The city's doctor established they were when a line-of-duty disability was granted.

I expected the established system to protect me and my family in the event I was injured in the line of duty. It didn't. At least initially it didn't. I had to fight and suffer tremendous hardship for the benefits I've received and *still* continue to fight to this day for them. There are dozens of my colleagues who've had to do the same thing. Most were forced back to work because they couldn't afford to fight back.

If there's a takeaway from this chapter for the reader, it should be this: Don't trust anyone to give you anything in life. It's your personal responsibility to protect yourself. Remember that security is all a state of mind and if you rely on anyone—*especially* your government—to truly give a damn about you, then you are gravely mistaken.

Conclusion

There really is no justification for the abuse of power and misuse of the public's trust that I witnessed—and was a part of—for over twenty years as a city employee. Whether we stole a pack of gum from the station candy store, sold drugs out of the firehouse, or were a dirty cop on the take, we were all part of the problem. No amount of saving lives, or rescuing people, or charitable work, or Sunday confessionals, could make it right and clean the taint from our souls.

As time went on, the misdeeds of once great men and women began to be exposed and the years of corruption became difficult to keep hidden. We knew it was all wrong from day one, but everyone there was doing it and if we didn't follow suit, then shit just didn't go our way and we were shunned from the group. We were an outcast, cut off from the rest of the developed world, like a third world country, complete with economic sanctions imposed on us by our superiors and colleagues. As a new firefighter, barely old enough to purchase alcohol, I was thrown into a system that rewarded the abuse of power.

I was trained to disobey the core values of righteousness, honor, and integrity. I was ordered by my superiors to follow their examples of awful leadership and I hope we can all learn from my experiences. It's up to us to make the best of the circumstances we find ourselves in. The Buddha said, "Who's to say what's good and bad?"; it all brings us to the present moment. What will we do with it? Will we do our best? Will we make things better just because we were there? Through it all, I've found that we, as human beings, are the happiest in life when our actions are in line with our greatest image of ourselves.

The ancient Sumerians had separate symbols in their Cuneiform writing for the words *fate* and *destiny*. Zechariah Sitchin, one of my favorite authors, postulates that they believed fate was fluid, able to be changed by our thoughts and actions, and that destiny was unchangeable: even if we'd done things differently, the same outcome would eventually play itself out. It's curious that we still seek the same understanding today that the earliest civilizations did.

Lee and I still wrestle with it today. Could I have prevented the turn of events that ended my career? She'd seen it all play out years in advance and warned me about things like Darren's death, retiring three years ahead of schedule, and a police standoff at our house. Could she or I have changed any of it? Was it fate or destiny? Why have the sight if she couldn't do anything about it? She tends to relentlessly beat herself up over it.

As we wrap up this crazy adventure, I've thought long and hard about the central theme of it. What is it exactly? What's the message I'm conveying here? While it's certainly open for interpretation, I would offer that it's awareness. Awareness of the things going on all around us. Awareness of what our first responders are *actually* going through. Awareness that everyone is in the process of either climbing up to the metaphorical peak of the soul's evolutionary mountain or sliding back down it. Lee likes to say the destination is the journey, and I prefer to say the journey is the destination, but here we go with the whole fate or destiny discussion again.

Maybe it's awareness of the fact there are people out there who can see everything about us. Which means the universe can see everything about us, too. Which means we'd best start living like someone's always watching and clean our act up. I sure did. I wouldn't even think an inappropriate thought because Lee could see that, too. One of the side effects of being married to a psychic medium is that I cleaned my life up really quick. It's also exceedingly difficult to surprise them with gifts or parties, but that's another story for another time.

Life, in my own limited opinion, for whatever that's worth, is about soul development. Did we get better at our relationships with the world around us? Relationships, I've found, are the most important things in life. Valuing *every* moment we find ourselves in. Knowing that it's happening by design to bring us exactly where we need to be. Living it with no regrets. Living our greatest life. Doing the right thing at the right time and always pushing for forward progress up the mountain of our soul's evolution. Learning lessons and breaking cycles of dysfunction.

So, there it is. People always seem to ask me: What's the worst thing you've ever seen as a firefighter? If you've trudged on this far, through hundreds of pages of unbelievable stories, I think you deserve to be the judge of that. The only thing I'm hopeful for is that I might have helped make a positive difference in someone's life. That, somehow, things were just a little bit better because I was there.

I'll most likely be prosecuted for a list of felonies and assorted misdemeanors after this thing comes out. But hopefully there's a statute of limitations and my defense attorney has frequent lunches with my judge. Perhaps I'll use a pen name and change all the names to aliases and nicknames to avoid sullying anyone's public image. At least you'll know the truth.

And if any of you find yourselves at a bar, or on a plane next to a firefighter, you'll know not to ask what the worst thing they've ever seen is. You'll be able to have a conversation about things like station life and firehouse cuisine, the subtle differences between straight stream and fog patterns. You'll know about Higbee notches and water hammers, and how you can do effective adult CPR by singing the song "Staying Alive" by the Bee Gees as a metronome while pumping away on those chest compressions.

You can speak the language now. In lay terms. Maybe not fluently like a career firefighter at FDIC, but you know enough to get you through the front door, order two beers and ask where the bathroom is: the basics. Hell, it may even be the start of a new career path for you. Although I wouldn't wish the emotional baggage and shortened life expectancy on anyone.

Hopefully, you have a new perspective on the crazy world around you. It's much bigger than it initially appeared to me to be. Along the way I've learned that pretty much everyone is high, and that everyone has a personal agenda. If they deny it, then remember my three favorite sayings: security is just a state of mind, always check your six, and chance favors the prepared mind... ol' buddy.

Smoke flew from the plane's landing gear as the wheels touched pavement at LAX. Trentin Quarantino had pulled some strings and we ended up sitting right next to each other, carrying our conversation through the entire flight. We exchanged business cards as we taxied from the runway to the gate.

"So, everything happens for a reason, right?" he asked.

"That's what they say," I offered.

"And your wife, she sees dead people, and they tell her all about the past, present, and future?" Trent confirmed.

"Yeah. She has her own epic saga for sure," I said, pulling our carry-ons from the overhead bin. "Pretty crazy, eh?"

"Certifiably. What are the odds?" he said, laughing and shaking his head.

"What?"

"That we'd meet. I've been searching for another story worth telling."

"And now you've found it?"

"I've found *them*. I'm gonna talk to some people and have my assistant call you tomorrow. We're gonna tell the world. Are you down?"

"Absa-fuckin-lutely." We shook hands and disembarked.

It was the beginning of a brave new adventure.

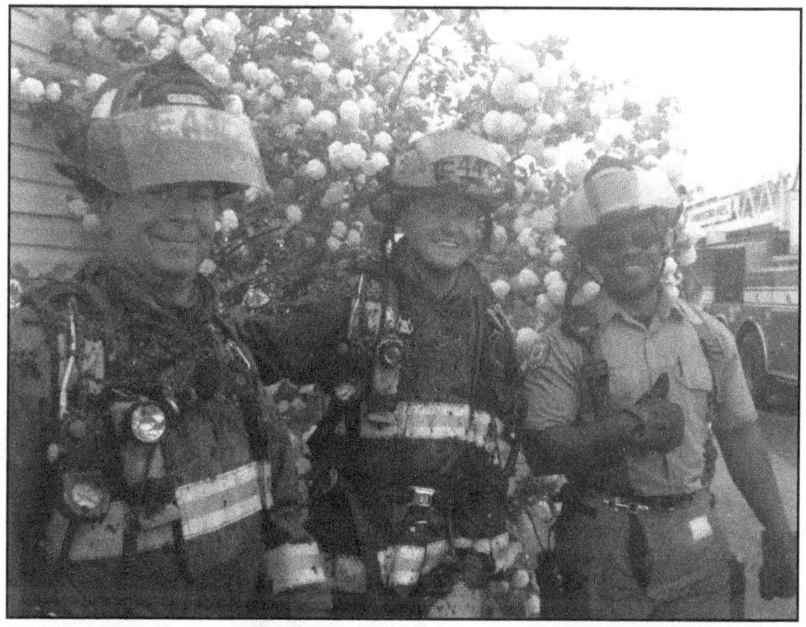

Acknowledgments

The author would like to thank his family for putting up with his bullshit and hardheadedness over the twenty plus years he was a professional firefighter. Thanks to Jack Daniels and Michelob Ultra for helping to recollect both the good times and the bad. Thanks to you, the reader, for plodding through to the end and for plunking down your hard-earned cash to buy this book. Hopefully you have a somewhat different perspective on the world we live in and feel like the read was a rather entertaining ride and worth the investment of time and money. May your days be filled with adventure, your nights with good company and romance, and may you never cease chasing the wonders of enlightenment and knowledge. Cheers!

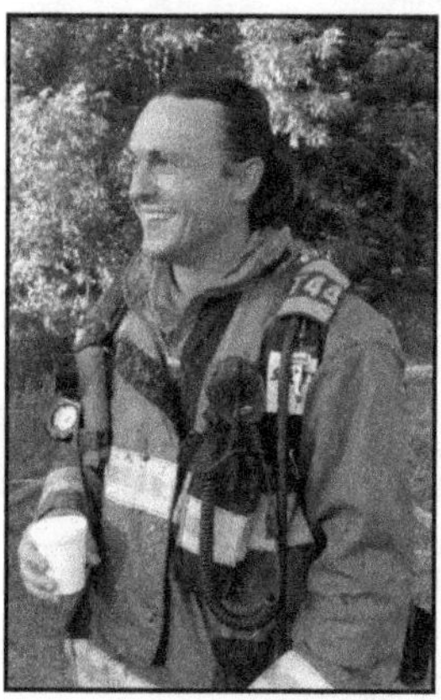

The author after the Golden Rose fire

About the Author

BRADLEY LILLY is the debut author of The Bravest - A Fireman's Tale He's served for over 20 years as a career Firefighter/EMT. He's a husband, father, author, football coach, entrepreneur, public speaker, and perpetual B.A.D. Original.

CPSIA information can be obtained
at www.ICGtesting.com
Printed in the USA
BVHW091924270922
648040BV00001B/1

9 798985 94672